Quality Work Environments for Nurse and Patient Safety

Quality Work Environments for Nurse and Patient Safety

Editor

Linda McGillis Hall, RN, PhD
Associate Professor, Faculty of Nursing, University of Toronto

Authors
(in chronological order)

Linda McGillis Hall, RN, PhD[1]

Diane Doran, RN, PhD[1]

Deborah Tregunno, RN, PhD[2]

Amy McCutcheon, RN, PhD[3]

Linda O'Brien-Pallas, RN, PhD[1]

Joan Tranmer, RN, PhD[4]

Ellen Rukholm, RN, PhD[5]

Allison Patrick, RN, MN[6]

Peggy White, RN, MN[7]

Donna Thomson, RN, MBA[8]

Funded by the Ontario Ministry of Health and Long-Term Care

[1] Faculty of Nursing, University of Toronto
[2] York University
[3] Vancouver Coastal Health
[4] Queen's University & Kingston General Hospital
[5] School of Nursing, Laurentian University
[6] George Brown College
[7] Ontario Ministry of Health & Long-Term Care
[8] St. Peter's Hospital

JONES AND BARTLETT PUBLISHERS

Sudbury, Massachusetts

BOSTON   TORONTO   LONDON   SINGAPORE

World Headquarters

Jones and Bartlett Publishers
40 Tall Pine Drive
Sudbury, MA 01776
978-443-5000
info@jbpub.com
www.jbpub.com

Jones and Bartlett Publishers
Canada
6339 Ormindale Way
Mississauga, ON L5V 1J2
CANADA

Jones and Bartlett Publishers
International
Barb House, Barb Mews
London W6 7PA
UK

ISBN-13: 978-0-7637-2880-9
ISBN-10: 0-7637-2880-2

Library of Congress Cataloging-in-Publication Data

Quality work environments for nurse and patient safety / editor, Linda McGillis Hall ; authors, Linda McGillis Hall ... [et al.].
     p. ; cm.
   Includes bibliographical references.
   ISBN 0-7637-2880-2
   1. Nursing—Practice.
   [DNLM: 1. Job Satisfaction. 2. Nurses—psychology. 3. Nursing Process. 4. Nursing Services—organization & administration. 5. Nursing Staff—supply & distribution. 6. Organizational Culture. 7. Outcome Assessment (Health Care)—organization & administration. WY 87 Q13 2004] I. Hall, Linda McGillis.
   RT86.7Q356 2004
   610.73—dc22
                            2004012077
6048

Production Credits
Acquisitions Editor: Kevin Sullivan
Production Manager: Amy Rose
Associate Production Editor: Karen C. Ferreira
Editorial Assistant: Amy Sibley
Marketing Manager: Ed McKenna
Associate Marketing Manager: Emily Ekle
Manufacturing and Inventory Coordinator: Amy Bacus
Composition: Paw Print Media
Design: Chiron, Inc.
Cover Design: Anne Spencer
Printing and Binding: Courier Stoughton
Cover Printing: Courier Stoughton

Printed in the United States of America
10 09 08 07 06   10 9 8 7 6 5 4 3 2

Acknowledgments

This book emerged from a grant funded by the Ministry of Health and Long-Term Care in Ontario, Canada, which involved a critical analysis of the literature on indicators that could be measured in the work environment of nurses. The request for this work came from the Expert Panel on Nursing and Health Outcomes, chaired by Dr. Dorothy Pringle, and the research was conducted by Dr. Linda McGillis Hall (principal investigator), Dr. Diane Doran, Dr. Deborah Tregunno, Dr. Amy McCutcheon, Dr. Linda O'Brien-Pallas, Dr. Joan Tranmer, Dr. Ellen Rukholm, Allison Patrick, Peggy White, and Donna Thomson. The opinions, results, and conclusions are those of the authors; no endorsement by the Ministry of Health and Long-Term Care is intended or should be inferred.

The authors would like to thank Cheryl Pedersen for her work with the copyediting and formatting of the book chapters.

Dedication

This book is dedicated to nurses—whose tireless commitment to the health of society cannot be overstated.

Contents

1

Indicators of Nurse Staffing and Quality Nursing Work Environments

Linda McGillis Hall

1.1 Introduction

The concerns nurses have about their worklife have evolved throughout the past decade. The Institute of Medicine (IOM) Committee on the Adequacy of Nurse Staffing in Hospitals and Nursing Homes identified the quality of nurses' worklife as a key issue (Wunderlich, Sloan, & Davis, 1996). A study conducted in 1995 identified "quality" worklife settings for nursing as those that place an emphasis on workplace safety, personal satisfaction and support, teamwork, a reasonable workload, and adequate physical surroundings (Villeneuve et al.,

1995). Work settings that promote nursing professional autonomy, greater control over the practice environment, and better physician–nurse relationships may have a positive influence on patient outcomes (Aiken, Smith, & Lake, 1994). Despite this knowledge, changes to health care internationally over the latter part of the 1990s have resulted in a number of new challenges for nursing leaders. In response to fiscal constraints and funding reductions, many health care settings restructured and downsized in an effort to reduce costs and improve the efficiency of services provided. These restructuring efforts, coupled with an impending nursing shortage, have prompted increased concern in the health care community regarding the quality of the worklife environment for nurses.

A number of recent initiatives have begun to address the work environment of nurses. The American Organization of Nurse Executives (AONE) released a report of insights from key informant interviews with nurse leaders and senior executives from 21 hospitals in 17 American states in May 2003 highlighting the improvements and innovations needed to create healthy work environments for nursing (AONE, 2003). Critical factors for achieving excellence in nursing work environments are: (a) leadership development and effectiveness, (b) empowered collaborative decision-making, (c) work design and service delivery innovation, (d) values-driven organizational culture, (e) recognition and reward systems, and professional growth and accountability (AONE). In Canada, an Advisory Committee on Health Human Resources (ACHHR, 2000) suggested that the quality of worklife for nurses is determined by a number of interrelated issues including "appropriate workload, professional leadership and clinical support, adequate continuing education, career mobility and career ladders, flexible scheduling and deployment, professional respect, protection against injuries and diseases related to the workplace, and good wages" (ACHHR, 2000, p. 10). A Canadian Nursing Advisory Committee (CNAC) was struck to develop recommendations for policy direction to improve the quality of nursing worklife at both the federal, provincial, and territorial level (ACHHR, 2002). The CNAC report identified 51 recommendations for policy direction for improving the quality of nurses' worklife under three broad categories. These categories are: (a) resolving operational workforce management issues that maximize the use of available resources, (b) creation of professional practice environments that attract and retain a healthy, committed workforce, and (c) monitoring of activities and generation of information to support a responsive, educated, and committed workforce. Issues in nurses' worklife identified in the report included workload, hours of work, retention, scheduling, salaries and benefits, scope of practice, respect from managers, nursing shortage, support for continuing education, abuse, and nurses' health (ACHHR, 2002). At the same time, a policy analysis conducted on the benefits of a healthy workplace for nurses, their patients, and the system in Canada identified issues related to workload, salary, support for education, nursing staff shortages, retention, and nurses' health and safety (Baumann et al., 2001). Most recently, the release of a new United States report by the Institute of Medicine (IOM) committee on transforming the work environment of nurses sought to identify key aspects of the work environment for nurses as well as potential improvements in health care working conditions that may have an impact on patient safety (Page, 2003). These initiatives highlight the need to determine indicators of the nursing work environment that are important measures of healthy workplaces that could form a link to outcomes experienced by patients.

This book provides a critical review and analysis of the literature on structural variables in work settings that can be considered indicators of the quality of nurses' worklife in health care settings. The indicators include staff mix ratios for full-time, part-time, and casual nursing staff; educational background of nursing staff; experience of nursing staff; team functioning; organizational climate and culture; span of control of unit manager; workload and productivity; level of autonomy and decision-making experienced by nurses; professional development opportunities; scope of nursing leadership role; use of overtime hours; and absenteeism hours. The goal of this analysis of the literature is to provide sound information related to measures that can be used for exploring the environments in which nurses work.

1.2 Objectives of the Literature Review

The specific objectives of the literature review are (a) to identify the essential characteristics or attributes defining each worklife concept through the development of a clear conceptual definition that provides the foundation for review of instruments for measuring it; (b) to identify the instruments (where applicable) or mechanisms that have been used to measure each of the worklife concepts in acute care, complex continuing care, long-term care, and home care settings; (c) to review the content validity of the instruments/mechanisms and assess their congruency with the essential characteristics of each worklife concept; (d) to critically review the instruments/mechanisms for reliability, validity, responsiveness to change, and sensitivity to nursing, organizational, and patient outcomes; and (e) to determine the extent to which each worklife concept has demonstrated sensitivity to nursing care and patient outcomes in acute care, complex continuing care, long-term care, and home care settings.

1.3 Methodology for the Literature Review

The literature review was conducted in four stages including: (a) literature search and selection of relevant empirical, conceptual, and practical data sources related to the worklife concept; (b) compilation of literature on each worklife concept; (c) extraction of data from literature on each worklife concept using guidelines to maintain consistency among team members; and (d) synthesizing literature on each worklife concept through aggregation of findings into a specific chapter.

The first step in the literature review consisted of identifying empirical references that discussed nurses' worklife related to the specific concept of interest. A comprehensive list of relevant articles, reports, and book chapters was generated using a computerized literature search. The literature databases that were accessed in the computerized literature search included CINAHL, Ebsco Research Databases, MEDLINE, Ontario Scholars Portal, OVID, PROQUEST, PSYCHLIT, and SOCIOFILE. The search strategy involved using general key words for each search. The general key words included nurses' worklife, quality of nurses' worklife, quality work environments, and nurses' work, as well as the specific key words identified by each chapter author for their particular quality work environment topic.

1.4 Framework for the Literature Review

The concept of nursing worklife has not been well defined in the literature. While some articles have proposed frameworks for examining nurses' worklife, no reports of their testing or evaluation are evident (O'Brien-Pallas & Baumann, 1992). A number of interrelated factors appear to influence nurses' worklife, as is evidenced in several recent reports. The literature review on nurse staffing and quality nursing work environments was guided by two frameworks: (a) the Quality of Nursing Worklife Issues Framework (O'Brien-Pallas & Baumann) and (b) the Nursing Role Effectiveness Model (Irvine, Sidani, & McGillis Hall, 1998).

1.4.1 *The Quality of Nursing Worklife Issues Framework*

O'Brien-Pallas and Baumann (1992) identified external and internal dimensions thought to influence the nurse and the nurses' work environment. The external dimensions involve: (a) demands placed by the client on the system such as demographic changes, the aging population, chronicity, shortened lengths of stay, technology, client empowerment and decision-making, and lobby groups; (b) health care policy such as funding, delivery of care, laws and regulations, constraints, and changing directions; and (c) the labor market, such as regional variations and demands of different nursing organizations. The internal dimensions involve: (a) individual factors such as work–home interplay, including job sharing, flexible schedules, day care, and part-time work; individual needs, including attitudes, self-image, mass media, job and career goals, life values, respect, recognition, and autonomy; (b) social/environmental and contextual factors such as climate, status role, management and decision-making style, communication, work team goals, interprofessional relations, decision-making, career advancement, physical environment, and organizational factors; (c) operations factors such as care delivery, work design, workload, work flow, staffing mix, schedules, shift work, work arrangements, degree of role specificity, technological demand and support, and equipment and materials; and (d) administration factors such as institutional policies, wage and salary benefits, promotional career ladders, budget reports, performance appraisals, philosophy of management, and recruitment programs.

1.4.2 The Nursing Role Effectiveness Model

Irvine et al. (1998) developed the Nursing Role Effectiveness Model to identify the contribution of nurses' roles to outcome achievement based on the structure, process, and outcome model of quality care (Donabedian, 1980). The structure component consists of nurse, patient, and organizational variables that influence the processes and outcomes of care. Nurse variables entail professional characteristics such as experience, knowledge, and skill levels, which can influence the quality of nursing care. Patient variables include personal and health- or illness-related characteristics such as age, type and severity of illness, and co-morbidities that impact either the delivery of care or the achievement of outcomes. Organizational variables focus on staffing and nursing assignment patterns, which directly impact the delivery of nursing care.

Together these models guided the selection of variables to be included in this literature review and analysis. The following nurse staffing and quality nursing work environment variables were examined.

1. Nurse staffing variables:

    a. Proportion of registered nurses

    b. Nursing hours per patient day (HPPD)

    c. Ratio of registered nurses to patients

    d. Mix of nursing staff

    e. Percentage of full-time, part-time, or casual staff

    f. Number of full-time equivalents (FTEs)

    g. Level of education and experience

2. Quality nursing work environment variables:

    a. Overtime utilization

    b. Absenteeism

   c. Level of autonomy and decision-making

   d. Professional development opportunities

   e. Scope of the nursing leadership role

   f. Span of control of nurse manager

   g. Team relationships (communication and coordination)

   h. Organizational culture and climate

   i. Workload and productivity

1.5 Summary

This book presents the findings from the comprehensive literature review on each of the nurse staffing and quality nursing work environment variables identified. An introduction to each concept is provided, followed by a definition and discussion of the theoretical underpinnings of the concept. Next, factors that influence the variable are outlined and linkages between the variables and outcome achievement are presented. Issues in the assessment of the variables and evidence concerning approaches to variable measurement are then outlined. Measures or instruments used to measure each variable are presented with detailed discussion of the reliability and validity of each. Finally, implications and future research are outlined.

1.6 References

Advisory Committee on Health Human Resources. (2000). *The nursing strategy for Canada: Report of the Advisory Committee on Health Human Resources.* Retrieved April 14, 2003, from http://www.hc-sc.gc.ca/english/pdf/nursing.pdf

Advisory Committee on Health Human Resources. (2002). *Our health, our future: Creating quality workplaces for Canadian nurses. Final report of the Canadian Nursing Advisory Committee.* Retrieved April 14, 2003, from http://www.hc-sc.gc.ca/english/for_you/ nursing/cnac_report/index.html

Aiken, L. H., Smith, H. L., & Lake, E. T. (1994). Lower medicare mortality among a set of hospitals known for good nursing care. *Medical Care, 32*(8), 771–787.

American Organization of Nurse Executives. (2003). *Healthy work environments, Volume II: Striving for excellence.* Retrieved March 29, 2004, from http://www.hospitalconnect.com/ aone/keyissues/hwe_excellence.html

Baumann, A., O'Brien-Pallas, L., Armstrong-Stassen, M., Blythe, J., Bourbonnais, R., Cameron, S., et al. (2001). *Commitment and care: The benefits of a healthy workplace for nurses, their patients, and the system.* Ottawa, ON, Canada: The Canadian Health Services Research Foundation.

Donabedian, A. (1980). *Explorations in quality assessment and monitoring: Vol. 1. The definition of quality and approaches to its assessment.* Ann Arbor, MI: Health Administration Press.

Irvine, D., Sidani, S., & McGillis Hall, L. (1998). Finding value in nursing care: A framework for quality improvement and clinical evaluation. *Nursing Economic$, 16*(3), 110–116, 131.

O'Brien-Pallas, L., & Baumann, A. (1992). Quality of nursing worklife issues: A unifying framework. *Canadian Journal of Nursing Administration, 5*(2), 12–16.

Page, A. (2003). *Keeping patients safe: Transforming the work environment of nurses.* Washington DC: National Academy Press.

Villeneuve, M., Semogas, D., Peereboom, E., Irvine, D., McGillis Hall, L., Walsh, S., et al. (1995). *Worklife concerns of Ontario nurses in 1993.* (Working Paper No. 95-11). Hamilton, ON, Canada: Nursing Effectiveness, Utilization, and Outcomes Research Unit.

Wunderlich, G. S., Sloan, F. S., & Davis, C. K. (1996). *Nursing staff in hospitals and nursing homes: Is it adequate?* Washington DC: National Academy Press.

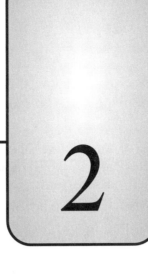

Nurse Staffing

Linda McGillis Hall

2.1 Introduction

Nurse staffing and the care provided by nursing personnel are central to the provision of quality patient care in the health care system. Since the 1970s, nurse researchers have examined nurse staffing from the perspective of scheduling and productivity. The move to explore nurse staffing in relation to patient outcomes emerged in the late 1990s following the release of a key report in the United States by the Institute of Medicine (IOM) Committee on the Adequacy of Nurse Staffing in Hospitals and Nursing Homes that served as a catalyst for much of the research conducted in this area (Wunderlich, Sloan, & Davis, 1996). Commissioned to explore whether there was a need to increase the number of nurses in hospitals and nursing homes to enhance patient care quality as well as the quality of nurses' worklife, the committee identified that few studies existed in this area and suggested a need for empirical evidence regarding the relationship between the quality of patient care and nurse staffing levels and staff mix. This resulted in a number of meetings throughout 1996 designed to explore the research needs in this area.

The American Academy of Nursing held an invitational meeting in June 1996 to identify outcome indicators currently shown to be sensitive to organizational factors in care delivery as well as indicators for further measurement development and to develop research and policy recommendations (Mitchell, Heinrich, Moritz, & Hinshaw, 1997). As well, a meeting was held in July 1996 involving the American Agency for Health Care Policy and Research (AHCPR), the Division of Nursing of the Health Resources and Services Administration (HRSA), and the National Institute of Nursing Research (NINR) to explore methodological issues and research questions related to nurse staffing, quality of care in hospitals, and selected outcomes (Agency for Health Care Policy and Research [AHCPR], 1997). Following these initiatives, in November 1996 a national research agenda was developed including key research questions and grant funding programs on nurse staffing and the quality of care in the United States (AHCPR). An international conference on hospital reform and outcomes research was also held in November 1996. This conference was aimed at assessing the feasibility of collaborative international research on the impact of hospital restructuring on nurse staffing and patient outcomes (Aiken & Sochalski, 1997). Beginning in the late 1990s, the results of many of these research activities emerged in the published literature and form the basis for the discussion in this chapter (Aiken, Clarke, Cheung, Sloane, & Silbur, 2003; Aiken, Clarke, & Sloane, 2002; Aiken et al., 2001; Aiken, Clarke, Sloane, Sochalski, & Silbur, 2002; American Nurses Association, 1997, 2000; Blegen, Goode, & Reed, 1998; Blegen & Vaughn, 1998; Cho, Ketefian, Barkauskas, & Smith, 2003; Kovner & Gergen, 1998; Kovner, Jones, Zhan, Gergen, & Basu, 2002; McGillis Hall & Doran, 2004; McGillis Hall et al., 2003; McGillis Hall, Doran, & Pink, 2004; Needleman, Buerhaus, Mattke, Stewart, & Zelevinsky, 2002; Sovie & Jawad, 2001).

This chapter:

- Reviews the way in which nurse staffing has been defined

- Examines the theoretical underpinnings of nurse staffing constructs

- Discerns the factors that influence nurse staffing

- Critically examines the empirical evidence linking nurse staffing to nursing, patient, and organizational outcomes

- Reviews the approaches to measurement of nurse staffing with regard to the reliability, validity, and sensitivity to nursing variables

- Concludes with a discussion of implications and future directions

A systematic search of the nursing and health databases yielded a variety of interpretations and applications of the nurse staffing construct. This review examined literature relating to theoretical and empirical work in the field of nurse staffing using the methodology outlined in Chapter One. The search yielded a total of 92 relevant sources, of which 65 met the criteria for inclusion in this chapter.

2.2 Definition of the Concept of Nurse Staffing

Early definitions suggested that nurse staffing involved "the provision of the appropriate amount and type of care by persons possessing the requisite skills to the largest number of patients possible in the most cost efficient and humanly effective manner consistent with desired patient outcomes and personnel needs for satisfaction" (U.S. Department of Health, Education, and Welfare [USD-HEW], 1978, p. 2). Nurse staffing involved "the numbers and kinds of personnel required to provide care to the patient or client" (Giovannetti, 1978, p. 2). Nurse staffing has also been described as the process of determining the appropriate number and mix of nursing resources to meet the workload demand for nursing care on the patient care unit (Jelinek & Kavois, 1992).

These definitions include a number of elements that are necessary to capture in theoretical models or frameworks aimed at determining nurse staffing. These elements include appropriateness of the number of nursing staff, type or level of patient care required, skill level of the nursing staff, mix of the nursing staff, the number of patients cared for on the assignment, cost efficiency and effectiveness, and linkage to patient and nurse outcomes.

2.3 Theoretical Underpinnings of Nurse Staffing

Nurse staffing is situated within the study of outcomes research, often in frameworks that have emerged from Donabedian's (1966) conceptual model for quality health care practice. Three conceptual domains comprised this framework including: (a) assessment of structural variables involved in the care, (b) assessment of the process of care, and (c) assessment of the outcome of that care. Originally described as a framework for conceptualizing the dimensions of health care practice, Donabedian postulated that each of these core dimensions was a necessary condition of the one that followed. Structure is concerned with the setting or factors within the delivery system. Process is concerned with caregiver activities and behaviors, including nursing process. Outcome consists of the measurable results of the care. Measures of nurse staffing fall within the structural domain of Donabedian's framework.

Holzemer (1996) described a framework for examining nurse staffing based on Donabedian's (1966) work. The Outcomes Model for Healthcare Research (Holzemer, 1994) involves a matrix model with a horizontal and vertical axis. The horizontal axis includes input, process, and outcomes variables, while the vertical axis includes the client, provider, and the setting. Nurse staffing is captured within the provider input matrices and reflects nurses' experience, attitudes, and knowledge (Holzemer, 1994).

More recently, Mitchell, Ferketich, and Jennings (1998) developed a model that expands Donabedian's (1996) framework beyond linear relationships to incorporate multiple directions and relationships between the model components. Components of the model include the system, client, interventions, and outcomes. System involves the structure and process variables such as organization size, ownership, skill mix, client demographics, and technology. Client characteristics include client health, demographics, and disease risk. Interventions are the clinical processes and activities that contribute to the outcome. Finally, outcomes include measures that capture the results of care structures and processes (e.g., achievement of appropriate self-care, demonstration of health promoting-behaviors, health-related quality of life, perception of being well cared for, and symptom management; Mitchell et al.). Nurse staffing is found in the system component of this model.

The Nursing Role Effectiveness Model developed by Irvine, Sidani, and McGillis Hall (1998) explores the contribution of nurses' roles to outcome achievement based on Donabedian's (1966) structure, process, and outcomes framework. The model proposes relationships between different roles that nurses assume and the outcomes of nursing care including the influence of structure on nurses' role and outcomes. Structure consists of nurse, patient, and organizational variables that influence patient care. Nurse variables include experience, knowledge, and skill levels. Patient variables include personal and health-related characteristics (e.g., age, type and severity of illness, and co-morbidities) that can affect the delivery of care or outcome achievement. Organizational variables include staffing and nursing assignment patterns. Process consists of nurses' independent, medical care related, and interdependent roles. Outcomes include prevention of complications such as injury or nosocomial infections; clinical outcomes such as symptom control; knowledge of the disease, its treatment, and management of side effects; functional health outcomes (e.g., physical, social, cognitive, and mental functioning and self-care); satisfaction with care; and cost. Measures of nurse staffing fall within the structural dimension of this model.

Nurse staffing has also been conceptualized within the context of systems theory. Jelinek (1969) described a patient care systems model comprising inputs and outputs that can be affected by workload, the environment, and organizational factors. Inputs refer to resources involved in patient care (e.g., personnel and physical facility). Organizational factors capture the form of organization used in delivering patient care through rules and policies, the degree of work specialization, and the type of supervision. Workload factors explore the workload that patients impose on the personnel and physical resources (e.g., number of patients and patient conditions). Environmental factors include factors that may affect patient care such as medical staff organization, other hospital departments, and services. Finally, outputs describe patient outcomes in terms of the quantity and quality of patient care delivered. Nurse staffing is captured within the inputs component of this model.

Mark, Salyer, and Smith (1996) proposed a theoretical model for nursing systems outcomes research using an adaptation of structural contingency theory. Structural contingency theory includes the concepts of context, structure, and effectiveness, implying that the context within which the organization exists is an important factor to consider (Mark et al.). Contextual variables comprise both hospital and unit characteristics. The hospital characteristics include teaching status, organizational size, organizational life cycle, and technology; while the unit variables include skill mix, education, nursing unit life cycle, and technology. Structural variables in this model are decentralization, autonomy, nurse-physician collaboration, and quality of support services. Finally, effectiveness variables included are medication administration errors, patient falls, patient satisfaction, job satisfaction, turnover, perceived team performance, and cost efficiency. The authors point out that the effectiveness variables are examples of outcomes that may be of interest to researchers, but should not be considered exclusive or of most importance in the study of outcomes research. Measures of nurse staffing fall within the contextual dimension of this model.

In summary, substantial theoretical evidence suggests that nurse staffing is an important parameter to capture in the study of outcomes research. Theoretical approaches to nurse staffing have evolved from models that describe traditional linear relationships (Donabedian, 1966) to models that are dynamic (Mitchell et al., 1998) and that capture the context of the nursing work environment (Mark et al., 1996). Much of the current work in this area has emerged from Donabedian's structure, process, outcomes model, but expands on this framework to incorporate multiple dimensions (Holzemer, 1994, 1996; Irvine et al., 1998; Mitchell et al.). Research conducted in the future should further test these models for sensitivity in the nursing work environment.

2.4 Factors that Influence Nurse Staffing

A number of individual factors that can influence nurse staffing have been identified in the literature. Utilizing an expert panel, the American Nurses Association (ANA, 1999b) has developed nine principles for nurse staffing that should be considered in decision-making related to nurse staffing. These principles were categorized into three groups of factors that influence nurse staffing including: (a) patient care unit related, (b) staff related, and (c) organization related.

2.4.1 Patient Care Unit Related

The ANA (1999b) suggested that appropriate staffing levels reflect the analysis of individual and aggregate unit patient care needs such as the number of patients on the unit and patient complexity level. As well, the geography of the unit work environment and technology utilized on the unit in the provision of patient care are important factors to consider in nurse staffing. Recent studies have substantiated that nurse staffing is affected by patient complexity (Mark, Salyer, & Wan, 2000; McGillis Hall et al., 2004) and technology (Mark et al.).

Patient physical and psychosocial factors including age, functional status, communication ability, cultural and linguistic diversities, severity and urgency of the admission condition, scheduled procedures, the ability to meet health care requisites, availability of social supports, and other needs are also important considerations in nurse staffing (ANA, 1999b). Evidence of the impact of nurse staffing on patient functional status and social functioning has been reported in the literature (McGillis Hall et al., 2003).

2.4.2 Staff Related

The literature provides evidence of a number of specific nurse characteristics that have been identified as important to consider in staffing decisions. These include experience with the specific patient population, level of nurses' experience (e.g., novice to expert levels), education and preparation (e.g., certification), language capabilities, tenure on the unit, level of control in the practice environment, degree of involvement in quality initiatives, immersion in activities such as nursing research that add to the body of nursing knowledge, involvement in interdisciplinary and collaborative activities regarding patient needs in which the nurse takes part, and the number and competencies of clinical and nonclinical support staff that the registered nurse must collaborate with and supervise (ANA, 1999b). The needs of the patient population form the basis for determining the clinical competencies required for nurses (ANA).

2.4.3 Organization Related

The ANA (1999b) principles of nurse staffing stress the importance of considering the unit functions necessary to support the delivery of quality patient care. These involve a wide variety of factors including effective and efficient support services; access to timely relevant information that is accurate and linked to patient outcomes; orientation programs and ongoing competency assessment mechanisms; technological preparation; adequate time for collaboration, care coordination, and supervision of unregulated workers; processes to facilitate transitions during mergers; mechanisms for reporting unsafe conditions; and a logical method for determining nurse staffing levels and skill mix (ANA).

Some of these organizational variables have been linked to nurse staffing and outcomes in recent research reports. As part of the International Hospital Outcomes Research Consortium study examining nurse staffing, organization, and outcomes in 711 hospitals in five countries, results of a survey of 43,329 nurses indicated concern with the adequacy of staffing and support services, management responsiveness to concern, workforce management policies, opportunities for involvement in decision-making, and acknowledgement of nurses' contribution to patient care (Aiken et al., 2001). In a later report of data from a subgroup of nurses in this study, Aiken, Clarke, and Sloane (2002) found that organizational support for nursing and nurse staffing were related to nurses' perceptions of the quality of care provided. Similarly, McGillis Hall and Doran (2004) reported that the staffing models utilized on a unit can present a challenge for unit-based communication and the coordination of care.

2.4.4 Summary

In summary, a number of factors have been found to influence nurse staffing from the patient, staff, and organizational perspectives. These factors often serve as variables explored in research studies that have sought to identify the links between nurse staffing and patient, nurse, and organizational outcomes. A detailed analysis of these studies follows.

2.5 Linking Nurse Staffing to Outcome Achievement

Thirty-nine empirical studies linking nurse staffing to nursing, patient, and organizational outcome achievement were identified in the literature. The majority of the empirical studies reviewed here investigated nurse staffing in relation to patient outcome achievement on medical-surgical patients or units in acute care hospitals. Fewer studies were found that examined nurse staffing in relation to nurse or organizational outcomes.

2.5.1 Nurse Staffing and Nurse Outcomes

Four empirical studies in this review assessed the relationship between nurse staffing and outcomes experienced by nurses. These studies examined a wide range of nursing outcomes including job satisfaction, job stress, job pressure, job threat, burnout, and role tension.

Aiken et al. (2001) examined nurse staffing, organization of care, and outcomes in 711 acute care hospitals across five countries. A 1998 survey of 43,329 nurses identified that 33–41% of nurses working in four of the five countries including the United States, Canada, England, and Scotland reported job dissatisfaction. Similarly, 30–40% of nurses from these countries had high burnout scores. Lower scores were reported by nurses from the Germany sample.

McGillis Hall and Doran (under review) conducted a study aimed at determining the links between nurse staffing and patient, system, and nursing outcomes on adult medical, surgical, and obstetrical units within 19 teaching hospitals in Ontario, Canada. A total of 1,116 nurses participated in this study. Although none of the nurse staffing variables were significantly related to the nursing outcomes studied, a number of the work environment variables were found to be predictors of the nurse outcomes in this study. Nurses' perceptions of the quality of care at the unit-level were found to have a statistically significant positive influence on nurses' job satisfaction, and a statistically significant negative influence on nurses' job pressure and job threat. Nurses who had a positive perception of the nursing leadership on their unit had higher job satisfaction and lower perceptions of job pressure, job threat, and role tension.

As part of a larger international study, Aiken, Clarke, Sloane, Sochalski, and Silber (2002) explored the relationship between nurse-to-patient ratios and nursing job satisfaction and burnout in 168 Pennsylvania hospitals. Nurses in hospitals with higher nurse-to-patient ratios "were more likely to experience burnout and job dissatisfaction" (Aiken et al., p. 1987).

Mark, Salyer, and Wan (2003) also examined the impact of professional nursing practice on organizational outcomes in a large study of 68 southeastern United States hospitals on 136 general medical-surgical units. One of the outcomes explored by the authors under the domain of organizational outcomes was nurses' work satisfaction, which can be considered a nurse outcome. No relationship was found between nursing skill mix and nursing satisfaction.

2.5.2 Nurse Staffing and Patient Outcomes

The majority of empirical studies found in the literature assessed the relationship between nurse staffing and adverse patient outcomes. These 29 studies examined a wide range of patient outcomes including mortality, length of stay, pressure ulcers, pneumonia, postoperative infections, urinary tract infections, medication errors, falls, upper respiratory tract infections, venous thrombosis or pulmonary embolism after major surgery or invasive vascular procedure, shock or cardiac arrest, upper gastrointestinal bleeding, hospital-acquired sepsis, deep venous thrombosis, central nervous system complications, pulmonary failure and metabolic derangement, and patient satisfaction. Only one study explored the relationship between nurse staffing and positive patient outcomes that may have resulted from the process of nursing care. An overview of the 19 large substantive empirical studies is presented in this chapter.

Scott, Forrest, and Brown (1976) examined hospital structural factors in relation to mortality and morbidity in 17 United States hospitals using data collected in 1973. The ratio of registered and graduate nurses to practical and vocational nurses working on surgical wards was the measure of nurse staffing utilized in this study. A higher ratio of RNs was significantly associated with lower mortality. Greater RN experience was positively related to care quality, although the relationship was not statistically significant.

Shortell and Hughes (1988) used 1983 to 1984 Health Care Financing Administration (HCFA) data from 214,839 patients to study hospital characteristics associated with patient mortality rates. The proportion of nursing staff that were RNs was unrelated to mortality.

Hartz et al. (1989) examined the association between hospital 30-day mortality rates and hospital characteristics in 3,100 U.S. hospitals using 1986 data obtained from the HCFA. The unit of analysis for this study was the hospital, and the data were obtained from general medical-surgical hospitals in the dataset. Corresponding data for these hospitals were obtained from the 1986 American Hospital Association's (AHA) annual survey of hospitals. Nurse staffing variables examined in this study included the number of registered nurses in the hospital divided by the hospital's average daily census, and the percentage of nurses in the hospital who were RNs (Hartz et al.). Lower mortality rates were found in hospitals with a higher proportion of RN staff.

Al-Haider and Wan (1991) examined hospital characteristics that were associated with patient mortality rates using 1984 HCFA data and found that the proportion of nursing staff that were RNs was unrelated to mortality.

Aiken, Smith, and Lake (1994) examined the mortality rates of 39 magnet hospitals in comparison to 195 control hospitals using 1988 HCFA and AHA data. Magnet hospitals had lower mortality rates and higher RN ratios than the control hospitals.

Shortell et al. (1994) examined the factors associated with risk-adjusted mortality and length of stay, nursing turnover, technical quality of care, and the ability to meet family members' needs in 42 intensive care units (ICUs) selected from 1,691 hospitals in the United States. The nurse staffing variable utilized in this study was the average nurse-to-patient ratio on each intensive care unit. Data were collected for each shift from the nursing director of the ICU. No relationship was found between nurse staffing and the outcomes of risk-adjusted mortality or length of stay. The study authors suggested that this may have been due to the low variance in nurse staffing ratios among the study units (Shortell et al.).

The American Nurses Association (1997) conducted a pilot study exploring the impact of nursing on patient outcomes using data from three American states from 1992 to 1994. Nurse staffing was measured using two variables: total nursing hours per Nursing Intensity Weight and RN hours as a percentage of all nursing hours. Higher levels of nurse staffing were related to shorter length of patient stay. Patient adverse outcomes of pressure ulcers, pneumonia, urinary tract infections, and postoperative infections were statistically significantly inversely related to RN skill mix and nurse staffing per acuity-adjusted day (ANA).

In a follow-up report released by the ANA in March 2000, similar findings were reported. Higher staffing levels (i.e., licensed hours per acuity-adjusted day) were associated with shorter length of stay. As well, patient outcomes including secondary bacterial pneumonia, postoperative infections, pressure ulcers, and urinary tract infections were reported to be lower in hospitals with higher registered nurse skill mixes and with greater staffing levels in some cases (ANA, 2000).

Blegen et al. (1998) examined the hours of care provided by all nursing personnel and the proportion of those hours of care provided by registered nurses in relation to patient outcomes across 42 patient care units in a U.S. hospital. Units involved in the study included medicine, surgery, obstetric/gynecology, pediatric, critical care, psychiatric, eye/ear/nose, urology, orthopedic, and neurosciences. The patient outcomes examined through multivariate regression analysis included medication errors, patient falls, urinary and respiratory tract infections, skin breakdown, patient complaints, and mortality. An RN proportion of up to 87.5% was negatively related to unit rates of medication errors, while, for some unexplained reason, a higher RN proportion led to higher unit rates. As well, the rates of decubiti were lower on units with higher RN proportions as were the rates of patient complaints (Blegen et al.). Conversely, the total hours of patient care provided by a mix of care providers (e.g., nursing assistants, licensed practical nurses [LPNs], RNs) was associated with higher rates of decubiti, complaints, and deaths.

In another study of 39 medical-surgical, intensive care, obstetric, and skilled care patient care units in 11 U.S. hospitals, Blegen and Vaughn (1998) examined two nurse staffing variables including "all hours of care per patient day" and "the proportion of those hours of care delivered by RNs" in relation to adverse patient outcomes (p. 198). The adverse outcomes explored included medication errors, patient falls, and cardiopulmonary arrests. On units where there was a higher proportion of RNs, lower rates of medication administration errors per 10,000 doses were reported, as well as lower rates of patient falls. As RN proportion on the unit increased from 50% to 85%, medication error rates decreased. However, as the RN proportion increased from 85% to 100%, medication error rates increased. This finding is similar to that reported by Blegen et al. (1998) in a single site study.

The relationship between hospital-level nurse staffing and adverse patient occurrences was also explored in a study of 506 hospitals across 10 states in the United States (Kovner & Gergen, 1998). The measure of nurse staffing employed in this study was the number of full-time equivalent (FTE) RNs working in the hospital and outpatient departments per adjusted patient day (RNAPD). The adverse outcomes examined were categorized as nurse-sensitive and non-nurse sensitive by the researchers. Nurse-sensitive adverse outcomes included venous thrombosis or pulmonary embolism after major surgery or invasive vascular procedure, urinary tract infections after major surgery, and pneumonia after major surgery or invasive vascular procedures. Outcomes considered as non-nurse sensitive included after major surgery pulmonary compromise, acute myocardial infarction, and gastrointestinal hemorrhage or ulceration, as well as mechanical complications because of device, implant, or graft. Data on hospital characteristics were obtained from the 1993 AHA Annual Survey of Hospitals and matched with the Nationwide Inpatient Sample from the AHCPR. A statistically significant negative relationship was found between the number of FTE RNs per adjusted inpatient day and urinary tract infections and pneumonia after major surgery (Kovner & Gergen). As well, a statistically significant negative relationship was also reported between RNAPD and thrombosis and pulmonary compromise after surgery.

Sovie and Jawad (2001) examined the impact of restructuring on patient outcomes in 1997 and 1998 on medical and surgical units in 29 university teaching hospitals in the United States. Patient outcomes examined included falls, nosocomial pressure ulcers, urinary tract infections, and patient satisfaction. Higher levels of RN hours worked per patient day were associated with lower fall rates and higher patient satisfaction with pain management (Sovie & Jawad). An increase in the hours worked per patient day by all staff was associated with lower urinary tract infection rates.

The relationship between the amount of care provided by nurses at a hospital and patient outcomes was examined by Needleman and colleagues (2002) using 1997 hospital discharge data from 11 states. The unit of analysis for this study was the hospital, and the patient outcomes explored included length of stay, urinary tract infections, pressure ulcers, hospital-acquired pneumonia, shock or cardiac arrest, upper gastrointestinal bleeding, hospital-acquired sepsis, deep venous thrombosis, central nervous system complications, in-hospital death, failure to rescue (i.e., deaths following complications), wound infections, pulmonary failure, and metabolic derangement (Needleman et al.). For medical patients, hospitals that had a "higher proportion of hours of care per patient day that were provided by RNs" and a "greater absolute number of hours of care provided by RNs" (Needleman et al., p. 1715) reported shorter patient length of stay and lower rates of urinary tract infections and upper gastrointestinal bleeding. Hospitals with a "higher proportion of hours of care provided by RNs" (Needleman et al., p. 1715) also had lower rates of pneumonia, shock or cardiac arrest, and failure to rescue. For surgical patients, hospitals that had a "higher proportion of hours of care per patient day that were provided by RNs" (Needleman et al., p. 1715) were associated with lower rates of urinary tract infections. As well, hospitals with a "greater absolute number of hours of care provided by RNs" (Needleman et al., p. 1715) were associated with lower rates of failure to rescue.

Kovner et al. (2002) explored the impact of nurse staffing on patient adverse outcomes across 13 American states using secondary data from the Nationwide Inpatient Sample from 1990 to 1996. Nurse staffing variables included RN and LPN hours, while adverse events included venous thrombosis/pulmonary embolism, pulmonary compromise following surgery, urinary tract infections, and pneumonia—variables that showed a significant relationship to nurse staffing in an earlier study by some of these researchers. A statistically significant inverse relationship was reported between RN hours per adjusted inpatient day and pneumonia.

Aiken, Clarke, Sloane, Sochalski, et al. (2002) explored the relationship between nurse-to-patient ratios and patient mortality and failure to rescue in 168 Pennsylvania general hospitals from 1998 to 1999. Surgical patients in hospitals with higher nurse-to-patient ratios experienced 7% higher risk-adjusted mortality and failure-to-rescue rates.

Data from the Ontario sample of 75 hospitals involved in Aiken's international study (Sochalski, Aiken, & Fagin, 1997) were examined to determine if relationships existed between nurse staffing and mortality (Tourangeau, Giovannetti, Tu, & Wood, 2002). Nursing skill mix was measured "as RN inpatient earned hours proportionate to other inpatient nursing staff earned hours (RN, registered practical nurse, and unlicensed assistive personnel earned hours)" (Tourangeau et al., p. 77). A second variable was utilized to assess the dose of nurse staffing in relation to patient case weights. A higher RN skill mix was associated with lower 30-day mortality rates. No relationship was found between the dose of nurse staffing and mortality.

Mark et al. (2003) examined the impact of professional nursing practice on patient and organizational outcomes in 68 southeastern U.S. hospitals in a sample comprising 136 general medical-surgical units. The patient outcomes explored included patient satisfaction, rate of reported medication errors, and falls. No relationship was found between nursing skill mix and the adverse patient occurrences of medication errors and falls. However, nursing skill mix was associated with higher mean levels of patient satisfaction (Mark et al.)

The relationship between nurse staffing and adverse events, mortality, and medical costs was explored at the hospital level using 1997 surgical patient data obtained from 232 California hospitals (Cho et al., 2003). Adverse events examined in this study included patient fall/injury, pressure ulcer, adverse drug event, pneumonia, urinary tract infection, wound infection, and sepsis. Nurse staffing was measured using three variables representing the number of nurses at each hospital on medical/surgical acute care, medical/surgical intensive care, and coronary care units. The nursing variables were "all hours" of care, "RN hours" and "RN proportion." "All hours" was positively related with pressure ulcers, while "RN hours" and "RN proportion" had a significant inverse relationship with pneumonia (Cho et al.).

McGillis Hall et al. (2004) examined the relationship between nursing staff mix models and patient adverse events as part of a larger study exploring the links between nurse staffing and patient, nurse, and organizational outcomes for adult medical-surgical and obstetrical inpatients in 19 teaching hospitals in Ontario, Canada. Nursing staff mix and average nurse experience level were assessed to see if they were related to any of the patient safety outcomes. The lower the proportion of professional nursing staff employed on a unit, the higher the number of medication errors and wound infections. As well, the less experienced the nursing staff, the higher the number of wound infections on a unit.

It is evident that a number of studies have examined the unfavorable outcomes of nursing care such as the occurrence of adverse events including medication errors, patient falls, decubiti, nosocomial infections (ANA, 1997, 2000; Blegen et al., 1998; Blegen & Vaughn, 1998; Cho et al., 2003; Kovner & Gergen, 1998; Kovner et al., 2002; Mark et al., 2003; McGillis Hall et al., 2003;

Needleman et al., 2002; Sovie & Jawad, 2001), and mortality (Aiken, Clarke, Sloane, Sochalski, et al., 2002; Aiken et al., 1994; Al-Haider & Wan, 1991; Hartz et al., 1989; Scott et al., 1976; Shortell & Hughes, 1988; Tourangeau et al., 2002). Less attention has been placed on examining the intended effects of nursing care on the patient, such as the improvement or maintenance of physical, mental, or emotional functioning. McGillis Hall et al. (2003) also evaluated the impact of different nurse staffing models on the patient outcomes of functional status, pain control, and patient satisfaction with nursing care. A repeated measures study was conducted in all of the 19 teaching hospitals in Ontario, Canada. The sample comprised hospitals and adult medical-surgical and obstetrical inpatients within those hospitals. The nurse staff mix variable was measured at the unit-level, and patient outcomes were assessed at the individual level. The proportion of regulated nursing staff on the unit was associated with better functional independence measure scores and better social function scores at hospital discharge. In addition, a mix of staff that included RNs and unregulated workers was associated with better pain outcomes at discharge than a mix that involved RNs, registered practical nurses (RPNs), and unregulated workers. Finally, patients were more satisfied with their obstetrical nursing care on units where there was a higher proportion of regulated staff.

2.5.3 Nurse Staffing and Organizational Outcomes

Few studies have explored the relationship between nurse staffing and organizational outcomes. Of the six studies that were found, organizational outcomes included market characteristics such as levels of competition and geographical areas; hospital characteristics such as hospital size, teaching status, level of technology provided, type of admission, patient case mix, length of stay, nursing costs, and nursing turnover; and unit characteristics such as type of unit and type of nursing care delivery model.

Bloom, Alexander, and Nuchols (1997) conducted a study aimed at exploring the effects of different nurse staffing patterns on hospital efficiency using 1981 data from the AHA nursing personnel and hospital surveys. The four nurse staffing variables examined included the use of RNs from temporary agencies, part-time RNs, an RN-rich skill mix, and organizationally experienced RNs. The utilization of part-time RNs and experienced RNs reduced personnel, benefits, and nonpersonnel operating costs. In contrast, the use of temporary agency RNs increased nonpersonnel operating costs. A higher RN skill mix was not related to any of the measures of hospital costs.

Brewer and Frazier (1998) conducted a study of factors that influenced nurse staffing on 180 units in 34 hospitals in New York State in 1995. The study included pediatric, maternity, intensive care, and medical-surgical units. Nursing unit factors including the type of nursing unit and model of nursing care used on the unit were found to be significant predictors of nurse staffing. The authors reported that intensive care, pediatric, and maternity units had significantly higher RN staffing than medical, surgical, and gynecological units. As well, the use of a primary nursing care delivery model was associated with the use of approximately one-third more RNs per occupied bed (Brewer & Frazier).

Mark et al. (2000) explored the contribution of a number of market, hospital, and unit characteristics in predicting the skill mix for nursing in a study of 67 hospitals in the southeast United States in 1996. The study was conducted on general medical-surgical units. The ratio of filled RN positions to the total filled nursing staff positions on the unit was the measure of nurse staffing utilized in this study. Market characteristics such as higher levels of competition were associated with a higher skill mix, while larger metropolitan statistical areas were associated with a lower nursing skill mix. Hospital characteristics such as high-tech services and a larger percentage of managed care admissions were associated with a higher RN skill mix, while more regular stay admissions were associated with a lower RN skill mix on the units. The unit characteristic of increased patient complexity was associated with the use of a higher proportion of RNs.

Aiken, Clarke, and Sloane (2002) also explored the effect of nurse staffing and supports for nursing care on nurses' job satisfaction, burnout, and perceptions of quality of care across four countries. Data were obtained from 10,319 nurses working on medical and surgical units in 303 hospitals in the United States, Canada, England, and Scotland. The authors reported that nurses working in hospitals with limited support for nursing care were twice as likely to report job dissatisfaction and burnout. These hospitals in turn, were rated as providing low quality care (Aiken et al.).

Mark et al. (2003) also examined the impact of professional nursing practice on organizational outcomes in their study of 68 southeastern U.S. hospitals in a sample comprising 136 general medical-surgical units. The organizational outcomes explored included nursing turnover and average length of patient stay. No relationship was found between nursing skill mix and nursing turnover or patient length of stay.

McGillis Hall et al. (2004) examined the relationship between nursing staff mix models and nursing costs as part of a larger study conducted in 19 teaching hospitals in Ontario, Canada. Nursing staff mix was found to have a statistically significant negative influence on nursing hours, with staff mix models that included a lower proportion of professional nursing staff related to the utilization of more nursing hours. As well, patient complexity was found to be a significant predictor of nursing hours cost as more complex patients had a statistically significant positive influence on nursing hours utilization. This finding suggests that more complex patients utilize more nursing care resources. Further analysis of nursing hours utilization in relation to specific patient groups showed that the proportion of professional nursing staff in the staff mix model was negatively related to the nursing hours utilized for medical-surgical patients. Holding constant patient age and complexity, medical-surgical units with a lower proportion of professional nursing staff actually utilized more nursing hours.

Patient age and complexity were positively related to the nursing hours utilized for medical-surgical patients. More nursing hours were utilized for patients that were older and for patients with higher complexity levels.

2.5.4 Summary

In summary, the literature provides substantial evidence of a link between nurse staffing and patient, nurse, and organizational outcomes with evidence accumulating from research employing large data sets and multicenter studies. As well, a number of smaller studies have also generated similar results, although the ability to generalize their findings is limited (Barkell, Killinger, & Schultz, 2002; Bostrom & Zimmerman, 1993; Grillo-Peck & Risner, 1995; Heinemann, Lengacher, Van Cott, Mabe, & Swymer, 1996; Lengacher et al., 1994, 1996; Mularz, Maher, Johnson, Rolston-Blenman, & Anderson, 1995; Potter, Barr, McSweeney, & Sledge, 2003; Powers, Dickey, & Ford, 1990).

Strong evidence exists to link nurse staffing to patient adverse occurrences including pressure ulcers (ANA, 1997, 2000; Blegen et al., 1998), urinary tract infections (ANA, 1997, 2000; Kovner & Gergen, 1998; Needleman et al., 2002), pneumonia (ANA, 1997, 2000; Cho et al., 2003; Kovner & Gergen; Needleman et al.), postoperative wound infections (ANA, 1997, 2000; McGillis Hall et al., 2004), medication errors (Blegen et al.; Blegen & Vaughn, 1998; McGillis Hall et al., 2004), pulmonary compromise (Kovner & Gergen), thrombosis (Kovner & Gergen), falls (Sovie & Jawad, 2001), pain management (McGillis Hall et al., 2003; Sovie & Jawad), upper gastrointestinal bleeding (Needleman et al.), shock or arrest (Needleman et al.), failure to rescue (Aiken, Clarke, Sloane, Sochalski, et al., 2002; Needleman et al.), as well as patient satisfaction (Mark et al., 2003; McGillis Hall et al., 2003). One study has established a link between nurse staffing and functional status and social functioning at discharge (McGillis Hall et al., 2003).

Recent work has identified that organizational outcomes such as costs (Bloom et al., 1997; McGillis Hall et al., 2004), patient complexity (Mark et al., 2000; McGillis Hall et al.), level of technology (Mark et al.), care delivery model (Brewer & Frazier, 1998; McGillis Hall & Doran, 2004), and length of stay (ANA, 1997, 2000) are linked to nurse staffing.

However, a gap exists in examining the nursing work environment in relation to patient outcomes. While the importance of considering nurses' job satisfaction (Aiken et al., 2001; Aiken, Clarke, Sloane, Sochalski, et al., 2002; Mark et al., 2003; McGillis Hall et al., 2001) and burnout (Aiken et al., 2001; Aiken, Clarke, Sloane, Sochalski, et al.) have been identified, little or no work has explored other elements of the work environment, for example, level of autonomy and decision-making of nurses, organizational culture and climate, the interrelationships among nurses and team members, and relationships with unit managers and nurse leaders.

2.6 Issues in the Assessment of Nurse Staffing

Three important issues to consider in the assessment of nurse staffing emerged from the review of the literature including: (a) level of analysis, (b) specificity of the nurse staffing variable, and (c) multiple measures of nurse staffing.

2.6.1 Level of Analysis

The level of analysis of the nurse staffing variable utilized in research studies is an important area for consideration in study design. To a large extent, the majority of research to date has been conducted using a nurse staffing variable measured at the hospital level (Aiken, Clarke, Sloane, Sochalski, et al., 2002; Al-Haider & Wan, 1991; Hartz et al., 1989; Kovner & Gergen, 1998; Needleman et al. 2002; Scott, Forrest & Brown, 1976; Tourangeau et al., 2002). Aiken, Clarke, Sloane, Sochalski, et al. calculated hospital-level nurse staffing as a mean score for the patient load of all RNs reporting patient loads between 1 and 20 in their last shift of work. Al-Haider and Wan measured RN ratios as the number of RNs per 100 nurses in a hospital. Hartz et al. used a nurse staffing measure that captured the number of registered nurses in the hospital divided by the hospital's average daily census and the percentage of nurses in the hospital who were RNs. Kovner and Gergen (1998) measured nurse staffing as the number of FTE RNs working in the hospital and outpatient departments per adjusted patient day. Needleman et al. examined nurse staffing at the hospital level capturing inpatient nursing care providers per adjusted patient day.

Nurse staffing is often measured in relation to patient days or case mix indices, which further complicates this issue. Blegen and Vaughn (1998) suggested that "patient acuity scores, considered only at the hospital level, mixed patients from different types of units and with different levels of need for nursing care" (p. 197). Mark et al. (2003) suggested that the relationship between the organization of the nursing unit and outcomes could best be seen at the level of the nursing unit. In an earlier study, these authors suggested that nurse staffing "is likely to exert its most direct influence on patient outcomes at the nursing unit rather than hospital level" (Mark et al., 2000, p. 553).

All of the nurse staffing variables examined are unique despite being calculated at the hospital level of analysis. The challenge with hospital-level measures of nurse staffing is that they often reflect averages representing the overall aggregate of nurse staffing within the hospital. The use of nursing staff ratios obtained from hospital-level data that includes all nursing personnel regardless of whether they are involved in direct patient care has been challenged by some researchers (Blegen et al., 1998; Blegen & Vaughn, 1998). A more accurate measure of nurse staffing is one that incorporates unit-based direct inpatient nursing care providers only. Adjustments for inpatient case mix and acuity are ideal, although this level of detail is not often available at the unit level.

2.6.2 *Specification of Nurse Staffing Variables*

Several studies have identified that measures of overall staffing levels that include care providers other than registered nurses in the staff mix are associated with adverse occurrences (Blegen et al., 1998; Blegen & Vaughn, 1998; Cho et al., 2003; Kovner & Gergen, 1998; McGillis Hall et al., 2003; Sovie & Jawad, 2001). Kovner and Gergen suggest that the particular type of health care worker (e.g., RNs) may have less to do with outcomes than the overall staff involved in the care.

Blegen et al. (1998) found that units that employed a greater number of overall nursing personnel had higher rates of decubiti ulcers. Similarly, Cho et al. (2003) found that hospitals employing higher levels of all types of nursing care providers were associated with an increase in pressure ulcers. In contrast, Sovie & Jawad (2001) reported that an increase in the hours worked per patient day by all staff was associated with lower urinary tract infection rates. McGillis Hall et al. (2003) found that a staff mix that comprised a higher proportion of regulated professional nursing staff (RNs and registered practical nurses) was associated with better functional independence measure scores and better social function scores at hospital discharge, as well as lower rates of medication errors and wound infections. Unruh (2003) found that hospitals with fewer licensed nurses (RNs and LPNs) experienced a greater incidence of decubitus ulcers and pneumonia.

2.6.3 *Multiple Measures of Nurse Staffing*

These somewhat paradoxical findings point to the need for measures of nurse staffing to go beyond simply capturing the percentage or proportion of RNs involved in patient care delivery. There is some suggestion that higher levels of professional nursing staff contribute to improved patient outcomes (McGillis Hall et al., 2003). Future work is needed to assess the association between staff mix models that employ higher proportions of unregulated workers as part of the "all types of nursing care providers" and patient outcomes.

Researchers who have attempted to employ multiple measures of nurse staffing in their studies have identified that other nurse staffing variables may also be related to the outcomes reported (Cho et al., 2003; Kovner & Gergen, 1998). When nurse staffing variables are highly correlated, the one that is least predictive of the outcomes being studied may be dropped from the analysis. Kovner and Gergen found collinearity between the RNs per adjusted inpatient day (RNAPD) and non-RNAPD variables in their study. When the variables were switched for further analysis and non-RNAPD was utilized in the model, the relationship between non-RNAPD and urinary tract infections and thrombosis after major surgery was significant, but at a level that was five-fold smaller than that reported when RNAPD was used in the analysis (Kovner & Gergen). The authors also reported collinearity between the nursing ratio variable that described the nursing skill mix in the study hospitals and RNAPD. Similarly, when skill mix was employed in the model rather than RNAPD, a small significant relationship was reported between the skill mix and pneumonia after surgery. Blegen et al. (1998) reported collinearity between the two nurse staffing variables "all hours of care" and "RN proportion." When all hours of care was added to the regression model, the direction of the relationship between RN proportion and each outcome variable remained negative but the size increased. "Higher total hours of care from all nursing personnel on the unit (all hours) were associated with a higher incidence of negative outcomes, but higher RN proportion was related to lower incidence of negative outcomes" (Blegen et al., p. 47). Tourangeau et al. (2002) reported moderate correlations between the two nurse staffing measures employed in their study—nursing skill mix and dose of nurse staffing—and used nursing skill mix in the model reported.

These conflicting results highlight the need for researchers to explore nurse staffing in a variety of ways in research studies, beyond single variables focused on RN staffing alone. However, the importance of having distinctly different measures of nurse staffing is also apparent.

2.7 Evidence Concerning Approaches to Measuring Nurse Staffing

No instruments exist to measure nurse staffing, thus evidence of the reliability, validity and sensitivity of measures is not possible. Nurse staffing has been assessed with methods that focus on numerical assessments of the staffing complement as well as methods that capture the mix of the staff employed in the organization or unit. As well, demographic characteristics of the nursing staff have also been considered. In the discussion of approaches to measurement, the review will focus first on the numerical assessment strategies for nurse staffing and staff mix, and then on specific demographic methods. The discussion summarizes these methods, providing a description of the methods for calculating and capturing these data, and evidence concerning utility of the method.

2.8 Measures of Nurse Staffing

Measures of nurse staffing include numerical assessments such as: (1) the proportion of registered nurses, (2) nursing hours per patient day (HPPD), (3) ratio of registered nurses to patients, (4) number of full-time equivalents (FTEs),

(5) percentage of full-time, part-time and casual, (6) mix of nursing staff, and demographic characteristics including (7) education and experience.

2.8.1 Proportion of Registered Nurses

The measure of the proportion of RNs within the staff mix has been calculated at both the hospital and unit-level in different studies. Depending on the level of analysis, the mechanism for determining RN proportion has been developed in a variety of ways.

A nurse staffing variable considered to be representative of direct nursing care hours provided to patients was utilized by Blegen et al. (1998). The calculation for this variable occurred in two stages. First, direct nursing care hours were derived as *RN Hours = Hours of direct patient care by RNs/Patient days of care on the unit*. Following this, the proportion of RN was calculated as *RN Proportion = RN hours per patient day on unit/All nursing hours per patient day on unit*. Direct patient care captured staff assigned to provide care to the patients on the unit. Data for this variable were obtained from hospital payroll and human resources databases (Blegen et al).

In a second study, Blegen and Vaughn (1998) determined the proportion of RNs differently. Data were obtained from each of the 11 hospitals in the study. The hours of care variable utilized in this study were calculated based on the number of full-time equivalents provided to the researchers by the hospital:

> Each hospital submitted the hours of care (or FTEs) delivered to patients by RNs, LPNs, and nursing assistants. FTEs were converted to hours using 500 hours per quarter for one FTE. Some hospitals submitted total annual hours; for these, 25% of the total hours were assigned to each quarter of the year. To calculate the hours of care per patient day variable, hours of patient care for each unit provided by all levels of personnel were added within each quarter and then divided by the patient days for that unit in that quarter. To calculate the RN proportion, the hours of care from RNs were divided by the total hours for all nursing care personnel. (p. 198)

Mark et al. (2000, 2003) defined skill mix as the proportion of nursing staff on a study unit that were registered nurses. Thus, "the proportion of RNs to the total complement of nursing staff" was used to determine the unit-level skill mix of nursing staff. Mark et al. (2000) collected data on the number of FTE nursing staff and the number of FTE RNs that were on the study units. Following this, the proportion of RNs was calculated in the following manner: *RN Proportion (Nursing skill mix) = Filled RN positions on unit/Total filled nursing staff positions on unit*.

Needleman et al. (2002) calculated all of the hours of nursing care provided per inpatient day, as well as the proportion of hours of nursing care that were provided by each category of nursing staff. The hours of nursing care per day were adjusted through the creation of a nursing case mix index for each hospital. The researchers used "estimates of the relative level of nursing care needed by patients in each diagnosis-related group to construct a nursing case mix index for each hospital" (Needleman et al., p. 1716). The hours of nursing care per inpatient day were then divided by this index to calculate the adjusted number of nursing hours of care per day (Needleman et al.).

2.8.2 Nursing Hours per Patient Day (HPPD)

The measure of nursing hours per patient day is a numerical calculation that divides the nursing hours available on a unit by the number of patients on the unit. A nurse staffing variable that represented all hours of care per patient day at the unit level was utilized in a study by Blegen et al. (1998). The calculation for this variable was *All Hours = Monthly hours of direct patient care by RNs, LPNs, and nursing assistants/Patient days of care on the unit for the month.*
Kovner and Gergen (1998) measured nurse staffing:

> ...as the number of FTE RNs working in the hospital and outpatient departments per adjusted patient day. Adjusted patient day included the number of patient days in the hospital, the number of patient days in the hospital's nursing home, and an adjustment for the number of outpatient visits that reflected the percentage of the hospital budget devoted to the outpatient departments as a part of the total facility's budget. (p. 316)

Cho et al. (2003) calculated nurse staffing by summing the number of nurses working on three types of patient care units in the hospital—medical-surgical acute care, medical-surgical intensive care, and coronary care. Next, three distinct nurse staffing variables were created. First, "all hours" represented the total productive hours worked by all nursing personnel per patient day. Second, "RN hours" reflected the total productive hours by RNs per patient day. Finally, the "RN proportion" variable represented the skill mix of nursing hours calculated as RN hours divided by all hours.
   The HPPD measure provides some indication of the hours of care available for patient care, but does not identify whether the hours utilized are adequate or appropriate for the level and complexity of patient care on the unit. As well, this measure does not address whether the mix of nursing personnel is appropriate for patient care. The ANA (1999b) suggested that "there is a critical need to either retire or seriously question the usefulness of the concept of nursing hours per patient day (HPPD)" (p. 2). A number of researchers have moved beyond simple calculations of HPPD by adjusting the nursing hours reported for case mix and patient complexity. The challenge remaining for future research is whether this hospital-level adjustment is sensitive to unit-level nurse staffing.

2.8.3 Ratio of Registered Nurses to Patients

The concept of nurse-to-patient ratios has emerged in recent literature following the move toward mandated nursing ratios in some states in the United States. Specifically, California passed legislation that took effect in July 2003 establishing minimum nurse staffing levels for RNs and licensed vocational nurses (LVNs) employed in hospitals (Spetz, Seago, Coffman, Rosenoff, & O'Neil, 2000). It has been projected that some California hospitals may experience increased expenditures for RN staffing once the ratios are implemented (Spetz et al.). To date, the use of nursing ratios in research has been synonymous with either RN proportion or HPPD. For example, the ratio of FTE RNs divided by the total number of FTE nursing staff was explored as a variable for skill mix by Kovner & Gergen (1998). One study utilized data collected from 10,184 Pennsylvania nurses to estimate the impact of the nurse staffing levels proposed in California on nurse burnout and job dissatisfaction (Aiken, Clarke, Sloane, Sochalski, & Silber, 2002). The authors determined that a 7% increase in 30-day mortality and failure-to-rescue would occur for each additional patient added to the nursing ratio.

2.8.4 Number of Full-Time Equivalents (FTEs)

One measure of nurse staffing involves a count of the number of full time equivalents (FTEs) that an organization or a unit has. This counting can be further broken down by category of worker (e.g., registered nurse FTEs, registered practical nurse FTEs, unregulated worker FTEs). The challenge with this measure is that it captures the number of positions allocated to the area, but does not account for the number of staff that make up these positions. For example, an FTE can be made up of a variety of workers, sometimes comprised of part-time and casual hours, to add up to 1.0 FTE. Thus, simply reporting the number of FTEs provides a somewhat inaccurate estimate of the actual number and types of staff employed in an organization or unit.

While FTEs have been used in a number of the research studies examined in this analysis of the literature, they have not been used as a single variable. Most researchers have linked the number of FTEs to the total number of nursing staff employed (Blegen & Vaughn, 1998; Kovner & Gergen, 1998; Mark et al., 2000). If FTEs are to be used as a measure of nurse staffing, a more accurate measurement may be to capture several components of what makes up an FTE. First, it is important to understand what types of workers comprise an FTE. Specifically, is one RN FTE comprised of RNs only, or are several lesser-skilled staff (e.g., LPNs and or unregulated workers) being used to "underfill" the FTE, creating a higher number of personnel in the staffing model? Second, what percentage of FTE hours is made up of full-time, part-time, and/or casual staff? This type of measurement addresses the degree of "casualization" of the nursing workforce.

2.8.5 Percentage of Full-Time, Part-Time, or Casual Staff

The debate surrounding the "casualization" of the nursing workforce has led to interest in assessing the percentage of full-time, part-time, and casual nursing staff in organizations or patient care units. In Canada, a 2002 report of statistical data on nursing employment using data obtained from provincial nursing registries identified that the percentage of nurses employed on a casual basis has been declining over the past five years (Canadian Institutes of Health Information [CIHI], 2002). In 1997 the casual employment rate was 18.3%, followed by 18.6% in 1998, 18.2% in 1999, 14.8% in 2000 and 12.8% in 2001 (CIHI). Similarly, full-time nursing employment percentages have steadily increased from 49.8% in 1997 to 53.2% in 2001, while only a slight increase in part-time nursing employment was noted, from 31.8% in 1997 to 34% in 2001 (CIHI). In a recent survey of 5,000 RNs identified as working part-time or casual in Ontario, 54.6% indicated that there were not any circumstances that would encourage them to move to full-time employment (Registered Nurses Association of Ontario, 2003). This finding is similar to that reported in a study of 1,116 nurses in Ontario (McGillis Hall et al., 2002). Media reports from nurses themselves have also suggested that nurses choose to work part-time (Cadesky, May 10, 2003).

Current interest in understanding the percentage of full-time, part-time, and casual nursing staff relates to the potential impact that these types of staffing models may have on patient, nurse, and organizational outcomes. To date, no empirical literature exists that links the number or percent of full-time, part-time, and casual nursing staff to outcomes.

2.8.6 Mix of Nursing Staff

Staff mix, the combination of different categories of health care workers that are employed for the provision of direct patient care to patients, has been employed in a number of studies (McGillis Hall et al., 2002, 2003; McGillis Hall, 2004; Unruh, 2003). Staff mix models can comprise regulated professional staff (RNs and registered practical nurses), or regulated and unregulated staff (RNs and unregulated workers); (McGillis Hall, 1997, 2004; McGillis Hall et al., 2002, 2003). As well, staff mix has been described as licensed nursing staff (RNs and LPNs; Unruh, 2003). The ANA (1999a) identifies staff mix as the "mix of RNs, LPNs, and unlicensed staff caring for patients in acute care settings" (p. 5).

2.8.7 Level of Education and Experience

The level of nurses' education (e.g., certificate-prepared, diploma-prepared, baccalaureate-prepared) as well as their amount of experience (e.g., overall in nursing, within an organization, on a particular unit, in a specific role) have emerged as important variables to consider when exploring the links between nurse staffing and outcome achievement. The impact of the individual nurse characteristics of education and experience on patient outcomes has been described in several recent empirical studies.

In a report of a secondary analysis of study data obtained from two studies exploring nurse staffing and patient outcomes, the level of nurses' experience was related to adverse patient occurrences with patient care units that employed more experienced nurses found to have lower medication errors and fall rates (Blegen, Vaughn, & Goode, 2001). Similar findings were reported by McGillis Hall et al. (2004), who found that the less experienced the nursing staff, the higher the number of wound infections on a unit. O'Brien-Pallas et al. (2002) reported that clients cared for by baccalaureate-prepared registered nurses (RNs) "had 1.8 times better odds of having improved knowledge scores and 2.2 times better odds of having improved behavior scores" (p. 17) in relation to their health condition. Doran et al. (under review) reported that baccalaureate preparation of nurses, nurses' experience level, and team nursing were related to the documentation of nursing interventions, which in turn predicted improvements in functional status and symptom distress and patients' perceived health benefit from nursing care. As well, Tourangeau et al. (2002) reported lower 30-day mortality rates on units where nurses had more years of unit experience. Most recently, Aiken et al. (2003) reported that hospitals where there were higher proportions of nurses with baccalaureate degrees had lower rates of surgical mortality and failure to rescue.

2.8.8 Summary

In summary, a number of variables have been identified in the literature that effectively measure nurse staffing. All of these variables have demonstrated relationships between nurse staffing and patient outcomes, while some have also successfully linked nurse staffing to organizational and nursing work outcomes. Continued efforts to refine the variables used to measure nurse staffing will help resolve some of the issues identified in previous research.

2.9   Implications and Future Directions

This review of the literature has identified that while the early findings of studies exploring the links between nurse staffing and patient outcomes have produced variable results, the majority of these were in earlier studies that focused on the outcome of patient mortality. For the most part, recent studies provide substantial evidence that higher levels of registered nurse staffing are linked to more positive patient outcomes. Some other challenges related to the inconsistent results in the studies included in this review may be a result of the unit of measurement utilized for nurse staffing and issues related to aggregation of nurse staffing and patient outcomes data to the hospital level.

It is increasingly evident that hospital-level nurse staffing and hospital-level patient case mix and complexity data may not effectively capture the impact of nurse staffing on patient outcomes that occur at the unit level. Kovner and Gergen (1998) identified that the homogeneous relatively simple patient diagnoses utilized in the samples for calculating adverse outcomes may bias study results as patients with multiple diagnoses, who may respond differently to nurse staffing, are excluded from the analysis. Future research should focus on more effectively capturing unit-level data to link nurse staffing to patient outcomes.

Some studies reported that as the proportion of RNs utilized in the staff mix increased beyond a certain level, less positive patient outcomes were observed (Blegen et al., 1998; Blegen & Vaughn, 1998). Studies reporting this finding identified that the units with the highest proportion of RNs were intensive care units. In the Blegen and Vaughn study, 25% of the 39 units studied had an RN proportion over 35%. It is possible that units with a higher proportion of RNs were the intensive care units, where medication administration may be more frequent than on a medical-surgical or skilled-care unit. The authors suggest that there may be "increased vigilance and therefore more reporting" of errors on these units, the patients on these units may be more "severely ill" and requiring more complex medications, thus leading to greater opportunities for error, and "units with higher RN proportions have less total personnel than needed for optimal patient care" (Blegen & Vaughn, p. 202). Further work is needed to determine what factors may have contributed to these results.

More recently, research has begun to move beyond exploring the relationships between nurse staffing and patient outcomes to predicting the change to patient outcomes that would occur with a change in nurse staffing. Kovner and Gergen (1998) reported that an increase of 0.5 RN hours per patient day would be associated with a 4.5% decrease in urinary tract infections, a 4.2% decrease in pneumonia, a 2.6% decrease in thrombosis, and a 1.8% decrease in pulmonary compromise after surgery. Cho et al. (2003) reported that an increase of one hour of RN care was associated with a decrease of 8.9% in the odds of pneumonia. These studies move the state of the science on nurse staffing beyond the establishment of links between nurse staffing and patient outcomes to estimating the staffing changes needed to achieve more positive outcomes. This is the work that may be of greatest interest to administrators and policy makers.

In the United States, substantial interest has evolved in the concept of mandated nurse staffing ratios. Future research exploring the outcomes experienced by patients cared for within systems employing mandated nurse-to-patient ratios will add to the state of the science regarding nurse staffing and outcome achievement.

This review of the literature of nurse staffing suggests that measures of nurse staffing should capture the proportion of RNs, the staffing mix, the proportion of full-time, part-time, and casual staff, and the level of education and experience of the nursing staff. Recent research has begun to examine the impact of nurse staffing in relation to the intended effects of nursing care. Further work is needed to determine the potentially positive contributions that nurses make to patient outcomes. Research that predicts estimates of the staffing changes necessary to achieve more positive patient outcomes should form the next step in this field of research. Further refinement of the unit of measurement for nurse staffing is needed. Unit-level measures of nurse staffing that are accurately adjusted for patient complexity should be employed in future research in this area.

A number of frameworks and theoretical models have been advanced that could guide the study of nurse staffing and outcomes research. While this area of study remains relatively new, it is important for further work to be conducted that tests the sensitivity of these models to the nursing work environment to further validate the proposed relationships. One of the key issues identified in the 1996 report by Wunderlich et al. was the importance of considering nurses' worklife in future research efforts. It is of interest to note that the majority of work to date has focused on determining the relationship between nurse staffing and patient outcomes. With the exception of Aiken's program of research, little attention has been paid to issues in the nursing work environment. Future work should focus on aspects of the nurses' worklife and the nursing work environment that can influence patient and organizational outcomes.

2.10 References

Agency for Health Care Policy and Research, the Division of Nursing of the Health Resources and Services Administration, and the National Institute of Nursing Research. (1997). *Nurse Staffing and Quality of Care in Health Care Organizations Research Agenda*. Retrieved February 27, 2003, from the AHCPR Web site: http://www.ahcpr.gov/fund/nursagnd.htm

Aiken, L. H., Clarke, S. P., Cheung, R. B., Sloane, D. M., & Silbur, J. H. (2003). Educational levels of hospital nurses and surgical mortality. *Journal of the American Medical Association, 290*(12), 1617–1623.

Aiken, L. H., Clarke, S. P., & Sloane, D. M. (2002). Hospital staffing, organization, and quality of care: Cross-national findings. *International Journal for Quality in Health Care, 14*(1), 5–13.

Aiken, L. H., Clarke, S. P., Sloane, D. M., Sochalski, J. A., Busse, R., Clarke, H., et al. (2001). Nurses' reports on hospital care in five countries. *Health Affairs, 20*(3), 43–53.

Aiken, L. H., Clarke, S. P., Sloane, D. P., Sochalski, J., & Silber, J. H. (2002). Hospital nurse staffing and patient mortality, nurse burnout, and job dissatisfaction. *Journal of the American Medical Association, 288*(16), 1987–1993.

Aiken, L. H., Smith, H. L., & Lake, E. T. (1994). Lower Medicare mortality among a set of hospitals known for good nursing care. *Medical Care, 32,* 771–787.

Aiken, L. H. & Sochalski, J. (1997). Hospital restructuring in North America and Europe: Patient outcomes and workforce implications. *Medical Care Supplement, 35*(10), OS1–OS152.

Al-Haider, A. S. & Wan, T. T. (1991). Modeling organizational determinants of hospital mortality. *Health Services Research, 26*(3), 303–323.

American Nurses Association. (1997). *Implementing Nursing's Report Card: A Study of RN Staffing, Length of Stay and Patient Outcomes.* Washington DC: American Nurses Association.

American Nurses Association. (1999a). *Nursing-sensitive quality indicators for acute care settings and ANA's safety and quality initiative.* Retrieved September 28, 2003, from: http://nursingworld.org/readroom/fssafe99.htm

American Nurses Association. (1999b). *Principles of Nurse Staffing.* Washington DC: Author.

American Nurses Association. (2000). *Nurse Staffing and Patient Outcomes in the Inpatient Hospital Setting: Report.* Washington DC: Author.

Barkell, N. P., Killinger, K. A., & Schultz, S. D. (2002). The relationship between nurse staffing models and patient outcomes: A descriptive study. *Outcomes Management, 6*(1), 27–33.

Blegen, M. A., Goode, C. J., & Reed, L. (1998). Nurse staffing and patient outcomes. *Nursing Research, 47*(19), 43–50.

Blegen, M. A. & Vaughn, T. (1998). A multisite study of nurse staffing and patient occurrences. *Nursing Economic$, 16*(4), 196–203.

Blegen, M. A., Vaughn, T., & Goode, C. J. (2001). Nurse experience and education. *Journal of Nursing Administration, 31*(1), 33–39.

Bloom, J., Alexander, J., & Nuchols, B. (1997). Nurse staffing patterns and hospital efficiency in the United States. *Social Science and Medicine, 44*(2), 147–155.

Bostrom J., & Zimmerman J. (1993) Restructuring nursing for a competitive health care environment. *Nursing Economic$, 11*(1), 35–41.

Brewer, C. S. & Frazier, P. (1998). The influence of structure, staff type, and managed-care indicators on registered nurse staffing. *Journal of Nursing Administration, 28*(9), 28–36.

Cadesky, T. (2003, May 10). Nurses who want part-time work being left out. *Toronto Star.* Retrieved May 10, 2003 from www.thestar.com

Canadian Institutes of Health Information. (2002). *Supply and Distribution of Registered Nurses in Canada, 2001.* Ottawa, ON: Canadian Institutes of Health Information.

Cho, S. H., Ketefian, S., Barkauskas, V. H., & Smith, D. G. (2003). The effects of nurse staffing on adverse events, mortality, and medical costs. *Nursing Research, 52*(2), 71–79.

Donabedian A. (1966) Evaluating the quality of medical care. *Millbank Memorial Fund Quarterly, 44*(3), 166–206.

Doran, D. M., Sidani, S., McGillis Hall, L., O'Brien-Pallas, L., Pestryshen, P., Hawkins, J., et al. (Under review). The relationship between baccalaureate education, nurse experience, practice patterns and patient outcome achievement. *Image: Journal of Nursing Scholarship.*

Giovannetti, P. (1978). *Patient Classification Systems in Nursing: A Description and Analysis.* DHEW Publication No. HRA 78-22. Washington, DC: U.S. Government Printing Office. July 1978.

Grillo-Peck, A. M., & Risner, P. B. (1995). The effect of a partnership model on quality and length of stay. *Nursing Economic$, 13,* 367–374.

Hartz, A. J., Krakauer, H., Kuhn, E. M., Young, M., Jacobsen, S. J., Gay, G., et al. (1989). Hospital characteristics and mortality rates. *New England Journal of Medicine, 321,* 1720–1725.

Heinemann, D., Lengacher, C.A., Van Cott, M.L., Mabe, P., & Swymer, S. (1996). Partners in patient care: Measuring the effects on patient satisfaction and other quality indicators. *Nursing Economic$, 14*(5), 276–285.

Holzemer, W. L. (1994). The impact of nursing care in Latin America and the Caribbean: A focus on outcomes. *Journal of Advanced Nursing, 20,* 5–12.

Holzemer, W. L. (1996). The impact of multiskilling on quality of care. *International Nursing Review, 43*(1), 21–25.

Irvine, D., Sidani, S. & McGillis Hall, L. (1998). Linking outcomes to nurses' roles in health care. *Nursing Economic$, 16*(2), 58–64, 87.

Jelinek, R. C. (1969). An operational analysis of the patient care function. *Inquiry, 6*(1), 51–58.

Jelinek, R. C. & Kavois, J. A. (1992). Nurse staffing and scheduling: Past solutions and future directions. *Journal of the Society for Health Systems, 3*(4), 75–82.

Kovner, C. & Gergen, P. J. (1998). Nurse staffing levels and adverse events following surgery in U.S. hospitals. *Image: Journal of Nursing Scholarship, 30*(4), 315–321.

Kovner, C., Jones, C., Zhan, C., Gergen, P.J., & Basu, J. (2002). Nurse staffing and postsurgical adverse events: An analysis of administrative data from a sample of U.S. hospitals, 1990–1996. *Health Services Research, 37,* 611–629.

Lengacher C. A., Kent K., Mabe, P. R., Heinemann D., Van Cott M. L., & Bowling, C. D. (1994). Effects of the partners in care practice model on nursing outcomes. *Nursing Economic$, 12*(6), 300–308.

Lengacher C. A., Mabe, P. R., Heinemann, D., Van Cott, M. L., Swymer, S., & Kent, K. (1996). Effects of the PIPC model on outcome measures of productivity and costs. *Nursing Economic$, 14*(4), 205–213.

Mark, B. A., Salyer, J., & Smith, C. (1996). A theoretical model for nursing systems outcomes research. *Nursing Administration Quarterly, 20*(4), 12–27.

Mark, B. A., Salyer, J., & Wan, T. T. (2000). Market, hospital and nursing unit characteristics as predictors of nursing unit skill mix. *Journal of Nursing Administration, 30*(11), 552–560.

Mark, B. A., Salyer, J., & Wan, T. T. H. (2003). Professional nursing practice: Impact on organizational and patient outcomes. *Journal of Nursing Administration, 33*(4), 224–234.

McGillis Hall, L. (1997). Staff mix models: Complementary or substitution roles for nurses. *Nursing Administration Quarterly, 21*(2), 31–39.

McGillis Hall, L. (2004). Nursing staff mix models and outcomes. *Journal of Advanced Nursing, 44*(2), 217–226.

McGillis Hall, L., & Doran, D. (2004). Nurse staffing, care delivery model and patient care quality. *Journal of Nursing Care Quality, 19*(1), 27–33.

McGillis Hall, L., & Doran, D. (Under review). Nurse staffing and quality work environments. *Research in Nursing & Health.*

McGillis Hall, L., Doran, D., Baker, G. R., Pink, G., Sidani, S., O'Brien-Pallas, L., et al. (2003). Nurse staffing models as predictors of patient outcomes. *Medical Care, 41,* 1096–1109.

McGillis Hall, L., Doran, D., & Pink, G. (2004). Nurse staffing models, nursing hours and patient safety outcomes. *Journal of Nursing Administration, 34*(1), 41–45.

McGillis Hall, L., Irvine, D., Baker, G. R., Pink, G., Sidani, S., O'Brien-Pallas, L., et al. (2002). Nurse staffing and work status in medical, surgical and obstetrical units in Ontario teaching hospitals. *Hospital Quarterly, 5*(4), 64–69.

Mitchell, P. H., Ferketich, S., & Jennings, B. M.. (1998). Quality health outcomes model. *Image: Journal of Nursing Scholarship, 30,* 43–46.

Mitchell, P. H., Heinrich, J., Moritz, P., & Hinshaw, A. S.(1997). Outcome measures and care delivery systems conference. *Medical Care Supplement, 35,* NS1–NS130.

Mularz, L. A., Maher, M., Johnson, A. P., Rolston-Blenman, B., & Anderson, M. A. (1995). Theory M: A restructuring process. *Nursing Management, 26,* 49–52.

Needleman, J., Buerhaus, P., Mattke, S., Stewart, M., & Zelevinsky, K. (2002). Nurse-staffing levels and the quality of care in hospitals. *New England Journal of Medicine, 346,* 1715–1722.

O'Brien-Pallas, L., Irvine Doran, D., Murray, M., Cockerill, R., Sidani, S., Laurie-Shaw, B., et al. (2002). Evaluation of a client care delivery model, Part 2: Variability in client outcomes in community home nursing. *Nursing Economic$, 20,* 13–23.

Potter, P., Barr, N., McSweeney, M. & Sledge, J. (2003). Identifying nurse staffing and patient outcome relationships: A guide for change in care delivery. *Nursing Economic$, 21*(4), 158–166.

Powers, P. H., Dickey, C. A., & Ford, A. (1990). Evaluating an RN/Co-worker model. *Journal of Nursing Administration, 20*(3), 11–15.

Registered Nurses of Ontario. (2003). Survey of Casual and Part-time Registered Nurses in Ontario. May 2003.

Scott, W. R., Forrest, W. H., & Brown, B. W. (1976). Hospital structure and postoperative mortality and morbidity. In S.M. Shortell and M. Brown (Eds.), *Organizational research in hospitals* (pp. 72–89). Chicago: Blue Cross Association.

Shortell, S. M. & Hughes, E. F. (1988). The effects of regulation, competition, and ownership on mortality rates among hospital inpatients. *New England Journal of Medicine, 318,* 1100–1107.

Shortell, S. M., Zimmerman, J. E., Rousseau, D. M., Gillies, R. R., Wagner, D. P., Draper, E. A., et al. (1994). The performance of intensive care units: Does good management make a difference? *Medical Care, 32,* 508–525.

Sochalski, J., Aiken, L. H., & Fagin, C. M. (1997). Hospital restructuring in the United States, Canada and Western Europe. An outcomes research agenda. *Medical Care, 35,* OS13–OS25.

Sovie, M. D. & Jawad, A. F. (2001). Hospital restructuring and its impact on outcomes. *Journal of Nursing Administration, 31,* 588–600.

Spetz, J., Seago, J.A., Coffman, J., Rosenoff, E., & O'Neil, E. (2000). *Minimum Nurse Staffing Ratios in California Acute Care Hospitals.* Oakland, CA: California Health-Care Foundation.

Tourangeau, A. E., Giovannetti, P., Tu, J. V., & Wood, M. (2002). Nursing-related determinants of 30-day mortality for hospitalized patients. *Canadian Journal of Nursing Research, 33*(4), 71–88.

Unruh, L. (2003). Licensed nurse staffing and adverse events in hospitals. *Medical Care, 41,* 142–152.

U.S. Department of Health, Education, and Welfare. (1978) *Methods for Studying Nurse Staffing in a Patient Care Unit. A Manual to Aid Hospitals in Making Use of Personnel.* Public Health Service, Health Resources Administration, Bureau of Health Manpower, Division of Nursing. DHEW Publication No. HRA 78-3. Washington, DC: U.S. Government Printing Office. May 1978.

Wunderlich, G. S., Sloan, F. S., & Davis, C. K. (1996). *Nursing Staff in Hospitals and Nursing Homes: Is It Adequate?* Washington, DC: National Academy Press.

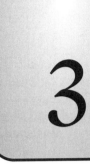

3

Teamwork—
Nursing and the
Multidisciplinary Team

Diane Doran

3.1 Introduction

Providing effective health care to patients in today's environment involves *teams* of health care providers interacting and delivering care for the purpose of achieving desired outcomes. The quality of health care depends on how well members of the team communicate, coordinate care, and negotiate their interdependencies in practice to achieve a cohesive treatment plan for patients. Accumulated evidence from several studies has demonstrated that the quality of team interactions, communication, and care coordination are important determinants of each team member's ability to influence improvements in the quality of care (Higgins & Routhieaux, 1999; Irvine Doran et al., 2002) and to achieve positive patient outcomes (Doran, McGillis Hall, et al., 2002; Doran, Sidani, Keatings, & Doidge, 2002; Knaus, Draper, Wagner, & Zimmerman, 1986). With the mounting evidence of the importance of effective teamwork for the quality of health care, there is a need to examine concepts relevant to teamwork and their role in creating quality nursing work environments.

This chapter:

- Reviews the literature on teamwork in nursing with the aim of understanding how improvements in team functioning in nursing can contribute to the quality of nurses' work environments

- Identifies the essential characteristics or attributes defining the team concepts

- Identifies the instruments (where applicable) or mechanisms that have been used to measure team concepts in acute care, complex continuing care, long-term care, and home care settings

- Reviews the content validity of the instruments or mechanisms

- Assesses the congruency of the instruments or mechanisms with the essential characteristics of each team concept

- Critically reviews the instruments or mechanisms for reliability, validity, responsiveness to change, sensitivity to nursing, and patient outcomes

3.2 Theoretical Underpinnings and Definition of the Team Concepts

The essence of teamwork is collaboration as evidenced by the definition of *team* proposed by Drinka and Ray (1987) and the definition of *teamwork* proposed by Brill (1976). Drinka and Ray defined team as "multiple health disciplines with diverse knowledge and skills who share an integrated set of goals and who utilize interdependent collaboration that involves communication, sharing of knowledge and coordination of services to provide services to patients and their caregiving systems" (p. 44). Brill defined teamwork as "that work which is done by a group of people who possess individual expertise, who are responsible for making individual decisions, who hold a common purpose and who meet together to communicate, share and consolidate knowledge from which plans are made, future decisions are influenced, and actions determined" (p. 10).

These definitions suggest that teamwork is a composite term made up of several subconcepts. These include concepts such as communication, coordination, and shared decision-making. Furthermore, teamwork and collaboration are essentially synonymous concepts. The Oxford dictionary defines collaboration as "to work jointly" (Bissett, 2000) and team as "two or more persons working together" (Bisset). It defines teamwork as "organized cooperation" (Hawkins, 1979).

3.2.1 Collaboration

Collaboration has been defined as the "interaction between nurses and physicians with trust, respect, and joint contributions of knowledge, skills, and value to accomplish the goal of quality patient care" (Krairiksh & Anthony, 2001, p. 17). Baggs, Ryan, Phelps, Richeson, and Johnson (1992) defined collaboration as "open discussion between nurses and physicians and shared responsibility for problem solving and decision making" (p. 19). Most definitions emphasize the joint contributions of persons in a relationship of mutual respect and trust, as evidenced by the following: collaboration is a "process whereby nurses and physicians work together in the delivery of quality care, jointly contributing in a balanced relationship characterized by mutual trust" (Alt-White, Charns, & Strayer, 1983, p. 8). For nurses, doctors, and allied health professionals sharing responsibility for the care of a patient, collaboration has been taken to mean sharing of information, coordination of work, and joint decision-making on aspects of patient care (Doran, Sidani, Keatings, & Doidge, 2002; Irvine, Sidani, & McGillis Hall, 1998; Zwarenstein & Bryant, 2003).

3.2.1.1 Defining Characteristics

Henneman, Lee, and Cohen (1995) proposed the following defining attributes of collaboration based on a concept analysis: joint venture, cooperative endeavor, willing participation, shared planning and decision-making, contribution of expertise, shared responsibility, and nonhierarchical relationships. Collaboration requires sharing of power, with power based on knowledge and expertise rather than on role or title (Henneman et al.). The authors suggested that empirical referents included multidisciplinary rounds, the use of "we" versus "I" statements, dialogue between members of the team, and high scores on collaborative practice scales. Weiss and Davis (1985) identified the following key features of collaboration: (a) the active and assertive contribution of each party, (b) receptivity and respect of the other party's contributions, and (c) a negotiating process that builds upon the contribution of both parties to form a new way of conceptualizing the problem.

Effective collaboration should lead to changes in team members' communication of information, opinions, and feelings; sharing of tasks, decision-making, and goals; power dynamics (i.e., visible expressions of power, such as more equal verbal participation in decisions); mutual respect (Zwarenstein & Bryant, 2003); and more effective coordination of care.

3.2.2 Communication

Communication is the process by which information is exchanged between a sender and a receiver. It occurs verbally and nonverbally. Communication plays an important role in the quality of health care because health care organizations are characterized by high levels of direct client contact. Provider-to-provider and provider-to-client interactions are key to the performance of work in health care organizations (Doran, McGillis Hall, et al., 2002). Timely and accurate communication is essential to the nurses' ability to coordinate the activities of health disciplines involved in patient care. It is also essential to the health care team's ability to respond to a sudden change in the patient's condition when it arises. Communication contributes to the continuity of care because nurses who work rotating shifts need to share information about the patient so that the plan of care can be maintained and modified as needed (Doran, McGillis Hall, et al.).

An effective communicator must have an understanding of how others learn that includes consideration of differences in how others perceive and process information (e.g., analytic versus intuitive, abstract versus concrete, verbal versus written). Furthermore, the achieved or ascribed credibility of the sender effects how the message will be received, with "trust" being most significant (Shortell, 1991).

Lingard, Reznick, Espin, Regehr, and DeVito (2002) used rhetorical theory to investigate communication patterns in the operating room. As described by the authors, a fundamental principle of rhetoric is that all communication has effects—intended and actual.

Similarly, communication is motivated by the need to identify with an audience in order to overcome difference and achieve the common ground required for a productive exchange. Forgoing such identification requires recognition of the elements of division and negotiation of shared interests (Lingard et al., p. 233).

Lingard et al. described communication in the operating room as a "complicated dance" (p. 233) that maintains relationships and minimizes tension while still achieving goals.

3.2.3 Coordination

Coordination has been defined as the management of interdependencies among tasks (Malone & Crowston, 1994). Longest (1974) defined coordination as "the process of assembling and synchronizing differentiated activities so that they function effectively in the attainment of the organization's objectives" (p. 65). Coordination "means integrating or linking together different parts of an organization to accomplish a collective set of tasks" (Van De Ven, Delbecq, & Koenig, 1976, p. 322). Organizational design theory suggests that coordination can be achieved through a variety of formal and informal coordinating mechanisms. Marsh and Simon (1958), Van De Ven and associates, and Trist (1977) were among the early theorists to describe coordination in organizations. According to Marsh and Simon, there are two general ways in which organizations can be coordinated: (a) by programming or (b) by feedback. Coordination by programming is exemplified by such integrating mechanisms as the use of pre-established plans, schedules, forecasts, formalized rules, policies and procedures, and standardized information and communication systems (Van De Ven et al.). In health care organizations, coordination by programming occurs through routines or protocols to codify best practices (Gittell, 2002). More recently, protocols have evolved into clinical pathways, which combine protocols used by different members of the care provider team into a single document, outlining the tasks to be completed and decisions to be made by each professional group, and the sequence in which they are to be performed (Gittell).

Coordination can also be achieved by standardization of skills, which involves the specification of the skills or information required to perform work. Often this is achieved through specification of minimum levels and types of education, certification as evidence of meeting minimum qualifications, or on-the-job training (Young et al., 1997, 1998). Nursing organizations rely heavily on coordination by standardization of skills through skills certification and delegated acts. There is some evidence in the literature that overlapping roles, achieved through a degree of role blurring, facilitates coordination of work (Gittell, 2000). Preuss (1997) found that overlapping task boundaries in nursing units were associated with improved information quality and reduced frequency of medication errors. Gibbon and colleagues (2002) suggested that it is better to have some role overlap and blurring of disciplinary boundaries than to have patients falling through care gaps.

Coordination by feedback is the mutual adjustment of work activities and patient care based on new information (Van De Ven et al., 1976). Coordination by feedback occurs through personal interaction or through group/team meetings. Team meetings give participants the opportunity to coordinate tasks directly with one another. Meetings in the health care setting take the form of patient rounds (Gittell, 2002).

Gittell (2002) proposed the term *relational coordination* to capture the notion of coordination through personal interaction. She argued that while coordination is facilitated by formal organizational design elements, such as those described above, coordination is more fundamentally a process of interaction among participants. "Relational coordination reflects the role that frequent, timely, accurate, problem-solving communication plays in the process of coordination, but it also captures the oft-overlooked role played by relationships" (Gittell, 2002, p. 1410). Gittell suggested that coordination is carried out through relationships of shared goals, shared knowledge, and mutual respect. In addition to these relationship characteristics, Van Ess Coeling and Cukr (2000) suggested that coordination involves recognizing alternative perspectives and a willingness to assume power and yield power appropriately.

3.3 Factors that Influence Teamwork

Because teamwork is a multidimensional construct, it is important to consider each dimension when developing an understanding of the factors that contribute to or influence teamwork. These will each be discussed in turn.

3.3.1 Factors Contributing to Team Collaboration

Henneman et al. (1995) identified personal, group dynamics, and environmental variables as antecedents to collaboration. The personal antecedents were identified by Henneman et al. as individuals' educational preparation, maturity, and prior experience working in similar situations. In addition, they suggested that it is important for individuals to have a clear understanding and acceptance of their own role and level of expertise. Confidence in one's ability as well as recognition of the boundaries of one's discipline are critical to this understanding (Henneman et al.). Personal expectations also motivate collaboration approaches. In one study, nurses' expectations about the physician's intention to collaborate influenced their own intentions to resolve conflict in a collaborative manner (Keenan, Cooke, & Hillis, 1998).

Factors at the group level play an important role in the promotion of collaboration. Group-level factors that promote collaboration include excellent communication skills, respect, sharing, and trust. For instance, effective communication allows team members to negotiate constructively with one another (Henneman et al., 1995).

Some theorists have suggested that before an interdisciplinary team can establish the open communication, flexibility in leadership, and coordination of efforts necessary for effective functioning, it must pass through a sequence of developmental stages (Farrell, Schmitt, & Heinemann, 2001). In the early stages of development, interpersonal conflicts, communication blocks, and poor process skills impair the quality of patient care. A critical factor that leads to movement from an undeveloped state to a more advanced stage of group development is the negotiation of a team culture that the members internalize. The shared culture includes a set of unambiguous, consensually approved expectations about decision-making, about each member's rights and responsibilities in his or her professional role, and about the procedures for working together (Farrell et al.).

Collaboration requires flexibility in roles as opposed to clearly demarcated role boundaries. For instance, Farrell et al. (2001) suggested that among mature teams, roles are assigned based on knowledge and skill, allowing for role blending. "Thus, a nurse may fill in for a social worker in providing support to a patient's family; and the social worker may in turn take on administrative responsibilities that would ordinarily be carried out by the nurse" (Farrell et al., p. 284). In their study of 111 interdisciplinary geriatric teams from 34 Veteran Affairs Medical Centers, they found that team members' diverse perceptions of each member converged in the later stages of team development. Team development was operationally defined as how confused or uncertain members were about team members' roles and the team's norms and goals (Farrell et al.).

An environment with a team orientation, reward systems that recognize group accomplishments, and organizational values that support participation have been identified as environmental antecedents to collaboration (Henneman et al., 1995). In addition, collaboration is fostered in environments that offer support systems, autonomy, freedom of expression, and interdependence (Henneman et al.). Structural features that mitigate against team collaboration include the distribution of doctors through varying parts of the hospitals, the use of agency nurses, and the lack of formal and informal team meetings (Meerabeau & Page, 1999).

3.3.2 *Factors Contributing to Team Communication*

Shortell (1991) noted that among the barriers to effective communication are power or status relationships, differing frames of reference, and the use of unfamiliar terminology among professions. Disciplinary jargon and different frames of reference that lead to misunderstanding (Roelofsen, The, Beckerman, & Lankhorst, 2002) may be a product of a team subculture and/or professional groups' socialization. In an audit of interprofessional communication problems, Fox (2000) found miscommunication occurred more frequently among individuals who had little experience of the team culture. Familiarity with the team culture helped individuals to understand the jargon and nuances of team communication. Furthermore, work experience and role clarity contributed to improved communication among team members (Fox). Dreachslin, Hunt, and Sprainer (1999) used a focus group methodology to investigate communication problems in patient-centered care teams. Poor communicators were identified by others as team members who tend to give orders rather than make requests, engage in one-way rather than two-way communication, lack the technical competence required to understand or perform a task, exhibit unpredictability in mood or behavior, or consider themselves as superior to other team members. Factors such as management style, interpersonal dynamics, attitudes toward the patient-centered care model, and lack of sufficient task and relationship skills on the part of some team members contributed to communication breakdown (Dreachslin et al.).

Patel, Cytryn, Shortliffe, and Safran (2000) conducted an observational study of team interaction in a primary care ambulatory setting. Communication within disciplines flowed hierarchically from the director of medicine and faculty physicians to research fellows, residents, and interns. The hierarchical structure did not apply between different disciplines—for example between medicine, nursing, and mental health (Patel et al.). Communication styles approached equality for issues requiring the clinical expertise of individuals in domains (disciplines) other than their own. For example, physicians were observed to consult with nurses for patient monitoring and continuity of care (Patel et al.). Communication between nurses and physicians accounted for about 88% of all communication observed by the investigators. Trainees, such as medical residents and interns, communicated less with team members than did the faculty physicians. Patel et al. proposed that a possible explanation for this was that the trainees had not yet developed the same level of expertise in providing care in a team context or were simply less familiar with the other team members because their tenure in the unit was short lived.

3.3.3 Factors Contributing to Coordination of Care

In some organizations, formalized roles have been developed to facilitate coordination of work across functional units or professional groups. "Boundary spanners," also known as cross-functional liaisons, are individuals whose primary task is to integrate the work of other people (Gittell et al., 2000). Project manager, case manager, and discharge planner are common boundary-spanning roles (Gittell et al.). Nurses play a coordinating role by virtue of their 24-hour, 7-day-a-week presence on the patient care unit in acute care, long-term care, complex continuing care, and to a large extent, home care. The primary nursing care delivery model, in which patients are assigned to a single nurse for the duration of their stay, is designed to facilitate the coordination of the care of the patient from the beginning to the end of the stay (Gittell et al.).

Gittell (2000) found relational coordination was facilitated by cross-functional liaison roles, work role flexibility, greater reliance on information technology to coordinate work, cross-functional performance measurement, smaller spans of supervisory control, and selection of individuals for teamwork.

An observational study of collaboration among trauma resuscitation teams found coordination breakdowns occurred in four forms: (a) conflicting plans, (b) inadequate support in crisis situations, (c) inadequate verbalization of problems, and (d) lack of task delegation. The video recordings in the study showed that team coordination was achieved in most situations with minimum explicit, verbal communication. When team coordination broke down, it often occurred in situations where there was a lack of explicit communication (Xiao & Mackenzie, 1998).

3.3.4 Summary

Providing effective health care to patients involves *teams* of health care providers interacting and delivering care to achieve desired outcomes. The quality of health care depends on how members of the team communicate, coordinate care, and negotiate differences in practice to achieve a cohesive treatment plan for patients. Collaboration among health care providers necessitates the joint contribution of persons in a relationship of mutual respect and trust. Communication is the process by which information is exchanged among health care providers. It is essential to maintaining continuity and coordination of effort. Coordination involves the integration of individual effort and care decisions to achieve coherence in patient care. Coordination is achieved both through programmed means such as care plans and clinical pathways, and through personal interaction among care providers. Effective collaboration, communication, and coordination require an environment with a team orientation, reward systems that recognize group accomplishments, and organizational values that support participation.

Studies have investigated the impact of teamwork on the quality of nurses' work environment, nurse outcomes, the quality of care, and patient outcomes. Of the studies reviewed, nine were conducted in an acute care setting, three in ambulatory care, one in an emergency room setting, one in a rehabilitation setting, one in palliative care, and one in a community setting. Those studies that examined the relationship between different aspects of team collaboration and the quality of nurses' work environment and nurse outcomes are discussed below. Following this, the studies that examined the impact of team collaboration on the quality of care and patient outcomes are discussed.

3.4 Linking Team Collaboration to the Quality of Nurses' Work Environment

There is evidence from the research literature that the quality of teamwork affects nurses' worklife. For instance, in a study of 42 intensive care units (ICUs) in the United States, Shortell et al. (1994) found that more effective interaction among caregivers on the ICU teams was significantly associated with lower nurse turnover. Caregiver interaction was operationally defined as the culture, leadership, coordination, communication, and conflict management abilities of the unit. The American Association of Critical Care Nurses' Demonstration Project also found high nurse-physician collaboration and the use of coordinating mechanisms to be factors in obtaining increased nurse satisfaction (Mitchell, Armstrong, Simpson, & Lentz, 1989). A third study of 446 nurses from 46 patient care units found a strong inverse relationship between collaboration and perceptions of organizational stress (Alt-White, Charns, & Strayer, 1983).

3.5 Linking Team Collaboration to Patient Outcome Achievement

In response to growing concern about patient safety and in recognition of the need for a systems approach to ensuring safe care, attention has been focused on methods to improve teamwork practices to reduce error (Kohn, Corrigan, & Donaldson, 2000). In the United States, communication failures among team members have been uncovered at the root of 60% of sentinel events reported to the Joint Commission on Accreditation of Healthcare Organizations (Joint Commission on Accreditation of Healthcare Organizations, May 2003).

The effectiveness of team collaboration has been observed to produce higher quality patient and system outcomes (Argote, 1984; Gittell et al., 2000; Knaus et al., 1986; Shortell et al., 1994; Young et al., 1997, 1998). For instance, one study of 298 nurses' reports of the impact of collaboration on their practice found that nurse-physician collaboration had a positive effect on nurses' caregiving decisions (Krairiksh & Anthony, 2001). In a sample of 5,030 patients in intensive care units, Knaus et al. (1986) found differences in death rates were related to the quality of the interaction and communication between physicians and nurses. A subsequent study of 17,440 ICU patients found caregiver interaction comprising group culture, leadership, communication, coordination, and conflict management abilities was significantly associated with low risk-adjusted length of stay and higher technical quality of care (Shortell et al.). The American Association of Critical Care Nurses Demonstration Project found high nurse-physician collaboration and the use of coordinating mechanisms to be factors in obtaining desired patient outcomes (Mitchell et al., 1989). Baggs et al. (1992) used the Decision About Transfer (DAT) Scale to measure collaborative decision-making between nurses and physicians in medical intensive care units. The nurses' reports of collaboration with physicians were significantly and positively associated with desired patient outcomes and the predicted risk of negative outcomes decreased in collaboration situations (Baggs et al.). Negative outcomes were either re-admission to the medical intensive care unit or death during the same hospital admission. This study found further that collaboration became more essential as the complexity of the patient-care situation increased. Young et al. (1997) found Veteran Affairs Hospitals that achieved lower-than-expected risk-adjusted mortality among surgical services used a greater number and greater variety of coordinating practices than hospitals that achieved higher-than-expected risk-adjusted mortality. The group of surgical services using coordination by feedback and coordination by programming had the best perceived quality of care. This group also had the lowest morbidity (Young et al., 1998). In a study involving 878 patients and 338 health providers from nine US hospitals, relational coordination among members of cross-functional care provider groups was associated with improved quality of care, postoperative freedom from pain, and reduced lengths of hospital stay (Gittell, 2002; Gittell et al., 2000). In looking more closely at the beneficial attributes of relational coordination, Gittell found postoperative freedom from pain and functioning was associated with the frequency of communication, shared goals, shared knowledge, and mutual respect.

Two studies were located that had evaluated an intervention designed to improve coordination among health care teams. These studies yielded mixed results. In a randomized controlled trial (RCT) set in an American academic hospital, an intervention involving daily multidisciplinary rounds resulted in significantly reduced hospital charges and shortened average length of hospital stay, but no difference between the intervention and control unit in mortality rates or of the type of care to which patients were discharged (e.g., long-term care or home;

Curley, McEachern, & Speroff, 1998). Another RCT involving four-times-per-week rounds held in a Thai academic hospital found no significant difference in length of stay and mortality outcomes for the intervention versus control group unit (Jitapunkul et al., 1995).

3.6 Issues in the Assessment of Nurses' Teamwork

Despite the importance of team interactions for the quality of health care, this is an area of health care research that is still relatively new with very few rigorously designed studies that have evaluated the effects of interprofessional interventions on teamwork (Zwarenstein, Reeves, Barr, Hammick, Koppel, & Atkins, 2003). For this reason, we are just beginning to build an understanding of some of the issues in assessing teamwork among nurses and other members of the health care profession. Some of the assessment issues that are arising from the current research base include: (a) how is the team defined, and from whose perspective; (b) how are multiple and sometimes, contradictory perspectives of teamwork reconciled; and (c) at what level of analysis should teamwork be assessed?

The first issue concerns how the team is defined. An underlying assumption of most approaches to assessing team concepts, like communication and coordination, is that team members have a common understanding of the term *team*. However, a review of the literature suggested that, in some cases, this assumption has not been confirmed. Cott (1998) conducted an observational study of multidisciplinary teamwork within a long-term care setting. As the study progressed, it became apparent that although all of the staff members valued teamwork, staff in different structural positions held different perceptions of meanings of teamwork because they were engaged in different kinds of teamwork. Staff in lower structural positions did not share the same meaning of teamwork as staff in higher structural positions. When the direct caregiving staff defined the team, it included the other nursing staff on their shift and specifically, those nursing staff with whom they were paired. They did not feel engaged with the multidisciplinary professionals, nor did they consider themselves part of a larger multiprofessional team (Cott). The direct caregiving staff rarely attended multidisciplinary rounds, nor were they expected to be part of team decision-making (Cott). This research suggested two areas that need to be addressed when assessing perceptions of teamwork. First, in order to avoid ambiguities, which could result in measurement error, the term team needs to be carefully defined for the respondents with attention to who constitutes the team. Second, it is probably useful to distinguish between the nursing team and multidisciplinary team, and study both in nursing organizations.

A second and somewhat related issue in the assessment of teamwork concerns the mounting evidence that members on the same team do not, in fact, share a common view of their teamwork. In fact, research into health professionals' relationships showed discord and disagreement among disciplinary groups (Lingard et al., 2002). Several studies have revealed an absence of consensus between physicians, nurses, and other health professionals with regard to issues of teamwork, particularly in relation to describing team communication and coordination of care (Lingard et al.; Weiss & Davis, 1985). For these reasons, individuals interested in studying teams need to account for multiple perspectives in making team concepts operational and in their measurement approach. Strategies for dealing with multiple perspectives are discussed below.

A third issue in assessing teamwork follows from the first two issues and concerns the level of analysis and analytic method for representing group versus individual effects. Researchers of team behavior are typically interested in the team as the level of analysis. However, they often rely on individuals to gain an understanding of the team phenomenon. This is especially true when quantitative measures, such as questionnaires, are used to assess team level concepts. An alternative to the quantitative method is the use of observational or qualitative methods to study team interaction patterns (Cott, 1998; Lingard et al., 2002; Patel et al., 2000). In this case, the unit of observation is the whole team or part of the team (e.g., when an interaction among a dyad or triad is studied) and the issue of resolving individual differences in perspective does not arise.

Investigators have addressed the issue of multiple perspectives in a couple of ways when quantitative methods are used to measure team phenomena utilizing individual group members' perceptions. One way that has been commonly seen in the literature is to represent the team level phenomenon as an average of the scores of the individual members (Shortell et al., 1994). This strategy ignores the level of divergence in perspective among team members by giving equal weight to all views. Alternatively, investigators have dealt with diverse perspectives of group phenomena by representing the group phenomena as a function of the strength of congruence among team members' perspectives. For example, in a study of relational coordination, each dimension of relational coordination was computed as the percentage of cross-functional connections that were strong (e.g., 4 or 5 on a 5-point scale) on the expectation that groups are more clearly distinguished by the percentage of strong connections than by the average strength of connections (Gittell, 2002). In the literature, the argument for one approach over the other is not strong, and in at least one study reviewed, the two methods yielded similar findings (Gittell).

When quantitative methods are used to assess team phenomena, it is necessary to address the issue of how to weight the perspectives of different professional groups when it is not possible to obtain the perspective of all team members and/or when there are differences in response rates across disciplines. In order to obtain an unbiased estimate of the team phenomenon under these circumstances, researchers have weighted the individual questionnaire responses to reflect the interdisciplinary composition of care providers on the team to correct for differences in response rates across disciplines (Gittell et al., 2000).

When studying variables that are measured at two levels, the group and the individual, it is necessary to establish that there is a group-level effect by demonstrating that two people in the same group are more similar than two people who are members of different groups (Florin, Giamartino, Kenny, & Wandersman, 1990). This is done through a multivariate analysis of variance, using a measure called the intraclass correlation coefficient. An intraclass correlation coefficient close to 1 indicates there is a strong group effect.

3.7 Evidence Concerning Approaches to Measuring Teamwork

Teamwork has been assessed with multidimensional measures that target multiple concepts such as communication, coordination, and decision-making, as well as measures that target one component of teamwork, such as questionnaires that assess only coordination or communication. In the discussion of approaches to measurement, the review will focus first on multidimensional instruments of teamwork and then on measures that have been developed to assess specific team concepts. These instruments are summarized below providing a description of the intended target audience, domains of measurement, method of administration, evidence concerning reliability and validity, and sensitivity to change (see Table 3.1).

3.8 Multidimensional Measures of Teamwork

3.8.1 Caregiver Interaction Questionnaire

The Caregiver Interaction Questionnaire developed by Shortell et al. (1994) measures leadership, communication, coordination, and problem-solving/conflict management. Each item is measured using 5-point Likert scales (1 = strongly disagree, 5 = strongly agree). Separate questionnaires were developed for nurses and physicians. Nursing and physician leadership are measured by two 8-item scales involving the extent to which leaders emphasize standards of excellence, communicate clear goals and expectations, respond to challenging needs and situations, and are in touch with unit members' perceptions and concerns. Shortell et al. reported Cronbach's alphas for both the nursing leadership scale and the physician leadership scale as .88. Convergent validity was demonstrated between nursing and physician leadership and team satisfaction oriented culture and open-collaborative, problem-solving approaches. McGillis Hall et al. (2001) used the Nursing Leadership Scale in a study of nurses from 19 Ontario teaching hospitals and found a significant relationship between nursing leadership and nurses' job satisfaction, job pressure, job threat, and role tension.

Table 3.1 Nursing Measures of Team Health Care

Instrument Author/Date of Publication	Target Population	Domains	Method of Administration	Reliability	Validity	Sensitivity to Nursing
Communication Instruments						
Communication and Cross-Functional Cooperation (Pinto & Pinto, 1990)	Hospital project teams developing a new program.	Intraproject communication; 15 items; 6-point Likert scale; cross-functional cooperation; 15 items; 7-point Likert scale.	Self-administered.	ICR: α = .96 for cross-functional cooperation.	Construct: three pretests were conducted to valid constructs.	None stated.
Verbal Aggressiveness (Infante & Wigley, 1986)	Students.	Verbal aggressiveness (communication); 30 items; 5-point response scale.	Self-administered.	ICR: α = .81; TRR: α = .81.	Concurrent: assessed and showed good validity (no details provided); predictive: assessed but no details provided.	Sensitivity to change, administered to a number of different groups over a four-week period and test-retest of the Scale showed good stability. r = .82, t = <1.
Coordination Instruments						
Relational Coordination Instrument (Gittell et al., 2000)	Health care providers.	Relational coordination (communication and relationship); 7 items; 5-point Likert scale.		ICR: α = .717 - .840 for individual domains α = .844 for overall measure of relational coordination (Gittell et al., 2000; Gittell, 2002).		
Patterns of Coordination (Young et al., 1998)	Surgical service teams.	Patterns of coordination (programming and feedback); 14- to 15-items (three versions of questionnaire); 5-point response scale.	Self-administered.	ICR: α between .68 and .87 for the three versions; TRR: r = .68 to .93.	Construct: aggregation of scores from three professions into a service score was validated with one-way analysis of variance ($p \leq .05$).	

r = correlation coefficient
α = Cronbach's alpha coefficient
ICR Internal Consistency Reliability
TRR = Test Re-test Reliability
IRR = Inter-rater Reliability

Table 3.1 (continued)

Instrument Author/Date of Publication	Target Population	Domains	Method of Administration	Reliability	Validity	Sensitivity to Nursing
Patterns of Coordination (continued)					Convergent and discriminate: tested using multitrait scaling for the two scales of coordination (i.e., programming and feedback); testing supported the two scales.	
Formalization on health care (Hetherington, 1991)	Health care settings.	Formalization, complexity, coordination, climate for change, quality of care and morale; number of items not specified; 6-point Likert scale.	Self-administered to in-patient medical care unit staff.	Showed good reliability among physicians, nurses and technicians (no details provided).	Construct: multiple regression analysis show that quality of care measures are one construct; predictive: assessed by factor analysis.	
Teamwork Questionnaire (O'Neil Jr. et al., 2003)	Technical support personnel.	Cognitive teamwork dimension: coordination (2 items), decision making (2 items), leadership (4 items); 4-point Likert scale.	Self-administered.	ICR: α = 69-.83 for total questionnaire; α = .75-.84 for cognitive teamwork dimension.	Construct validity: t-tests show difference between teamwork questionnaire for areas of high or low performance ($p < .05$); for cognitive teamwork dimension and the total scale, t-tests show teamwork skills are exhibited more in participants who more frequently worked in teams ($p < .05$).	

r = correlation coefficient

α = Cronbach's alpha coefficient

ICR Internal Consistency Reliability

TRR = Test Re-test Reliability

IRR = Inter-rater Reliability

Table 3.1 (continued)

Instrument Author/Date of Publication	Target Population	Domains	Method of Administration	Reliability	Validity	Sensitivity to Nursing
			Collaboration Instruments			
Decision About Transfer Scale (Baggs et al., 1992)	Nurses and physicians.	Collaboration, satisfaction and alternatives in decisions to transfer from the ICU; 3 items, each measuring one above concept; 7-point Likert scale for collaboration and 4-point Likert scale for alternatives.	One questionnaire designed specifically for nurses, another for physicians; self-administered.	No testing done.	Content: conducted extensive literature review; face: pre-tested by ten ICU nurses. Criterion: residents and nurses were given the Collaborative Practice Scales (Weiss, 1985) while nurses also filled out Index of Work Satisfaction (Stamps, 1986). Both instruments have established high validity and reliability.	
Collaboration Practice Scale (Weiss & Davis, 1985)	Nurses and physicians.	Nurses: direct assertiveness of professional expertise and active clarification or mutual responsibilities; 9 items, 6-point Likert scale. Physicians: acknowledgement of nurse's contribution to patient care and consensus development with nurses; 10 items; 6-point Likert scale.	Self-administered.	ICR: α = .80 (nurses); α = .84 (physicians); TRR: α = .83 (nurses); α = .85 (physicians).	Construct: results from factor analysis support existence of different domains; concurrent: compared with two validated measures: Health Role Expectations Index (Weiss and Davis, 1983) and Management of Differences Exercise (Kilmann and Thomas, 1977); predictive: results from peer evaluations positively correlated with instrument.	

r = correlation coefficient
α = Cronbach's alpha coefficient
ICR Internal Consistency Reliability
TRR = Test Re-test Reliability
IRR = Inter-rater Reliability

Table 3.1 (continued)

Instrument Author/Date of Publication	Target Population	Domains	Method of Administration	Reliability	Validity	Sensitivity to Nursing
		Multidimensional Instruments				
Organizational Assessment in ICU : Caregiver Interaction (Shortell et al., 1991)	Health care personnel.	All are measured on 5-point Likert scale; leadership 8-item scale (one for nurses, one for physicians); communication: openness, accuracy, timeliness, effective communication and satisfaction; 25 items for nurses and 26 items for physicians; coordination: within unit (5 items), between unit (4 items) and relationships between units (4 items); problem-solving/conflict management: open, collaborative problem solving (4 items), arbitration (3 items), avoidance strategy (3 items) and forcing approach (3 items) (Filley, 1975).	Self-administered.	ICR: all α > .70 (Shortell 1994); leadership α = .87 (nursing), α = .88 (physician); communication (α = .64); coordination (α = .75).	Content: interviewed hospital staff to validate questionnaire; convergent and discriminate: assessed by correlation matrices analysis.	
Group Interaction Scale (Watson & Michaelsen, 1988; Watson et al., 1991)	Teams.	Expectation & integration, power struggle, organization, non-involvement, communication & participation.	Self-report.	Watson & Michaelsen reported α = .68 to .88; Doran et al. (2002) reported α = .85 and .86 for a two factor structure, measuring functional and dysfunctional interaction.	Construct: in a study of health care teams—group interaction predicted successful quality improvement teams (Doran et al., 2002).	Significant improvement in group interactions were observed after a CQI team intervention (Doran et al., 2002).

r = correlation coefficient

α = Cronbach's alpha coefficient

ICR Internal Consistency Reliability

TRR = Test Re-test Reliability

IRR = Inter-rater Reliability

Table 3.1 (continued)

Instrument Author/Date of Publication	Target Population	Domains	Method of Administration	Reliability	Validity	Sensitivity to Nursing
Team Climate Inventory (TCI) (Anderson & West, 1998)	Work group.	Vision, participation, interaction frequency, support for innovation, task orientation.	Self-report.	Reliability coefficients in a sample of health care teams 0.84 to 0.94.	The TCI predicted innovativeness among hospital management.	
Modified Operating Room Management Attitudes Questionnaire (Flin, 2003)	Operating room management teams (modified from Hemreich, 1997).	Section 1: Leadership-structure, information sharing; teamwork; work values and organizational climate; 60 items; 5-point Likert scale. Section 2: rate perception of quality of teamwork and cooperation/ communication they experienced. 8 groups listed. Section 3: 5 questions relating to error management; 5-point Likert scale. Section 4: Open-ended questions on effectiveness.	Self-administered.	ICR: α = .18-.54.		

r = correlation coefficient

α = Cronbach's alpha coefficient

ICR Internal Consistency Reliability

TRR = Test Re-test Reliability

IRR = Inter-rater Reliability

Communication is measured along a number of dimensions including openness, accuracy, timeliness, understanding, and satisfaction. There were high correlations among the dimensions. As a result, Shortell et al. (1994) used only the timeliness dimension in their ICU study and reported a Cronbach's alpha of .64. Doran, McGillis Hall et al. (2002) reported a Cronbach's alpha of .86 in a study of 74 nursing teams from 19 Ontario teaching hospitals. Coordination between units is measured by a 4-item scale relating to the unit's ability to coordinate its work with other units. Shortell et al. reported a Cronbach's alpha of .75. Problem-solving/conflict management is a four-item scale of open collaborative problem-solving, the extent to which physicians and nurses work actively to make sure that all available expertise is brought to bear on a problem and the goal of arriving at the best possible solution. The Cronbach's alpha was .82 (Shortell et al.). A Cronbach's alpha for the caregiver interaction composite index was .89. Construct validity of the composite index was evidenced in a significant relationship between caregiver interaction and lower risk-adjusted length of stay, lower nurse turnover, and higher technical quality of care (Shortell et al.).

3.8.2 Group Interaction Scale

Watson and Michaelsen (1988) developed the Group Interaction Scale to measure effective and ineffective group interactions. The scale measures five dimensions of group interaction: expectation and integration, power struggle, organization, noninvolvement, and communication and participation (i.e., everyone has a chance to express themselves). In a study of university students, the scale demonstrated a 65% and 80% accuracy rate in differentiating effective and ineffective problem-solving groups over two measurement points and internal consistency reliability of its subscales (alpha coefficients ranging from .68 to .78 at Time 1, and from .82 to .88 at Time 2) (Watson & Michaelsen). Irvine Doran et al. (2002) used the Group Interaction Scale in a study of 24 health care teams and found that health care teams that were successful in implementing changes in practice that led to improved outcomes or processes of care demonstrated more effective functional group interactions. Factor analysis of the Group Interaction Scale in this study demonstrated two factors, one measuring functional group interactions and a second measuring dysfunctional group interactions. Cronbach's alpha for the two factors was .85 and .86 (Irvine Doran et al.).

3.8.3 Team Climate Inventory

Anderson and West (1998) developed the Team Climate Inventory (TCI) to measure work group climate for innovation. The construction of the inventory was based on a 4-factor theory of group innovation consisting of vision, participative safety, task orientation, and support for innovation. Anderson and West defined vision as "an idea of a valued outcome which represents a higher order and a motivating force at work" (p. 240). Twelve items were constructed to measure vision, assessing the team members' views on the clarity, sharedness, attainability, and value of team objectives. Participative safety was defined as "a single psychological construct in which the contingencies are such that involvement in decision-making is motivated and reinforced while occurring in an environment which is perceived as personally non-threatening" (Anderson & West, p. 240). For the purpose of measurement, the construct of participative safety was subdivided into two components—team participation and safety. Team participation is measured with 15 items to which respondents are asked to respond on a 5-point strongly disagree or strongly agree scale. Safety is measured by nine items, rated on a 5-point response scale. Task orientation was defined as "a shared concern with excellence of quality of task performance in relation to shared vision or outcomes" (Anderson & West, p. 240). This concept was also subdivided into two components—climate for excellence consisting of 10 items measured on a 7-point scale, and constructive controversy consisting of seven items measured on a 5-point scale. Support for innovation is "…the expectation, approval and practical support of attempts to introduce new and improved ways of doing things in the work environment" (Anderson & West, p. 240). Support for innovation consisted of eight items measured on a 5-point scale.

The 61-item version of the scale was pilot tested with 14 nursing teams in a hospital setting and with two hospital management teams. Five factors, rather than four, emerged in exploratory factor analysis, consisting of vision, participation, interaction frequency, support for innovation, and task orientation. These five factors were subsequently confirmed in a follow-up study involving community psychiatric teams, hospital management teams, oil company teams, primary health teams, and social service teams. Alpha coefficients ranged from .84 to .94. The inventory predicted innovativeness among hospital management teams. Gibbon et al. (2002) used a 44-item version of the TCI in a study evaluating two different approaches to facilitating teamwork for stroke rehabilitation teams consisting of the use of integrated pathways and the use of unified team notes. The results indicated that team attitudes were not strongly influenced by either intervention.

3.8.4 Operating Room Management Attitudes Questionnaire

The Operating Room Management Attitudes Questionnaire (ORMAQ) was developed to measure operating room staff attitudes toward teamwork and safety and to assess attitudes toward stress, hierarchy, teamwork, and error. The ORMAQ consists of 60 Likert attitude statements relating to eight themes: leadership-structure, confidence-assertion, information sharing, stress and fatigue, teamwork, work values, error, and organizational climate. A second section of the questionnaire assesses perceptions of the quality of teamwork and cooperation/communication. A third section contains five statements relating to error management. The ORMAQ was adapted for use in the United Kingdom and was tested in a sample of 222 anaesthetists from 11 Scottish hospitals (Flin, Fletcher, McGeorge, Sutherland, & Patey, 2003). The reliability analysis for the dimensions in this sample showed low reliabilities ranging from .18 to .54. Elsewhere in a U.S. sample, alpha coefficients have been reported as .55 to .85 (Flin et al.).

3.9 Instruments Measuring Specific Team Concepts

3.9.1 Relational Coordination

The Relational Coordination instrument developed by Gittell (2000) encompasses four communication dimensions including request, timely, accurate, and problem-solving, as well as three relationship dimensions including shared goals, shared knowledge, and mutual respect. The Relational Coordination questionnaire was developed and validated in the context of commercial airline flight departures (Gittell). It was adapted for use in a study of health care teams. The overall measure of relational coordination is a 7-item measure comprising each of the seven dimensions of relational coordination identified above (i.e., the four communication and three relationship dimensions). Cronbach's alpha in a study of health care teams ranged from .72 to .84. The Cronbach's alpha for the overall index was .85. The Relational Coordination instrument was sensitive to interagency differences in coordination. Construct validity in the health care sample was evidenced by significant relationships between relational coordination and improved quality of care, improved postoperative pain and functioning for patients undergoing joint arthroplasty, and shortened length of hospital stay. Evidence of use in studies other than those reported by Gittell was not found.

3.9.2 Coordination Approach Scale

Young et al. (1998) developed an instrument to measure two approaches to coordination of health care: programming approaches and coordination through feedback. The instrument was based on an earlier instrument developed by Alt-White et al. (1983). Clinical staff are asked to rate on a 5-point scale the extent to which specific activities or mechanisms provide them with information in performing their work. Examples of items that assess coordination by programming are use of protocols, pathways, and treatment plans. Feedback approaches to coordination are separated into group feedback such as interdisciplinary rounds and patient care conferences, and personal feedback such as one-to-one discussion. Different versions of the instrument exist for different professional groups. The Coordination Approach Scale has demonstrated test-retest reliabilities of .68 to .93. Cronbach's alphas ranging between .68 and .87 were reported (Young et al.). Construct validity was established through factor analysis. As further evidence of construct validity, coordination by programming and feedback were associated with higher perceived quality of care and lower surgical morbidity (Young et al.).

3.9.3 Collaborative Practice Scales

The Collaborative Practice Scales (CPS) were designed to measure collaborative practice behavior as it is reported by nurses and physicians. Collaborative practice was defined by the authors of the instrument as "interactions between nurses and physicians that enable the knowledge and skills of both professionals to synergistically influence the patient care being provided" (Weiss & Davis, 1985, p. 299). The CPS consists of two scales, one measuring practices of physicians and the other measuring practices of nurses. All items are measured on a 6-point scale. Factor analysis confirmed two factors in each scale, with alpha coefficients ranging from .72 to .77 and .80 to .85 for the total scale over repeated points of measurement. Test-retest reliability was high, .60 for the physician total CPS, and .79 for the nurse total CPS. Evidence of concurrent validity was not the same for the nurse and physician scales. Nurses' scores for all items of the CPS correlated highly with their scores on the Health Role Expectations Index; however, they showed no correlation with scores on another measure of collaborative behavior, the Management of Differences Exercise. Physician scores for the CPS did not correlate with their scores on the Health Role Expectations Index but correlated with the Management of Differences Exercise scores. CPS scores predicted physicians' collaborative practice as viewed by nurses but did not predict nurses' collaborative practice as viewed by physicians (Weiss & Davis). The CPS showed moderate correlations with a measure of nurse and physician collaborative decision-making concerning patient transfers from a medical intensive care unit (Baggs et al., 1992).

3.9.4 Decision About Transfer Scale

The Decision About Transfer (DAT) Scale was developed to measure collaboration and satisfaction with specific decisions to transfer patients out of the medical intensive care unit. Collaboration was defined as "open discussion between nurses and physicians and shared responsibility for problem solving and decision making" (Baggs et al., 1992, p. 19). The questionnaire was designed to be completed independently by nurses and medical residents. A single global question is asked about how much collaboration has been involved in making the decision to transfer a specific patient. Responses are in a Likert format, graded from 1 (no collaboration) to 7 (complete collaboration). Content and face validity was established. The DAT correlated moderately with scores on the Collaborative

Practice Scales, offering modest evidence of concurrent validity. The nurses' reports of collaboration with physicians were significantly and positively associated with desired patient outcomes and the predicted risk of negative outcomes decreased in collaboration situations (Baggs et al.). Negative outcomes were either re-admission to the medical intensive care unit or death during the same hospital admission.

3.9.5 Summary

Some instruments were designed for a specific purpose, such as assessment of cross-functional cooperation in hospital project teams (Pinto & Pinto, 1990). These instruments have questionable generalizability to other contexts. Without evidence of use in different types of settings and teams, it is difficult to determine their utility for evaluating the quality of nurses' work environment.

3.10 Implications and Future Directions

Effective health care involves teams of health care professionals working together to bring their skills to bear on a particular health problem or patient in order to achieve health care goals (Molnar Feiger & Schmitt, 1979). Conclusions in the literature suggest that team interaction, collaboration, communication, and coordination have an important effect on the quality of nurses' worklife and, more importantly, affect the quality of care and outcomes for patients.

While there is a long tradition of research into teams and work groups, there are very few rigorously designed trials investigating interprofessional interventions in health care teams. As a consequence, the instruments that have been developed to measure team concepts have not been well validated and evaluated in multiple health care settings. Very few examples were found of instruments that have been evaluated in more than one or two studies. Furthermore, with very few exceptions, the instruments have not been adequately evaluated in settings other than acute care.

Understanding teamwork in health care, finding methods to assess it, and effectively intervening to improve it are going to be increasingly important because of the complexity of patient care today. Therefore, the investigation of interprofessional teamwork is an important research agenda. There is a need for rigorously designed studies to evaluate interprofessional interventions that promote effective teamwork.

Some measures, such as the Organizational Assessment Inventory/Team Interaction Questionnaire (Shortell et al., 1994), have demonstrated good reliability and validity in a number of studies and warrant further evaluation in settings outside of hospitals for which they were developed.

There are several team assessment instruments, such as the Relational Coordination Instrument (Gittell, 2000), that have been adapted for use in health care from other industry settings. These instruments show promise, but have only had limited testing in the health care context, primarily in the acute care setting. Further testing of instruments that have demonstrated good reliability and validity in other settings, and/or have had only limited testing in health care is encouraged.

3.11 References

Alt-White, A. C., Charns, M., & Strayer, R. (1983). Personal, organizational and managerial factors related to nurse-physician collaboration. *Nursing Administration Quarterly, 8*, 8–18.

Anderson, N. R., & West, M. A. (1998). Measuring climate for work group innovation: Development and validation of the team climate inventory. *Journal of Organizational Behavior, 19*, 235–258.

Argote, L. (1984). Input uncertainty and organizational coordination in hospital emergency units. *Administrative Science Quarterly, 27*, 420–432.

Baggs, J. G., Ryan, S. A., Phelps, C. E., Richeson, J. F., & Johnson, J. E. (1992). The association between interdisciplinary collaboration and patient outcomes in a medical intensive care unit. *Heart & Lung, 21*(1), 18–24.

Bisset, A. (Ed.). (2000). *The Canadian Oxford Paperback Dictionary*. Don Mills, Canada: Oxford University Press.

Brill, N. (1976). *Teamwork: Working Together in the Human Services*. Toronto, Canada: Lippincott.

Cott, C. (1998). Structure and meaning in multidisciplinary teamwork. *Sociology of Health & Illness, 20*(6), 848–873.

Curley, C., McEachern, J. E., & Speroff, T. (1998). A firm trial of interdisciplinary rounds on the inpatient medical wards. *Medical Care, 36*(8, supplement), AS4–AS12.

Doran, D., McGillis Hall, L., Sidani, S., O'Brien-Pallas, L., Donner, G., Baker, G., et al. (2002). Nursing staff mix and patient outcome achievement: The mediating role of nurse communication. *The Journal of International Nursing Perspectives, 1*(2–3), 74–83.

Doran, D. M., Sidani, S., Keatings, M., & Doidge, D. (2002). An empirical test of the nursing role effectiveness model. *Journal of Advanced Nursing, 38*(1), 29–39.

Dreachslin, J. L., Hunt, P. L., & Sprainer, E. (1999). Communication patterns and group composition: Implications for patient-centered care team effectiveness. *Journal of Health Care Management, 44*(4), 252–268.

Drinka, T., & Ray, R. O. (1987). An investigation of power in an interdisciplinary health care team. *Gerontology and Geriatrics Education, 6*(3), 43–53.

Farrell, M. P., Schmitt, M., H., & Heinemann, G. D. (2001). Informal roles and the stages of interdisciplinary team development. *Journal of Interprofessional Care, 15*(3), 281–295.

Filley, A. C. (1975). *Interpersonal Conflict Resolution.* Glenview, IL: Scott, Foresman.

Flin, R., Fletcher, P., McGeorge, P., Sutherland, A., & Patey, R. (2003). Anaesthetists' attitudes to teamwork and safety. *Anaesthesia, 58*, 233–242.

Florin, P., Giamartino, G. A., Kenny, D. A., & Wandersman, A. (1990). Levels of analysis and effects: Clarifying group influences and climate by separating individual and group effects. *Journal of Applied Psychology, 20*(11), 881–900.

Fox, E. (2000). An audit of inter-professional communication within a trauma and orthopaedic directorate. *Journal of Orthopaedic Nursing, 4*, 160–169.

Gibbon, B., Watkins, C., Barer, D., Waters, K., Davies, S., Lightbody, L., et al. (2002). Can staff attitudes to team working in stroke care be improved? *Journal of Advanced Nursing, 40*(1), 105–111.

Gittell, J. H. (2000). Organizing work to support relational co-ordination. *International Journal of Human Resource Management, 11*(2), 517–539.

Gittell, J. H. (2002). Coordinating mechanisms in care provider groups: Relational coordination as a mediator and input uncertainty as a moderator of performance effects. *Management Science, 48*(11), 1408–1426.

Gittell, J. H., Fairfield, K., M., Bierbaum, B., Head, W., Jackson, R., Kelly, M., et al. (2000). Impact of relational coordination on quality of care, postoperative pain and functioning, and length of stay: A nine-hospital study of surgical patients. *Medical Care, 38*(8), 807–819.

Hawkins, J. M. (Ed.). (1979). *The Oxford Paperback Dictionary.* Oxford, England: Oxford University Press.

Helmreich, R. L. & Davies, J. M. (1996). Human factors in the operating room: Interpersonal determinants of safety, efficiency and morale. In A. A. Aitkenhead (Ed.), *Bailliere's Clinical Anaesthesiology: Safety and Risk Management in Anaesthesia* (pp. 227–296). London: Balliere Tindall.

Henneman, E. A., Lee, J. L., & Cohen, J. I. (1995). Collaboration: A concept analysis. *Journal of Advanced Nursing, 21*(1), 103–109.

Hetherington, R. W. (1991). The effects of formalization on departments of a multi-hospital system. *Journal of Management Studies, 28*(2), 103–141.

Higgins, S. E., & Routhieaux, R. L. (1999). A multiple-level analysis of hospital team effectiveness. *Health Care Supervisor, 17*(4), 1–13.

Infante, D. A. & Wigley, C. J. III. (1986). Verbal aggressiveness scale [VAS]. In K. Corcoran & J. Fischer (1987), *Measures for Clinical Practice: A Sourcebook* (pp. 351–353). New York: Free Press.

Irvine, D., Sidani, S., & McGillis Hall, L. (1998). Linking outcomes to nurses' roles in health care. *Nursing Economic$, 16*(2), 58–64, 87.

Irvine Doran, D., Baker, G., Murray, M., Bohnen, J., Zahn, C., Sidani, S., et al. (2002). Achieving clinical improvement: An interdisciplinary intervention. *Health Care Management Review, 27*, 42–56.

Jitapunkul, S., Aksaranugraha, S., Leenawat, B., Sornthonchartwat, B., Nuchprayoon, C., Chaiwanichsiri, D., et al. (1995). A controlled clinical trial of multidisciplinary team approach in the general medical wards of Chulalongkorn Hospital. *Journal Medical Association Thai, 78*(11), 618–623.

Joint Commission on Accreditation of Healthcare Organizations. (May 2003). *Sentinel Events Statistics:* Available from the Internet: http://www.jcaho.org/accredited+ organizations/hospitals/sentinel+events/sentinel&pl.event+statistics.htm

Keenan, G. M., Cooke, R., & Hillis, S. L. (1998). Norms and nurse management of conflicts: Key to understanding nurse-physician collaboration. *Research in Nursing & Health, 21,* 59–72.

Kilmann, R H., & Thomas, K W. (1977). Developing a forced choice measure of conflict-handling behaviour: The mode instrument. *Education and Psychological Measurement, 37,* 309-325.

Knaus, W. A., Draper, E. A., Wagner, D. P., & Zimmerman, J. E. (1986). An evaluation of outcome from intensive care in major medical centers. *Annals of Internal Medicine, 118,* 753.

Kohn, L. T., Corrigan, J. M., & Donaldson, M. S. (2000). *To Err is Human.* Washington DC: National Academy Press.

Krairiksh, M., & Anthony, M. K. (2001). Benefits and outcomes of staff nurses' participation in decision making. *Journal of Nursing Administration, 31*(1), 16–23.

Lingard, L., Reznick, R., Espin, S., Regehr, G., & DeVito, I. (2002). Team communication in the operating room: Talk patterns, sites of tension, and implications for novices. *Adad Medicine, 77,* 232–237.

Longest, B. B. J. (1974). Relationships between coordination, efficiency, and quality of care in general hospitals. *Hospital Administration, 19,* 65–86.

Malone, T. W., & Crowston, K. (1994). The interdisciplinary study of coordination. *ACM Computing Surveys, 26*(1), 87–119.

Marsh, J. G., & Simon, H. A. (1958). *Organization.* New York: Wiley, Meyer, Marshall W.

McGillis Hall, L., Doran, D. M., Baker, G. R., Pink, G. H., Sidani, S., O'Brien-Pallas, L., et al. (2001). *A Study of the Impact of Nursing Staff Mix Models and Organizational Change Strategies on Patient, System, and Nurse Outcomes.* Toronto, Canada: University of Toronto. ISBN 0-7727-3603-0.

Meerabeau, L., & Page, S. (1999). I'm sorry if I panicked you: Nurses' accounts of teamwork in cardiopulmonary resuscitation. *Journal of Interprofessional Care, 13*(1), 29–40.

Mitchell, P. H., Armstrong, S., Simpson, T. F., & Lentz, M. (1989). American Association of Critical-Care Nurses Demonstration Project: Profile of excellence in critical care nursing. *Heart & Lung, 18,* 219–237.

Molnar Feiger, S., & Schmitt, M. H. (1979). Collegiality in interdisciplinary health teams: Its measurement and its effects. *Social Science & Medicine, 13A,* 217–229.

O'Neil, H. F., Jr., Wang, S-L., Chung, G. K. W. K., & Herl, H. E. (2000). Assessment of teamwork skills using computer-based teamwork simulations. In H. F. O'Neil, Jr. & D. H. Andrews (Eds.), *Aircrew Training and Assessment* (pp. 245-276). Mahwah, NJ: Erlbaum.

Patel, V. L., Cytryn, K. N., Shortliffe, E. H., & Safran, C. (2000). The collaborative health care team: The role of individual and group expertise. *Teaching and Learning in Medicine, 12*(3), 117–132.

Pinto, M. B., & Pinto, J. K. (1990). Project team communication and cross-functional cooperation in new program development. *Journal of Product Innovation Management, 7,* 200–212.

Preuss, G. (1997). *The structuring of organizational information capacity: An examination of hospital care.* Academy of Management Proceedings.

Roelofsen, E. E., The, B. A-M., Beckerman, H., & Lankhorst, G. J. (2002). Development and implementation of the rehabilitation activities profile for children: Impact on the rehabilitation team. *Clinical Rehabilitation, 16,* 441-453.

Schaefer, H., & Helmreich, R. (1993). *The Operating Room Management Attitudes Questionnaire (ORMAQ). University of Texas Aerospace Crew Research Project Technical Report, 97-6.* Austin, TX: The University of Texas.

Shortell, S. M. (1991). *Effective Hospital-Physician Relationships.* Ann Arbor, MI: Health Administration Press.

Shortell, S. M., Zimmerman, J. E., Rousseau, D. M., Gillies, R. R., Wagner, D. P., Draper, E. A., et al. (1994). The performance of intensive care units: Does good management make a difference. *Medical Care, 32*(5), 508–525.

Stamps, P. L. & Peidmonte, E. B. (1986). *Nurses and work satisfaction: An index for measurement.* Ann Arbor, MI.: Health Administration Press Perspectives.

Trist, E. (1977). Collaboration in work settings: A personal perspective. *The Journal of Applied Behavioral Science, 13*(3), 268–278.

Van De Ven, A. H., Delbecq, A. L., & Koenig, R. J. (1976). Determinants of coordination modes within organizations. *American Sociological Review, 41,* 322–338.

Van Ess Coeling, H. & Cukr, P. L. (2000). Communication styles that promote perceptions of collaboration, quality, and nurse satisfaction. *Journal Nursing Care Quality 14*(2), 63–74.

Watson, W. E., & Michaelsen, L. K. (1988). Group interaction behaviors that affect group performance on an intellective task. *Group & Organizational Studies, 13,* 495–516.

Watson, W. E., Michaelsen, L. K., & Sharp, W. (1991). Member competence, group interaction, and group decision making: A longitudinal study. *Journal of Applied Psychology, 76,* 803–809.

Weiss, S. J., & Davis, H. P. (1985). Validity and reliability of the collaborative practice scales. *Nursing Research, 34,* 299–304.

Xiao, Y., & Mackenzie, C. F. (1998). *Collaboration in complex medical systems.* Paper presented at the RTO HFM Symposium on "Collaborative Crew Performance in Complex Operational Systems," Edinburgh, United Kingdom. ftp://ftp.rta.nato.int/pubfulltext/rto/mp/rto-mp-004/$mp-004-04.pdf.

Young, G. J., Charns, M. P., Daley, J., Forbes, M. G., Henderson, W., & Khuri, S. F. (1997). Best practices for managing surgical services: The role of coordination. *Health Care Management Review, 22*(4), 72–81.

Young, G. J., Charns, M. P., Desai, K., Khuri, S. F., Forbes, M. G., Henderson, W., et al. (1998). Patterns of coordination and clinical outcomes: A study of surgical services. *Health Services Research, 33*(5), 1211–1236.

Zwarenstein, M., & Bryant, W. (2003). Interventions to promote collaboration between nurses and doctors. *The Cochrane Library, 2,* 1–23.

Zwarenstein, M., Reeves, S., Barr, H., Hammick, M., Koppel, I., & Atkins, J. (2003). Interprofessional education: Effects on professional practice and health care outcomes. *The Cochrane Library, 1,* 1–12.

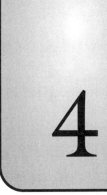

4

Organizational Climate and Culture

Deborah Tregunno

4.1 Introduction

Organizational climate and culture are increasingly recognized as important variables in the success or failure of change initiatives including quality improvement (Carman et al., 1996; Irvine Doran et al., 2002) and patient safety (Affonso & Doran, 2002; Baker & Norton, 2001). A key assumption in the literature is that the internal social psychological environment of organizations is related to individual meaning and organizational adaptation.

This chapter:

- Reviews the way in which organizational culture and climate have been defined

- Examines the theoretical underpinnings of the constructs

- Discerns the factors that influence organizational climate and culture

- Critically examines the empirical evidence linking nursing and patient outcomes

- Reviews the approaches to measurement with regard to the reliability, validity, and sensitivity to nursing variables

- Concludes with implications and future directions identified

A systematic search of the nursing and health databases yielded a variety of interpretations and applications of the organizational climate and culture constructs. The search yielded a total of 125 relevant sources, of which 72 met the criteria for inclusion in this chapter. As discussed below, there is an ongoing academic debate about the difference between climate and culture. Based on the work of Denison (1996), this chapter adopts the perspective that climate and culture are not strongly differentiated, and that they represent different but overlapping interpretations of the same phenomena. Further, this chapter focuses on quantitative assessments of organizational climate and culture in relationship to nurse, patient, and organizational outcomes.

4.2 Definition of the Concept of Organizational Climate and Culture

Organizational culture and climate have been described as perhaps the most difficult organizational concepts to define (Hatch, 1997). Both constructs examine a wide range of perceptions individuals hold about their work environment and how the context shapes behaviors.

4.2.1 Organizational Culture

Definitions of organizational culture emphasize its shared or social nature including a wide range of social beliefs, values, assumptions, symbols, ceremonies, and rituals that define an organization's character and norms. Although there is no single, widely agreed upon definition of organizational culture, there is consensus that it is holistic, historically derived, and socially constructed (Detert, Schroeder, & Mauriel, 2000). According to Edgar Schein (1991), organizational culture is the unconscious pattern of: Basic assumptions that a given group has identified, discovered, or developed in learning to cope with its problems of external adaptation and internal integration, and that have worked well enough to consider valid, and therefore, to be taught to new members as the correct way to perceive, think and feel as related to these problems (p. 3).

Hofstede (1998) notes that while culture is manifested in and measured from the verbal and/or nonverbal behavior of individuals, it is aggregated at the level of their organizational unit. Simply stated, "culture is a characteristic of the organization, not of individuals" (p. 479).

4.2.2 *Organizational Climate*

In contrast, definitions of organizational climate typically focus on general dimensions of the environment such as leadership, roles, and communication, or specific dimensions such as ethic climate (Olson, 1998) and safety climate (Neal, Griffin, & Hart, 2000). Moreover, organizational climate is regarded as a more superficial concept than organizational culture. Hofstede (1998) argues that "climate is more clearly linked with motivation and behavior than culture, which resides entirely at the organizational level" (p. 486). Denison (1996) suggests that organizational climate is "relatively temporary, subject to direct control, and largely limited to aspects of the organization that are consciously perceived by organizational members" (p. 624). More simply stated, organizational climate is how it "feels" to work in a particular environment, or the "atmosphere" of the workplace (Snow, 2002). Thus, while climate evolves out of the same elements as culture, it is shallower than culture; it forms more quickly and alters more rapidly (Moran & Volkwein, 1992).

4.3 Theoretical Underpinnings of Organizational Climate and Culture

The constructs of organizational climate and culture are not identical, and a clear understanding of the theoretical underpinnings of both organizational climate and culture is necessary to gain an understanding of the boundaries of each construct. Denison (1996) provides an excellent overview of the two constructs, highlights the similarities and differences, and explores practical implications particularly relevant to the study of nursing work environments.

Organizational climate refers to a specific situation and its link to the thoughts, feelings, and behaviors of organizational members (Denison, 1996). Thus, organizational climate is temporal, subjective, and often subject to direct manipulation by people with power and influence. The study of organizational climate preceded that of organizational culture. The concept of organizational climate has its roots in Lewin's (1951) studies of experimentally created social climates, which views the social world as three components comprising behaviors, the environment, and the person. The person, by definition, is analytically separated from the social context. The subjects of the social system, most often employees, are the primary focus of climate studies. Concerned with the impact that organizational systems have on groups and individuals, climate is reflected in members' overall perceptions and sense making of policies, practices, goals, and goal attainment in an organization. Thus, climate research focuses on aspects of the environment that are consciously perceived by organizational members.

Dependent on quantitative methods, climate research assumes that generalization across social settings is warranted. More recently, organizational researchers have developed specific measures of climate that are important for achieving certain organizational goals such as creativity (Ekvall, Arvonen, & Waldenstrom-Lindbald, 1983), ethical behavior (Olson, 1998), and patient safety (Sexton et al., under review). These measures conceptualize a particular type of social process and its influence on the behavior of organizational members and the achievement of defined organizational goals.

Organizational culture, in contrast, refers to an evolved context within which a situation may be embedded. Thus, it is rooted in history, collectively held and sufficiently complex to resist many attempts at direct manipulation (Denison, 1996). The study of organizational culture is rooted in the social construction perspective (Berger & Luckmann, 1966) and the symbolic interaction perspective (Mead, 1934), which assume that the individual cannot be analyzed separately from the environments, and that individuals are at the same time organizational subjects and agents. Thus, organizational culture literature focuses on the recursive interaction between the individual and the system. With its roots in anthropology, culture has primarily been studied using qualitative methods. Unlike climate, which focuses on members' perceptions of behaviors and practices that are more superficial, culture emphasizes the deep subconscious, implicit, underlying values and assumptions. Biased toward harmony, culture focuses on how individual behaviors reflect adherence to group norms.

4.4 Factors that Influence Organizational Climate and Culture

Although organizational climate and culture have been seen as relatively enduring, much of the climate and culture literature has focused on factors that influence cultural change including individual, organizational, and external factors. However, for all the interest in the dynamic nature of climate and culture, the crucial question of what factors have influenced organizational climate and culture has remained empirically poorly explored.

4.4.1 Individual

Climate and culture shape, and can be shaped by, individuals in the organization. Newcomers are especially important to an organization because they may bring with them expectations about culture when they join, and because culture is transmitted to new arrivals by established staff. Socialization of newcomers focuses on how individuals learn the beliefs, values, orientations, behaviors, and skills necessary to fulfill organizational roles (Fisher, 1986). Thus, socialization facilitates the transmission of organizational climate and culture to the newcomers in organizations (Ashforth & Saks, 1996). Individuals can also facilitate cultural change through leadership that clarifies values and develops a common organizational vision (Schein, 1991). For instance, Manley (2000a, 2000b) demonstrated how the social process of clinical nursing leadership facilitated a cultural transformation in a general intensive care unit over three years, contributing to clinical effectiveness, increased accountability, and clinical governance. This finding was consistent with the perspective that leadership that transforms practitioners' interpretations and experiences of health care influenced cultural change in an organization (Goodwin, 2000).

4.4.2 Organizational Features

Organizational climate and culture are shaped and articulated not just by individuals but also by organizational features. For instance, organizational structures, routines, command and control expectations, and operational norms influence the organization's culture (Langfield-Smith, 1995). Organizational features have a fundamental framing effect on individuals' expectations and perceptions, setting the context for the social construction of roles and relationships. Examinations of organizational structure have focused on how an organization's culture might facilitate or hinder the implementation of new models of care (e.g., Jones & Redman, 2000; Wakefield et al., 2001) as well as how new models have influenced the organizational and work group culture over time (e.g., Jones, DeBaca, & Yarbrough, 1997).

4.4.3 External

Organizational culture can also be influenced by factors external to the organization (Langfield-Smith, 1995). For instance, Bloor and Dawson (1994) illustrated how the stability of an organization's external environment influenced the degree to which professional subcultures maintained the status quo, refined and amended existing belief systems, or acted as a transforming influence within an organization. This finding was consistent with Schein's (1996) assertion that professional subcultures could complement, conflict, and counterbalance an organization's primary culture. At the organizational level of analysis, Liteinenko and Cooper (1994) demonstrated how the change in ownership status within the rapidly changing environment of the National Health Service influenced the workplace culture.

4.5 Linking Organizational Climate and Culture to Outcome Achievement

Nineteen empirical studies linking organizational climate or culture to patient, nursing, and organizational outcome achievement were identified in the nursing literature. Assessments of organizational culture were evidently favored in the empirical literature, since the majority of the empirical studies reviewed here investigated culture in relationship to outcome achievement. All but three of the studies were conducted in acute care hospitals.

4.5.1 Organizational Climate and Culture and Nurse Outcomes

The majority of the reviewed outcome studies assessed the relationship between organizational climate and culture and nursing outcome achievement. These studies examined a wide range of nursing outcomes including job satisfaction, work satisfaction, empowerment, professionalism, turnover, organizational commitment, and organizational fit.

Three studies examined the relationship between organizational climate and job satisfaction. Keuter, Byrne, Voell, and Larson (2000) identified a significant positive correlation between the aggregate measure of organizational climate using the Motivational and Organizational Climate Survey (Litwin & Stringer, 1968) and job satisfaction as measured by the Nurse and Work Satisfaction Index (Stamps, 1997). This study also found significant differences in three of the nine climate subscales (i.e., responsibility, standards, and structure) when comparing the culture profile of a medical unit and a cardiac intensive care unit of the same hospital. Kangas, Kee, and McKee-Waddle (1999) found that higher levels of job satisfaction, as measured by the Nurse Job Satisfaction Scale (Torres, 1988), were predicted by a supportive culture. These authors used the terms climate and culture synonymously. In this study, climate/culture was measured using a version of the Litwin and Stringer (1968) Organizational Climate Questionnaire that was modified by Wallach (1983). Tzeng, Ketefian, and Redman (2002) demonstrated a positive correlation between nursing job satisfaction (scale not specified) and organizational culture as measured by the Nursing Assessment Survey (Maehr & Braskamp, 1986).

One study examined the relationship between organizational culture and job satisfaction. Gifford, Zammuto, Goodman, and Hill (2002) explored the relationship between job satisfaction and culture type, as measured by the Competing Values Framework (Zammuto & Krakower, 1991). This study also examined the relationship between organizational culture and job involvement, empowerment, organizational commitment, and intent toward turnover. The researchers concluded that human relations culture type was positively related to job satisfaction, organizational commitment, job involvement, and empowerment, and negatively related to intent toward turnover.

Three studies examined the relationship between organizational culture and work satisfaction. McDaniel and Stumpf (1993) and Stumpf (2001) found a positive correlation between work satisfaction as measured by the Work Satisfaction Scale (Hinshaw, Smeltzer, & Atwood, 1987) and constructive culture defined by the Organizational Culture Inventory (Cooke & Lafferty, 1987). Both studies reported the absence of variation in culture types, which lead McDaniel and Stumpf to suggest the absence of a strong organizational culture in the study hospitals. McDaniel (1995) modified the Work Satisfaction Scale (Hinshaw et al.) to examine the relationship between culture and ethics work satisfaction. McDaniel defined ethics work satisfaction as opinions about one's work as it reflects ethics, including participation in ethical deliberations or decisions, and rules or actions regarding ethical conduct in practice. Moreover, McDaniel suggested that while employees preferred cultures in which norms and expectations were visible, one could work in a strong culture with explicit, yet *unethical* work norms. In this study, organizational culture was measured using the Organizational Culture Inventory (Cooke & Lafferty). Study findings indicated that ethics work satisfaction was positively and inversely related to constructive and passive-defensive culture types, respectively.

One study examined the relationship between nurse empowerment and organizational culture. Mok and Au-Yeung (2002) found a positive correlation between nurse empowerment as measured by Spreitzer (1995) and six climate subscales defined by the Motivational and Organizational Climate Survey (Litwin & Stringer, 1968).

One study examined the relationship between professionalism and organizational culture. Manojlovich and Ketefian (2002) found that strength of culture as measured by the Nursing Assessment Survey (Maehr & Braskamp, 1986) predicted nursing professionalism as measured by the Hall/Snizek Professionalism Scale. In this study, the authors found that the other four culture subscales— accomplishment, affiliation, power, and recognition—were not significant predictors of nursing professionalism.

Two studies examined the relationship between nurse turnover and organizational culture. In a national study of intensive care units, Shortell et al. (1994) found that a lower rate of nurse turnover was significantly correlated with caregiver interaction; a composite measure including organizational culture, leadership, communication, coordination, and conflict management. In this study, organizational culture was assessed using a modified version of the Organizational Culture Inventory (Cooke & Lafferty, 1987). The researchers also found that caregiver interaction was significantly correlated with higher provider evaluation of the technical quality of care provided in their critical care units. Seago (1996) examined the relationship between organizational culture as measured by the Organizational Culture Inventory (Cooke & Lafferty) and workplace stress, hostility, absenteeism, and turnover. There was little variation in the culture type, workplace stress, and hostility but high variability in absenteeism and turnover between the 67 units involved in the study. The study found a positive correlation between hostility and aggressive-defensive culture and between the psychological demand subscale of the Job Content Stress Scale (Karasek, 1979) and aggressive-defensive and passive-defensive culture types. Seago found no relationship between organizational culture and the other nurse outcomes.

One study examined the relationship between organizational commitment and organizational culture. Ingersoll, Kirsch, Merk, and Lightfoot (2000) considered the relationship between organizational culture, commitment to the organization, and organizational readiness in two tertiary care hospitals undergoing work redesign. Commitment and readiness were measured by the commitment/energy subscale and the innovativeness and cooperation subscale of the Pasmore Sociotechnical Systems Assessment Survey (Pasmore, 1988). The researchers found that commitment to the organization was positively associated with a constructive culture and with organizational readiness, while negatively associated with a passive-defensive culture.

One study examined the relationship between organizational culture and organizational fit. Luk, Chen, Yau, Tsang, and Leung (1998) used Harrison's Organizational Ideology Instrument (Harrison, 1992) to demonstrate the degree of organizational fit for six stakeholder groups (i.e., physicians, nurses, administrators, paramedical staff, support staff, and clerical staff) in one acute care hospital in Hong Kong. This study assessed the difference between organizational members' perceptions of the existing culture and their preferred culture type. Specifically, nurses assessed the existing culture type as role, which emphasized a well-designed system of roles in which performance was organized by structures and procedures, while they reported a preference for a supportive culture type, which emphasized mutual trust between individual staff members and management. The authors found no significant differences between the existing and preferred culture types across the six stakeholder groups.

4.5.2 Organizational Climate and Culture and Patient Outcomes

Two of the studies reviewed used Ekvall and colleagues' (1983) Creative Climate Questionnaire to examine the relationship between climate and patient outcome achievement. Norbergh, Hellzen, Sandman, and Asplun (2002) explored the relationship between creative climate and the content of daily life for people living with dementia in group dwellings. The results showed that residents in more creative climates spent twice as much of their time interacting with nurses, as compared to residents in climates that were less creative. Mattiasson and Andersson (1995) examined the differences in patient autonomy in nursing homes that demonstrated high and low creative climates, reporting higher levels of patient autonomy in organizations that report higher levels of creative climate.

Two studies examined the relationship between organizational culture and a variety of patient outcomes. Shortell and colleagues (1994) examined the relationship between organizational culture and critical care patient outcomes including lower risk-adjusted length of stay and a greater ability of staff to meet family needs. In this study, organizational culture was assessed using a modified version of the Organizational Culture Inventory (Cooke & Lafferty, 1987). Shortell et al. (2000) examined the influence of organizational culture on several outcomes for coronary artery bypass graft (CABG) patients in 16 hospitals including mortality, return to operating room, postoperative stroke, mediastinitis, postoperative atrial fibrillation, functional health status, and patient satisfaction. In this study, the Organizational Culture Inventory (Cooke & Lafferty) was used to assess organizational culture. Supportive group culture type was associated with higher six-month postoperative physical and mental functional status as measured by the RAND short form (SF-36; Ware, 1993). Overall, the authors concluded that a positive organizational culture appeared to have little influence on multiple endpoints of care for CABG patients.

4.5.3 Organizational Climate and Culture and Organizational Outcomes

Three of the studies reviewed used the Competing Values Framework (Zammuto & Krakower, 1991) to examine the relationship between work redesign and organizational culture. Jones and associates (1997) used a pre-post method to examine culture in relationship to the implementation of patient-focused care on two units with five caregiver groups in an acute care hospital. The findings indicated a dominant culture type for each unit at baseline; the dominant culture type changed in only one of the units, suggesting cultural stability over time. Only one significant difference in culture type across the four units was found at baseline, a difference that was not present in the postimplementation period. Different perceptions of organizational culture were found across the caregiver categories at baseline; however, there were no significant changes per caregiver group between the two time periods. Jones and Redman (2000) also used a pre-post method to examine changes in organizational culture associated with work redesign in three hospitals. Comparison of the pre-post culture types indicated that the hospital with a balanced culture preimplementation was more successful at work redesign than the hospitals with dominant baseline market and hierarchical cultures.

Wakefield et al. (2001) examined the relationship between culture type, quality improvement (QI), and the reporting of medication administration errors in six acute care hospitals. They reported that group culture was positively correlated with QI implementation and that hierarchical and rational culture types were negatively correlated with QI implementation as measured by the criteria outlined by the Malcolm Baldrige National Quality Award. Moreover, group culture and QI implementation were positively but not significantly correlated with nurses' estimates of the total percentage of medication administration errors reported.

Shortell and colleagues (2000) measured four organizational outcomes— length of stay, operating room time, postoperative intubation time, and cost of care—for CABG surgery patients in 16 hospitals. Findings indicated that supportive group culture was associated with shorter postoperative intubation time and longer operating room time.

One study examined the relationship between organizational culture and change in corporate governance. Liteinenko and Cooper (1994) examined the change in organizational culture pre- and posttrust status achievement in one health authority in the United Kingdom. In this study, Harrison's Organizational Ideology Questionnaire (Harrison, 1972) was used as a measure of organizational culture. The results indicated that the predominant culture remained similar over the study period but there was decreased posttrust emphasis on people-oriented support culture characteristics. The results also indicated greater pretrust variation between occupational groups.

In summary, one of the most striking features about the studies included in this review is the range of instruments used and outcomes assessed. Most of the studies reviewed examined the relationship between climate and culture and nurse outcomes such as job satisfaction. The majority of the studies reported in this chapter have employed correlational techniques. Moreover, most of the studies adopted a static perspective of climate and culture. This work was virtually silent to questions of what factors influenced organizational climate and culture in relationship to the outcomes of interest. Further, the lack of clarity between the climate and culture constructs, the use of multiple instruments, and other methodological concerns raise important questions about the ability to generalize many of the findings.

4.6   Issues in the Assessment of Organizational Climate and Culture

Four important issues to consider in the assessment of organizational climate and culture emerged from the review of the literature: (a) unit of analysis, (b) sample size, (c) instrument selection, and (d) overlapping interpretations.

4.6.1   Unit of Analysis

Organizational climate is defined as organizational members' perceptions of how they see their environment, thus, it is appropriately analyzed as an individual variable. However, since organizational culture is defined as something a group has, it seems reasonable that the unit of analysis would be the group level. Often data are reported at both the individual and group level without clearly distinguishing the differences (Seago, 1997). For instance, the unit of analysis in the studies by McDaniel (1995) and McDaniel and Stumpf (1993) was the individual, yet culture data were reported as a group finding. Moreover, if the group is the unit of analysis, it is important to consider issues of data aggregation. Seago described a variety of issues related to data aggregation and recommended (a) the use of the intraclass correlation to assess the reliability of group-level data, and (b) the use of hierarchical linear modeling to account for both the individual and group effects on individual outcomes. Of the studies reviewed, only Shortell et al. (1994) reported the appropriateness of group-level data aggregation.

4.6.2 Sample Size

Organizational theorists are also concerned with the degree to which various cultural dimensions are shared among organizational members. Also known as an integration perspective, analysis in this vein assumes a "strong" or "desirable" culture, characterized by organization-wide consensus and clarity. Thus, an important issue related to assessments of organizational culture is the question of sample size and the percentage of people in the group needed to provide an accurate picture of group culture. The studies reviewed illustrated a variety of approaches to the question of sample size. For instance, Seago (1997) reported a requirement of at least 25% of the staff members working over 20 hours a week from each nursing unit included in the study. In contrast, McDaniel and Stumpf (1993) reported using 250 randomly selected nurses from seven randomly selected hospitals. Shortell et al. (2000) reported on the influence of culture on patient outcomes in 16 hospitals, but did not discuss the appropriateness of the sample size.

While clear recommendations about required sample size were not found in the literature, the determination of sample size depended on the unit of analysis and statistical power. This is especially important in studies in which the group is the unit of analysis, because of the challenges associated with obtaining a large enough group sample size. Moreover, groups of different sizes may require different percentages of participants (Seago, 1997). Finally, because subcultures can exist within an organization, particularly in health care where there is a strong professional influence, it is important to select a sample that will allow analysis at the subgroup level as well as that of the whole organization.

4.6.3 Instrument Selection

The selection of instruments is an important issue in assessments of organizational climate and culture. As discussed below, a range of instruments are available, the selection of which depends on the purpose and focus of the investigation. Selection of climate instruments tends to be related to specific attitudes and values toward specific organizational dimensions such as safety, customer service, or information technology. Because the content of climate instruments can overlap with those of culture, clarity about the dimensions of interest is essential when assessing complex phenomena like organizational culture.

4.6.4 Overlapping Interpretations

While from a theoretical perspective, similarities and differences between the constructs of culture and climate are clear, the literature often reflects confusion about the terms, which has resulted in interchangeable use. Moreover, in the nursing literature, climate and culture are often entangled with the concept of practice environment, a term commonly used in nursing. For instance, Clarke, Sloan, and Aiken (2002) defined organizational climate in terms of administrative support for nursing practice and average nurse experience as measured by the Revised Nursing Work Index (NWI-R), a measure of attributes of the nursing practice environment (Aiken & Patrician, 2000). However, some observers such as Estabrooks and colleagues (2002) have argued that the NWI-R is conceptually distinct from organizational climate and culture, while others have stressed the relationship between the structures of interest in the NWI-R (i.e., administration, professional practice, and professional development) and organizational culture (Manley, 2000a). Even more confusing is the work by Kangas and associates (1999), who cite the magnet hospitals study to support the importance of examining the relationship between nurse job satisfaction and organizational culture, which is measured using a modified climate scale.

4.7 Evidence Concerning Approaches to Measuring Organizational Climate and Culture

There are generally two major approaches to measuring organizational culture. One involves typing organizations into particular taxonomies, which is usually accompanied by detailed descriptions of associated behaviors and values. Typing instruments identify organizations as belonging to one of several possible mutually exclusive categories. Typing allows respondents to understand the consequences of their type-category and compare their types with others. Ashkanasy, Broadfoot, and Falkus (2000) suggest that organizational typing is subject to three limitations. First, the implication that organizations of a particular type are similar, or should be similar, negates the unique nature of organizations and cultures. The second limitation is that typing implies discontinuous categories. The third limitation is that not all organizations conform to particular types, and others appear to be a mixture of types.

The second approach to measuring organizational culture involves the use of profiling instruments that measure the strengths or weaknesses of a variety of organizational members' beliefs and values. The different scores on several cultural dimensions describe culture by its position on a number of continuous variables. Thus, profiling surveys categorize organizations in terms of multiple categories that are not necessarily mutually exclusive. There are three approaches to profiling surveys: effectiveness, descriptive, and fit profiles. Effectiveness surveys assess the values related to high levels of organizational performance. Descriptive surveys measure values but do not attempt to make evaluations of effectiveness based on the profile of values. Fit profiles examine the congruence between individual beliefs and values and the organization. Most instruments can be formatted to create fit profiles. For instance, Liteinenko and Cooper (1994) use Harrison's Organizational Ideology Questionnaire to create fit profiles for occupational and clinical groups.

4.8 Nursing Measures of Organizational Culture

The only instruments included in this review are those that have been used in a study where the relationship between organizational culture and nursing, patient, or organizational outcomes was examined.

4.8.1 *Nursing Unit Culture Assessment Tool (NUCAT-2)*

The Nursing Unit Culture Assessment Tool (NUCAT-2) was developed specifically for use in nursing units (Coeling & Simms, 1993a). This 50-item instrument uses a 6-point scale that asks participants to indicate their "preferred behavior" and their "group's typical behaviors." The instrument is designed to measure the majority of group members' current and preferred behaviors. According to H. Coeling (2003, personal communication), data are to be examined on an item-by-item basis to support qualitative evaluations of culture; thus, psychometric properties of the instrument have not been published. While study results, including the work of Coeling and Simms (1993b) and Rizzo, Gilman, and Mersmann (1994) have demonstrated variation among nursing units, these findings have not been consistent. For instance, Goodridge and Hack (1996) reported such wide variation in responses (i.e., unspecified number of nursing units in one hospital) that meaningful differences in culture among units could not be detected.

4.8.2 *Nursing Assessment Survey*

The Nursing Assessment Survey (Maehr & Braskamp, 1986) is a 91-item instrument with three dimensions including culture, job satisfaction, and retention and 11 subscales (i.e., five culture, four job satisfaction, and two retention). Use of the Nursing Assessment Survey varied in the studies that were included in this review. For instance, Tzeng et al. (2002) used only one of the culture subscales (i.e., strength of culture) to demonstrate a relationship between organizational culture and nurse job satisfaction and patient satisfaction. In contrast,

Manojlovich and Ketefian (2002) used the five subscales as independent variables in their regression equation but found that strength of organizational culture was the only significant predictor of nursing professionalism. In both of these studies, culture was interpreted as an individual-level variable. Data on the sensitivity of the instrument to differences in culture across nursing units was not provided.

4.9 General Organizational Climate and Culture Measures

The only instruments included in this review are those that have been used in a study where the relationship between organizational climate or organizational culture and nursing, patient, or organizational outcomes was examined (see Tables 4.1 and 4.2).

4.9.1 Litwin and Stringer Organizational Climate Questionnaire (LSOCQ)

Three different versions of the Litwin and Stringer Organizational Climate Questionnaire (LSOCQ) were found in the literature (Litwin & Stringer, 1968). Keuter and associates (2000) used the original LSOCQ in their examination of the relationship between nurse satisfaction and organizational climate. While the 48-item instrument provides four climate subscales (i.e., standards, structure, responsibility, and support), an aggregate measure of climate was used to demonstrate a significant relationship between climate and nurse job satisfaction. The instrument differentiated between the two study units on three of the four climate subscales (i.e., standards, structure, and responsibility). Kangas et al. (1999) used a version of the LSOCQ modified by Wallach (1983) to examine the relationship between organizational climate and nurse job satisfaction. The modified 24-item instrument provided three climate subscales including bureaucratic, innovative, and supportive. The instrument did not differentiate between the climates of the three study units.

Mok and Au-Yeung (2002) also modified the Litwin and Stringer instrument to examine the outcome of nurse empowerment. In this study, the modified LSOCQ had 60 items and six climate subscales including leadership, work harmony, challenge, recognition, teamwork, and decision-making. This study was conducted in a single site acute care hospital. The modified instrument differentiated between the climates of the three staff groupings included in the study (i.e., top nursing managers, middle managers, and front-line nurses).

Table 4.1 Nursing Measures of Climate

Instrument Author/Date of Publication	Target Population	Domains	Method of Administration	Reliability	Validity	Sensitivity to Nursing
Creative Climate Questionnaire (CCQ) (Ekvall et al., 1983)	General application.	50 statements, 10 categories of work climate: challenge, freedom, idea-support, trust, liveliness or dynamics, playfulness or humor, debates, conflicts, risk-taking, and idea-time; 4-point Likert scale.	Self-administered.			Differentiated highest and lowest creative climate nursing homes (Mattiasson and Andersson, 1995).
Litwin and Stringer Organizational Climate Questionnaire (LSOCQ) (Litwin & Stringer, 1968)	General organizational application.	48 items, three categories: structure, support, and standards.	Self-administered.			Differentiated between nursing units (Keuter et al. 2000).
Modified Litwin and Stringer Organizational Climate (1968) (Mok & Au-Yeung 2002)	Modified for study group of hospital nurses.	50 items, six empirically derived domains: leadership work harmony challenge recognition teamwork, decision-making; 4-point Likert scale.	Self-administered.	Climate: leadership ($\alpha = 0.71$), work harmony ($\alpha = 0.78$), challenge ($\alpha = 0.70$), recognition ($\alpha = 0.74$), teamwork ($\alpha = 0.71$), decision-making ($\alpha = 0.70$).		Differentiated among three nursing staff groups: top nursing managers, middle nurse managers, & frontline nurses.
Modified Litwin and Stringer Organizational Climate (1968) (Wallach, 1983)	General application.	24 questions, three sub-scales: bureaucratic, innovative, supportive; 4-point Likert scale.	Self-administered.	Sub-scale reliability ranges from $\alpha = 0.57$ to $\alpha = 0.91$ (Koberg and Chusmi, 1987); details not provided.	Face; content; pilot study.	Differentiated between units (Kangas et al., 1999); significant correlation of climate and job satisfaction on four climate sub-scales: structure, support, standards, and professional status.

α = Cronbach's alpha coefficient

Table 4.2 Nursing Measures of Culture

Instrument Author/Date of Publication	Target Population	Domains	Method of Administration	Reliability	Validity	Sensitivity to Nursing
Competing Values Framework survey (CVF) (Zammuto & Krakower, 1991)	Assessment focuses on two dimensions: whether organization focuses attention inward toward internal dynamics of outward to external environment; preferences for flexibility versus control in organizational structuring; four culture types: clan, adhocracy, hierarchy, and market. Each organization usually has more than one of these types.	5 questions divide 100 points among four scenarios representing dimensions of performance: open systems, rational goal, internal process, and human relations; these dimensions reflect four descriptions of culture: group (human relations), developmental (open systems), hierarchical (internal process), and rational (rational goal).	Self-report.	Strong theoretical base; good reliability (Quinn & Spreitzer, 1991).	Face validity.	Provides a narrow classification of culture types: balanced culture type associated with successful work redesign (Jones and Redman, 2000), dominant culture type associated with outcome of interest (Shortell et al. 2000; Gifford et al. 2002).
Organizational Culture Inventory (OCI) (Cooke & Lafferty 1987	Shared norms and expectations that guide thinking and behavior.	120 items, 5-point scale, 12 thinking styles: humanistic-helpful, affiliative, approval, conventional, dependent, avoidance, oppositional, power, competitive, competence or perfectionist, achievement, and self-actualizing; three empirically derived factors: passive-defensive, constructive, and aggressive-defensive.	Self-report.	Range of internal consistency α = 0.67 to α = 0.92 (Cook & Szumal, 1991).	Good face validity; convergent and discriminate validity established (Cook & Szumal 1991).	Widely used for intra- and inter-organizational comparisons in health care; little variation among the nursing units and hospitals (McDaniel & Stumpf 1993); some items do not apply to nursing unit context.

α = Cronbach's alpha coefficient

Table 4.2 (continued)

Instrument Author/Date of Publication	Target Population	Domains	Method of Administration	Reliability	Validity	Sensitivity to Nursing
Harrison's Organizational Ideology Questionnaire (Harrison, 1972)	Assesses ideology of organization in terms of orientation to four types.	16 statements, 6-point Likert scale, four culture typology sub-scales: role, power, task, and support for individuals.	Self-report.			Differentiated between culture of professional groups and change in culture over time (Litcinenko & Cooper, 1994).
Nursing Unit Cultural Assessment Tool (NUCAT-2) (Coeling & Simms, 1993a)	Developed specifically for use in nursing units. Individual and group preferred behavior; rated as behaviors preferred by respondents in comparison to those that typically occur in their unit.	50 items, 4- or 6-point Likert scale; developed to assist with qualitative assessment of culture; lack of subscales limits assessment to one stakeholder group.	Self-report.	Little evidence to support reliability.	Construct validity established through qualitative studies; studies report on an item-by-item basis.	Differentiates between culture of nursing units; users are encouraged to use items separately (Coeling, personnel communication, 2003).
Nursing Assessment Survey (Maehr & Braskamp, 1986)		91 items, 11 subscales: five culture sub-scales: accomplishment (9 items), affiliation (9 items), power (5 items), recognition (9 items), and strength of culture (7 items); four job satisfaction sub-scales: accomplishment, recognition, power, and affiliation; two retention sub-scales: job satisfaction and organizational commitment.	Self-report.	Accomplishment ($\alpha = 0.80$), affiliation ($\alpha = 0.85$), power ($\alpha = 0.51$), recognition ($\alpha = 0.87$), and strength of culture ($\alpha = 0.82$).		Strength of culture related to professionalism (Manojlovich & Ketefian 2002), nurse satisfaction (Tzeng et al., 2002) and patient satisfaction (Tzeng et al., 2002).

α = Cronbach's alpha coefficient

4.9.2 Creative Climate Questionnaire (CCQ)

One instrument used to measure a specific aspect of organizational climate was found in the literature. The Creative Climate Questionnaire (Ekvall et al., 1983) was used in two studies to examine the relationship between climate and patient outcome achievement. The creative climate scale provides 10 categories of work climate, including challenge, freedom, idea-support, trust, liveliness/dynamics, playfulness/humor, debates, conflicts, idea-time, and risk-taking. Mattiasson and Andersson (1995) and Ekvall et al. found the instrument to be sensitive to differences in creative culture between patient care units and to patient outcomes.

4.10 Organizational Culture Measures

4.10.1 Organizational Culture Inventory (OCI)

The Organizational Culture Inventory (OCI; Cooke & Lafferty, 1987) was designed to be used in a variety of businesses and industries and has been demonstrated to have acceptable construct and content validity (Scott, Mannion, Davies, & Marshall, 2003). The OCI has 12 scales (i.e., achievement, self-actualizing, humanistic-encouraging, affiliative, approval, conventional, dependent, avoidance, oppositional, power, competitive, and perfectionistic) that are reflected in three empirically reliable factors (i.e., constructive [scales 1-4], passive-defensive [scales 5-8], and aggressive-defensive [scales 9-12]). The OCI has been used to examine organizational culture in a wide variety of settings; however, when used in the context of health care, little variation among nursing units within a hospital or among nursing units between hospitals has been found (Seago, 1997). For instance, both McDaniel and Stumpf (1993) and Stumpf (2001) did not find significant differences among culture types across the study units.

4.10.2 Competing Values Framework (CVF)

Competing Values Framework (CVF), which is designed to represent the balance of different cultures within the same organization, examines the underlying values and beliefs that inform those cultures (Zammuto & Krakower, 1991). The four culture types of developmental, human relations, hierarchical, and rational have a strong theoretical base and have demonstrated convergent and discriminant validity (Quinn & Spreitzer, 1991). The studies included in this review demonstrated two ways of approaching the question of organizational culture using the CVF. Because of the underlying theoretical assumption of the CVF, the first approach suggested that effective organizations will demonstrate a balance of the four culture types. One approach to analysis examines the relationship between the degree to which culture types are balanced and the outcome of interest. For instance, Jones and Redman (2000) found that hospitals with a balanced culture were more successful at work redesign than the hospitals with dominant culture types. Alternatively, analysis focused on examining the link between the dominant culture type and the outcome of interest. Gifford et al. (2002) provided data on only one of the four culture types in their examination of the relationship between culture and nurse quality of worklife. Shortell et al. (2000) also focused on one culture type in their study of coronary artery bypass surgery.

4.10.3 *Harrison's Organizational Ideology Questionnaire*

Harrison's Organizational Ideology Questionnaire (Harrison, 1972) consists of 16 statements ranked by respondents in terms of how representative they are of (a) the organization, and (b) the respondents' own attitudes and beliefs. The instrument provides four culture types including role, power, task, and support for individuals. Harrison's Organizational Ideology Questionnaire has demonstrated sensitivity to professional subcultures as well as to changes in culture type over time (Liteinenko & Cooper, 1994).

4.11 Implications and Future Directions

There appears to be consensus in the literature that organizational climate and culture are two of the most potential constructs available to researchers for understanding the human dynamics of organizations and their importance in shaping organizational life. This review of the current literature that explores the relationship between organizational climate and culture and nurse, patient, and organizational outcomes highlights a number of important issues and directions for future research. The challenge remains to strengthen the literature linking culture and climate to outcome achievement.

The main points of this chapter are summarized as follows:

- Organizational climate and culture are not strongly differentiated and the literature reflects confusion between the climate and culture constructs.

- Organizational climate research focuses on aspects of the environment that are consciously perceived by individual organizational members.

- Organizational culture emphasizes deep, subconscious, implicit underlying values and assumptions of a group.

- While there are differences between climate and culture, they share an interest in the relationship between organizational traits and members' interpretation and response to those traits.

- Organizational climate and culture evolve out of some of the same elements, but climate forms and alters more quickly.

- Organizational climate and culture are influenced by individual, organizational, and external factors.

- Much of the research on climate and culture focuses on nursing outcomes, especially job and work satisfaction.

- The evidence provides support for the benefits of examining organizational climate and culture in relationship to work redesign.

- The evidence illustrates many of the methodological challenges associated with establishing a relationship between organizational culture and patient outcomes.

- Several instruments for measuring organizational climate and culture are available. The instruments capture various domains on climate and culture. The instruments demonstrate acceptable reliability; however, there is limited evidence to support validity. Sensitivity to nursing varies across the instruments.

- The process by which organizational climate and culture are fashioned and refashioned remains largely unexplored.

Four main observations are derived from these points. First, nursing research continues to be limited by confusion and overlap in the constructs and by the instruments used to measure the constructs. Moreover, as interest in work environments increases, there is the potential for confusion with other concepts such as practice environment[1]. Researchers, therefore, need to be clear about the construct of interest when designing a study and selecting an instrument.

The second concern is limitation in the ability to compare climate and culture across settings and the impact on outcomes due to variation in measures and analytical approaches. While it is unlikely that a single instrument will provide valid and reliable assessments of organizational culture, further work is required to improve the validity and nursing sensitivity of some of the instruments described in this paper.

Third, the process by which organizational climate and culture change bears further consideration. Bate, Khan, and Pye (2000) proposed a model for managing organizational change that accounts for the relationship between culture,

---

[1]   Estabrooks et al. (2002) define practice environment as "a set of features that, when present, enable nurses to demonstrate professional practice characterized by decision-making autonomy, clarity of mission, and organizational responsiveness. These features are perceived by employees as desirable and reflect the standards and values commonly espoused in professional education, and they are also highly valued by leaders in the profession" (p. 265).

structure, and leadership that could serve as a framework to guide this field of study. This four-phase change model (i.e., cultural framing, soft structuring, hard wiring, and retrospecting) focuses on the process by which organizations utilize structural features to reframe organizational practices and relationships and culture. This framework may provide a structure to integrate research on structural components of the magnet hospitals, which have been positively linked to staff and patient outcomes, with research that explores factors that influence cultural change.

Finally, while a number of measures exist in the literature, selection of one measure for use in the nursing environment is problematic. This is more challenging with the overlapping interpretations of the climate, culture, and practice environment constructs found in this review. This literature and instrument review highlights the need to conduct content analysis of the instruments examined in this review (e.g., Organizational Culture Inventory, Nursing Unit Culture Assessment Tool–2, and the culture component of the Nursing Assessment Survey) and to compare these findings with elements explored in the practice environment measures (Revised Nursing Work Index). From a theoretical perspective, this review will provide insights into areas of overlap between the construct and provide a better understanding of the strengths and limitations of each instrument.

4.12 References

Affonso, D., & Doran, D. M. (2002). Cultivating discoveries in patient safety research: A framework. *The Journal of International Nursing Perspectives*, *2*(1), 33–47.

Aiken, L. H., & Patrician, P. A. (2000). Measuring organizational traits of hospitals: The revised nursing work index. *Nursing Research*, *49*,146–153.

Ashforth, B. E., & Saks, A. M. (1996). Socialization tactics: Longitudinal effects on newcomer adjustment. *Academy of Management Journal*, *39*(1), 149–178.

Ashkanasy, N. M., Broadfoot, L. E., & Falkus, S. (2000). Questionnaire measures of organizational culture. In N. M. Ashkanasy, C.P. Wilderom, & M. F. Peterson (Eds.), *Handbook of Organizational Culture & Climate*. Thousand Oaks, CA: Sage Publications Inc.

Baker, G. R., & Norton, P. G. (2001). Making patients safer! Reducing error in Canadian health care. *Healthcare Papers*, *2*(1), 10–31.

Bate, P., Khan, R., & Pye, A. (2000). Towards a culturally sensitive approach to organization structuring: Where organization design meets organization development. *Organization Science*, *11*(2), 197–211.

Berger, P., & Luckmann, T. (1996). *The Social Construction of Reality*. New York: Penguin.

Bloor, G., & Dawson, P. (1994). Understanding professional culture in organizational context. *Organization Studies*, *15*(2), 275–295.

Carman, J. M., Shortell, S. M., Foster, R. W., Hughes, E. F. X., Boerstler, H., O'Brien, J. L., et al. (1996). Keys for successful implementation of total quality management in hospitals. *Health Care Management Review, 21*(1), 48–60.

Clarke, P., Sloane, D., & Aiken, L. (2002). Effects of hospital staffing and organizational climate on needlestick injuries to nurses. *American Journal of Public Health, 92*(7), 1115–1119.

Coeling, H., & Simms, L. (1993a). Facilitating innovation at the nursing unit level through cultural assessment, part 1: How to keep management ideas from falling on deaf ears. *Journal of Nursing Administration, 23*(4), 46–53.

Coeling, H., & Simms, L. (1993b). Facilitating innovation at the unit level through cultural assessment, part 2: Adapting managerial ideas to the unit work group. *Journal of Nursing Administration, 23*(5), 13–20.

Cooke, R., & Lafferty, J. (1987). *Organizational Culture Inventory (OCI)*. Plymouth, MI: Human Synergistics.

Cooke, R. A., and Szumal, J. L. (1993). Measuring normative beliefs and shared behavioral expectations in organizations: The reliability and validity of the organizational culture inventory. *Psychological Reports, 72*, 1299–1330.

Denison, D. R. (1996). What is the difference between organizational culture and organizational climate? A native's point of view on a decade of paradigm wars. *Academy of Management Review, 21*(3), 619–654.

Detert, J., Schroeder, R., & Mauriel, J. (2000). A framework for linking culture and improvement initiatives in organizations. *Academy of Management Review, 25*(4), 850–863.

Ekvall, G., Arvonen, J., & Waldenstrom-Lindbald, I. (1983). *Creative Organizational Climate, Construction and Validation of a Measuring Instrument*. Stockholm: Fa-institute.

Estabrooks, C. A., Tourangeau, A. E., Humphrey, C. K., Hesketh, K. L., Giovannetti, P., Thomson, D., et al. (2002). Measuring the hospital practice environment: A Canadian context. *Research in Nursing & Health, 25*, 256–268.

Fisher, C. D. (1986). Organizational socialization: An integrative review. In K. M. Rowland & G. R. Ferris (Eds.), *Research in Personnel and Human Resources Management (Vol. 4, pp. 104–145)*. Greenwich, CT: JAI Press.

Gifford, B. D., Zammuto, R. F., Goodman, E. A., & Hill, K. S. (2002). The relationship between hospital unit culture and nurses' quality of worklife. *Journal of Healthcare Management, 47*(1), 13–27.

Goodridge, D., & Hack, B. (1996). Assessing the congruence of nursing models with organizational culture: A quality improvement perspective. *Journal of Nursing Care Quality, 10*(2), 41–48.

Goodwin, N. (2000). Leadership and the UK health service. *Health Policy, 51*, 49–60.

Harrison, R. (1972). How to describe your organization's culture. *Harvard Business Review, 5*(1), 119–128.

Harrison, R. (1992). *Diagnosing Organizational Culture*. New York: Pfeiffer.

Hatch, M. (1997). *Organization Theory: Modern, Symbolic and Postmodern Perspectives*. Oxford: Oxford University Press.

Hinshaw, S. A., Smeltzer, C. H., & Atwood, J. R. (1987). Innovative retention strategies for nursing staff. *Journal of Nursing Administration, 17*(6), 8–16.

Hofstede, G. (1998). Attitudes, values and organizational culture: Disentangling the concepts. *Organization Studies, 19*(3), 477–492.

Ingersoll, G., Kirsch, J., Merk, S., & Lightfoot, J. (2000). Relationship of organizational culture and readiness for change to employee commitment to the organization. *Journal of Nursing Administration, 31*(1), 11–20.

Irvine Doran, D. M., Baker, G. R., Bohen, J., Zahn, C., Sidani, S., & Carryer, J. (2002). Achieving clinical improvement: An interdisciplinary intervention. *Health Care Management Review, 27*(4), 42–56.

Jones, K. R., DeBaca, V., & Yarbrough, M. (1997). Organizational culture assessment before and after implementing patient-focused care. *Nursing Economic$, 15*(2), 73–81.

Jones, K. R., & Redman, R. W. (2000). Organizational culture and work redesign: Experiences in three organizations. *Journal of Nursing Administration, 30*(12), 604–610.

Kangas, S., Kee, C., & McKee-Waddle, R. (1999). Organizational factors, nurses' job satisfaction, and patient satisfaction with nursing care. *Journal of Nursing Administration, 29*(1), 32–42.

Karasek, R. A. (1979). Job demands, job decision latitude and mental strain: Implications for job re-design. *Administrative Science Quarterly, 24*, 285–308.

Keuter, K., Byrne, E., Voell, J., & Larson, E. (2000). Nurses' job satisfaction and organizational climate in a dynamic work environment. *Applied Nursing Research, 13*(1), 46–49.

Koberg, C. S., & Chusmir, L. H. (1987). Organizational culture relationships with creativity and other job-related variables. *Journal of Business Research, 15*, 397–409.

Langfield-Smith, K. (1995). Organizational culture and control. In A. Berry, J. Broadbent & D. Otley (Eds.), *Management Control Theories, Issues and Practices*. London: Macmillan.

Lewin, K. (1951). *Field Theory in Social Science*. New York: Harper & Row.

Liteinenko, A., & Cooper, C. (1994). The impact of trust status on corporate culture. *Journal of Management in Medicine, 8*(4), 8–17.

Litwin, G. H., & Stringer, R. A. (1968). *Motivation and Organizational Climate* (2nd ed.). Boston: Division of Research, Harvard University.

Luk, A., Chen, R., Yau, F., Tsang, E., & Leung, C. (1998). Assessment of the organization culture in a new hospital. *The Hong Kong Nursing Journal, 34*(3), 13–22.

Maehr, M. L., & Braskamp, L. A. (1986). *The Motivation Factor: A Theory of Personal Investment*. Lexington, MA: Lexington Books.

Manley, K. (2000a). Organizational culture and consultant nurse outcomes, part 1: Organizational culture. *Nursing Standard: Official Newspaper of the Royal College of Nursing, 14*(36), 34–38.

Manley, K. (2000b). Organizational culture and consultant nurse outcomes, part 2: Nurse outcomes. *Nursing Standard: Official Newspaper of the Royal College of Nursing, 14*(37), 34–39.

Manojlovich, M., & Ketefian, S. (2002). The effects of organizational culture on nursing professionalism: Implications for health resource planning. *Canadian Journal of Nursing Research*, *33*(4), 15–34.

Mattiasson, A., & Andersson, L. (1995). Organizational environment and the support of patient autonomy in nursing home care. *Journal of Advanced Nursing*, *22*(6), 1149–1157.

McDaniel, C. (1995). Organizational culture and ethics work satisfaction. *Journal of Nursing Administration*, *25*(11), 15–21.

McDaniel, C., & Stumpf, L. R. (1993). The organizational culture: Implications for nursing service. *Journal of Nursing Administration*, *23*(4), 54–60.

Mead, G. (1934). *Mind, Self and Society*. Chicago: University of Chicago Press.

Mok, E., & Au-Yeung, B. (2002). Relationship between organizational climate and empowerment of nurses in Hong Kong. *Journal of Nursing Management*, *10*, 129–137.

Moran, E., & Volkwein, J. (1992). The cultural approach to the formation of organizational climate. *Human Relations*, *45*(1), 19.

Neal, A., Griffin, M. A., & Hart, P. M. (2000). The impact of organizational climate on safety climate and individual behavior. *Safety Science*, *34*, 99–109.

Norbergh, K., Hellzen, O., Sandman, P., & Asplun, K. (2002). The relationship between organizational climate and the content of daily life for people with dementia living in a group-dwelling. *Journal of Clinical Nursing*, *11*(2), 237–246.

Olson, L. (1998). Hospital nurses' perceptions of the ethical climate of their work setting. *Image: The Journal of Nursing Scholarship*, *30*(4), 345–349.

Pasmore, W. A. (1988). *Designing Effective Organizations: The Sociotechnical Systems Perspective*. New York: John Wiley & Sons.

Quinn, R. E. & Spreitzer, G. M. (1991). The psychometrics of the Competing Values Culture Instrument and an analysis of the impact of organizational culture on quality of life. *Research in Organizational Change and Development*, *5*, 115–142.

Rizzo, J. A., Gilman, M. P. & Mersmann, C. A. (1994). Facilitating care delivery redesign using measure of unit culture and work characteristics. *Journal of Nursing Administration*, *24*(5), 32–37.

Schein, E. (1991). *Organizational Culture and Leadership*. San Francisco: Jossey-Bass.

Schein, E. (1996). Culture: The missing concept in organizational studies. *Administrative Science Quarterly*, *41*, 229–240.

Scott, T., Mannion, R., Davies, H. T., & Marshall, M. N. (2003). Implementing culture change in health care: Theory and practice. *International Journal for Quality in Health Care: Journal of the International Society for Quality in Health Care/ Isqua*, *15*(2), 111–118.

Seago, J. A. (1996). Work group culture, stress, and hostility. Correlations with organizational outcomes. *The Journal of Nursing Administration*, *26*(6), 39–47.

Seago, J. A. (1997). Organizational culture in hospitals: Issues in measurement. *Journal of Nursing Measurement*, *5*(2), 165–178.

Sexton, B. J., Helmreich, R. L., Rowan, K., Vella, K., Boyden, J., Neilands, T. B., et al. (Under Review). The Safety Attitudes Questionnaire: A psychometric validation. *Medical Care.*

Shortell, S. M., Jones, R. H., Rademaker, A. W., Gillies, R. R., Dranove, D. S., Hughes, E. F., et al. (2000). Assessing the impact of total quality management and organizational culture on multiple outcomes for care for coronary artery bypass graft surgery patients. *Medical Care, 38*(2), 207–217.

Shortell, S. M., Zimmerman, J. E., Rousseau, D. M., Gillies, R. R., Wagner, D. P., Draper, E. A., et al. (1994). The performance of intensive care units: Does good management make a difference? *Medical Care, 29*(8), 508–525.

Snow, J. (2002). Enhancing work climate to improve performance and retain valued employees. *Journal of Nursing Administration, 32*(7/8), 393–397.

Spreitzer, G. M. (1995). Psychological empowerment in the workplace: Dimensions, measurement, and validation. *Academy of Management Journal, 38*(5), 1442–1465.

Stamps, P. L. (1997). *Nurses and Work Satisfaction: An Index for Measurement, 2nd Ed.* Chicago: Health Administration Press.

Stumpf, L. R. (2001). A comparison of governance types and patient satisfaction. *Journal of Nursing Administration, 31*(4), 196–202.

Torres, G. (1988). A reassessment of instruments for use in a multivariate evaluation of a collaborative practice project. In O. L. Strickland & C. F. Waltz (Eds.), *Measurement of Nursing Outcomes, Volume 2. Measuring Nursing Performance: Practice, Education and Research.* (pp. 381–391). New York: Springer.

Tzeng, H. M., Ketefian, S., & Redman, R. (2002). Relationship of nurses' assessment of organizational culture, job satisfaction, and patient satisfaction with nursing care. *International Journal of Nursing Studies, 39,* 79–84.

Wakefield, B., Blegen, M., Uden-Holman, T., Vaughn, T., Chrischilles, E., & Wakefield, D. (2001). Organizational culture, continuous quality improvement, and medication administration error reporting. *American Journal of Medical Quality, 16*(4), 128–134.

Wallach, E. J. (1983). Individuals and organizations: The cultural match. *Training and Development Journal, February,* 20–36.

Ware, J. E. (1993). *SF-36 Health Survey: Manual and interpretation guide.* Boston: New England Medical Centre, The Health Institute.

Zammuto, R. F., & Krakower, J. Y. (1991). *Quantitative and Qualitative Studies of Organizational Culture, Volume 5.* Greenwich, CT: JAI Press.

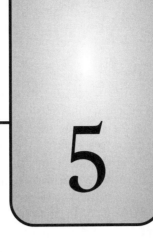

Span of Control

Amy McCutcheon

5.1 Introduction

Nurse managers have been found to have an impact on staff outcomes (Baumann et al., 2001; McGillis Hall et al., 2001; McNeese-Smith, 1993). In several nursing studies, the nurse manager's leadership style has been shown to be a key factor influencing nurses' job satisfaction (Decker, 1997; Loke, 2001; McNeese-Smith, 1995) and retention (Irvine & Evans, 1995; Lucas, 1991; Medley & Larochelle, 1995). A high level of support from managers was found to decrease nurses' feelings of emotional exhaustion (Stordeur, D'Hoore, & Vandenberghe, 2001) and to increase nurses' self-esteem (Bakker, Killmer, Siegriest, & Schaufeli, 2000). Furthermore, a participatory and supportive management style was identified as one of the key characteristics of magnet hospitals (Buchan, 1999; Scott, Sochalski, & Aiken, 1999). However, organizations such as hospitals are increasingly adopting structures with wider managerial spans of control (Pillai & Meindl, 1998; Spence Laschinger, Sabiston, Finegan, & Shamian, 2001) creating dramatic changes in the work environment including a reduction in the number of management positions. This reduction has resulted in nurse managers being responsible for several units and for motivating and evaluating a large number of staff, sometimes more than 100 staff members. Nurse managers, who are directly responsible for maintaining standards of care and developing staff, are less able to provide nurses with the traditional mentoring and coaching, and individual support and encouragement.

Spence Laschinger et al. (2001) found that nurses identified relations with management as a concern about their work conditions. The nurses stated that with additional units and staff numbers, managers are not able "to be really in touch with many situations . . . and that communication to staff was decreased" (Spence Laschinger et al., p. 10). Similarly, a study by Blythe, Baumann, and Giovannetti (2001) found that as a result of an increased span of control, relations between managers and nurses became distant and communications less frequent and more formal.

A few studies were found that demonstrated the effect of span of control on staff performance such as satisfaction and turnover, which have been shown to affect patient outcomes. However, no studies have as yet linked managers' span of control with patient outcomes.

This chapter reviews the available literature on span of control viewed as a concept affecting staff performance, and in turn, patient outcomes. This chapter:

- Reviews the concept of span of control

- Discusses the theoretical underpinnings of span of control

- Identifies the factors that influence span of control

- Critically examines the empirical evidence linking span of control to patient outcomes

- Considers the issues with the assessment of span of control

- Identifies approaches to measuring span of control

- Reviews the measures of span of control

- Outlines implications and directions for the future

The methodology used to identify, select, and systematically review the relevant literature is discussed in Chapter One. A systematic search of the nursing, health care, and management databases yielded a total of 469 empirical and conceptual articles addressing span of control. Thirty-five met the predetermined inclusion and exclusion criteria. The review of the six studies and one unpublished doctoral dissertation is presented in this chapter.

5.2   Definition of the Concept of Span of Control

Span of control pertains to the number of persons who report directly to a single manager, supervisor, or leader (Meier & Bohte, 2000) and includes the functions of planning, organizing, and leading (Hattrup & Kleiner, 1993). Span of control, which has been referred to as span of management, span of authority, or span of supervision, is considered a useful concept for measuring the closeness of contact between a manager and staff (Ouchi & Dowling, 1974).

5.3   Theoretical Underpinnings of Span of Control

Span of control is one of the three principles of management proposed by Gulick (1937) and Urwick (1956). They and other early management scholars postulated that the structural attributes of organizations affect performance and proposed that adherence to a core set of management principles would help organizations achieve high performance. The three management principles were division of labor, span of control, and unity of command. However, Gulick's and Urwick's beliefs were not developed by other researchers because Simon (1946) presented a very convincing critique of these principles of management.

Gulick (1937), and later Urwick (1956) postulated that individuals in management positions should oversee a relatively small number of employees to make the mentoring and monitoring of employees a less daunting task for the supervisor. A span of control of six individuals was recommended. It was postulated that the supervisor's direct relationships with individuals, the group, and cross relationships with other groups decreased in proportion to the addition of subordinates. Gulick added that as the number of employees per supervisor increased, so did the difficulty in monitoring the behavior of employees.

Simon (1946) identified two arguments against a narrow span of control. First, if the span of control has been limited and the supervisor has overseen a relatively small number of employees, the number of levels of hierarchy or layers of management in the organization would have increased. Second, a greater number of hierarchical levels resulted in a difficulty in vertical communication. However, these do not appear to be valid arguments in health care settings. In terms of the number of layers, the size of the hospital rather than the size of the patient care unit appears to determine the number of management layers. Medium to large hospitals have four layers (i.e., chief executive officer or president, vice president, director, and manager) while small hospitals have three layers (i.e., president or executive director, vice president or assistant executive director, and manager). In some cases, and contrary to Simon's argument, in the health care environment a wide span of control creates another management layer in the form of an assistant nurse manager. The difficulty in vertical communication is not as critical in patient care units or in teams that depend mainly on horizontal communications. Most of the daily communications by the patient care team, particularly the nursing staff, are horizontal not vertical. For example, nurses need to communicate with their colleagues and nurse managers more often than with the director of nursing or vice president.

Scholars uncritically accepted the arguments of Simon (1946), resulting in the principles of management not being pursued (Meier & Bohte, 2000). Researchers moved away from investigating the structural characteristics of organizations toward the study of organizational behavior (Hammond, 1990). More recently, using Gulick's (1937) and Urwick's (1956) principle of span of control, Meier and Bohte developed the theory of span of control, which provides a general statement about the relationship between span of control and performance. This theory proposed that there is a certain point at which the size of the span of control reaches its point to be effective, and increasing the size of the span of control beyond this point does not have additional value, and could even be harmful. In general, as spans of control increase, performance increases. However, performance gains resulting from increases in the span of control are subject to diminishing marginal returns. At even higher spans of control, additional subordinates may result in reduced, perhaps even an absence of, coordination, management, and supervision resulting in a decrease in the overall performance.

A limitation of the span of control theory is the assumption that narrow span of control means more time for managers to provide support and encouragement to their staff. However, the added time would not necessarily be spent with staff, and if spent with the staff, the quality of interaction would not necessarily be positive or beneficial to the staff, the unit, or the organization.

5.4 Factors that Influence the Manager's Span of Control

Stieglitz (1962), in his study of the Lockheed Company, identified factors that may be essential in determining an optimal span of control. These factors included similarity of the workers' functions, complexity of functions, geographic proximity of the workers, direction and control required by the workers, degree of coordination required of the workers, planning for future programs and objectives, and organizational assistance. Some of these factors have been found in the general management (Dewar & Simet, 1981; Van Fleet 1983; Van Fleet & Bedeian, 1977) and nursing literature (McCutcheon, 2003; Rodger, 2002).

5.4.1 Similarity and Complexity of Functions

Similarity and complexity of functions (Dewar & Simet, 1981; Stieglitz, 1962; Van Fleet & Bedeian, 1977) refer to the degree to which the functions performed by the staff are alike or different and the nature of the duties of staff taking into account the skills needed to perform satisfactorily. Numerous and complex functions require a number of different categories of staff. A manager responsible for various categories of staff must have knowledge of different professional standards and union contracts. Thus, the more categories of staff reporting to the manager, the more demands on the manager's time. This factor may be captured by using the number of staff categories reporting to the manager (McCutcheon, 2003).

5.4.2 *Geographic Proximity*

Geographic proximity (Stieglitz, 1962; Van Fleet & Bedeian, 1977) is the physical location of the staff reporting to the manager. Geographic proximity may be measured using the number and location of the units for which the manager is responsible (McCutcheon, 2003). The more units and the more dispersed the units are, the more time the manager spends going from one unit to another, creating more demand on the manager's time.

5.4.3 *Direction, Control, and Coordination*

Direction, control, and coordination (Stieglitz, 1962; Van Fleet, 1983; Van Fleet & Bedeian, 1977) refer to the degree of the manager's attention required to supervise the staff's work and coordination of unit activities. This variable may be measured by determining the unit unpredictability (Rodger, 2002). The more unpredictable the unit is, the more direction, control, and unit coordination are required. Thus, the greater the unit unpredictability, the more demands on the manager.

5.4.4 *Planning*

Planning refers to the complexity and time required to develop and evaluate programs and objectives (Stieglitz, 1962). The greater the complexity, the more of the manager's time and effort are required. The type of unit may provide for a measure of this variable (McCutcheon, 2003), since certain units need more planning than others.

5.4.5 *Organizational Assistance*

Organizational assistance pertains to the help received by the manager (Stieglitz, 1962; Van Fleet, & Bedeian, 1977). This variable may be measured by the number of resource staff who may or may not be reporting directly to the manager (McCutcheon, 2003). Resource staff who provide support to the unit decrease the workload of the manager and unit staff. Resource staff may provide support through various activities including orientation of new staff, development of self-teaching educational packages, and coordination of clinical inservices.

5.4.6 *Summary*

In summary, several factors that influence the manager's span of control have been identified in the literature. It is important that these factors are measured and considered when determining the manageable size of span of control, particularly in health care, for two reasons. First, managers' span of control has increased due to restructuring and mergers. A recent study showed an average span of control of 81 with a range of 36–258 for managers (McCutcheon, 2003). Second, several empirical studies (Gittell, 2001; Hechanova Alampay & Beehr, 2001; McCutcheon; Meier & Bohte, 2000) have demonstrated the effect of span of control on staff performance such as satisfaction and turnover, which have been shown to affect patient outcomes. These studies are discussed below.

5.5 Linking Managers' Span of Control to Outcome Achievement

No studies were found linking the manager's span of control to patient outcomes. However, several empirical studies demonstrated direct and moderating effects of span of control on staff performance, such as satisfaction and turnover, which have been associated with patient outcomes.

5.5.1 Direct Effect of Span of Control on Staff Performance

Three empirical studies in the management literature (Gittell, 2001; Hechanova Alampay & Beehr, 2001; Meier & Bohte, 2000) and one in the nursing literature (McCutcheon, 2003) were found demonstrating a direct effect of span of control on performance.

In a study involving airlines (n = 352 staff, 9 groups, mean span of control = 20), Gittell (2001) found that groups with broad span of control (M = 34) were significantly associated with lower levels of group performance compared to the groups with narrow span of control (M = 9). For example, Gittell found that groups with broad span of control had significantly less timely communication between group members and lower levels of problem solving. Hechanova Alampay and Beehr (2001) showed similar findings in a study of a chemical company (n = 531 staff, 24 teams, mean span of control = 47) that showed that wide span of control groups had significantly higher rates of unsafe behaviors (r = .43), and safety accidents (r = .44). Meier and Bohte (2000), in a study of schools (n = 678 schools; 2,712 students; mean student to teacher ratio = 14.5:1; range = 9–19), found that span of control had a significant impact on student performance. A reduction of one student per teacher improved student performance on reading and math tests by 0.78%.

In a doctoral study conducted in hospitals (n = 717 nurses, 51 patient care units, 41 managers, 7 hospitals), McCutcheon (2003) found that the wider the span of control, the higher the unit staff turnover rate. For every increase of 10 in the span of control, the predicted unit staff turnover rate increased by 1.6%.

5.5.2 Moderating Effect of Span of Control on Staff Performance Control

The moderating effect of span of control on the relationship between leadership and performance was found in three management studies and one nursing study. The study findings of Cogliser and Schriesheim (2000); Green, Anderson, and Shivers (1996); McCutcheon (2003); and Schriesheim, Castro, and Yammarino (2000) provided support for the argument that span of control may be an important leadership contingency variable. In a study conducted in libraries (n = 208 staff, 42 work groups, mean size = 6.4, range = 1–20), Green et al. found a significant negative relationship (r = -.22, p < .05) between work unit size and leader-member exchange. Cogliser and Schriesheim, in a study of libraries (n = 285 staff, 65 work groups, mean size = 10, range = 2–26), had similar findings, although they were not significant (r = -.08, p > .05). In a study conducted in banks (n = 150 staff, 75 managers, mean span = 11, range = 5–21), Schriesheim et al. found that span of control was a moderator of the relationship between leader-member exchange and commitment but not performance.

The study findings of Cogliser and Schreisheim (2000), and Green et al. (1996) suggest that when the work unit increases in size, there is less positive interaction between manager and staff. For instance, Green et al. found that as work unit size increased, relationships between managers and staff became less positive. Possibly, managers of large work units tend to have more time constraints and demands than managers of small work units. Unit size may limit the amount of time a manager may spend with staff. As a result, opportunities for interaction between managers and individual staff tend to be more limited, which in turn may limit the ability of managers to develop close and quality relationships with their staff.

McCutcheon (2003) showed that span of control had a significant effect on the relationship between leadership style and nurses' job satisfaction. Specifically, the wider the span of control, the less the positive effect of transformational and transactional leadership styles on nurses' job satisfaction. As well, the wider the span of control, the greater the negative effect of management by exception leadership style on job satisfaction. Management by exception managers are perceived as only available to monitor their staff to prevent mistakes (Bass, 1998). This tends to cause higher levels of anxiety and emotional exhaustion (Stordeur et al., 2001). As well, the manager's monitoring may be perceived as a lack of trust by staff. This in turn may decrease staff satisfaction.

5.5.3 Summary

In summary, although no studies were found that examined the relationship between span of control and patient outcomes, a few studies were found that demonstrated relationships between span of control and staff performance that have been linked to patient outcomes. Conducting studies that will examine the link between span of control and patient outcomes remains a challenge.

5.6 Issues in the Assessment of the Manager's Span of Control

Issues specific to the assessment of the manager's span of control were identified in the review of literature. These issues include: (a) can a numerical measure adequately determine span of control and (b) what is the desired scope of the measure of span of control?

5.6.1 Can a Numerical Measure Adequately Determine Span of Control?

The review of literature on span of control identified two streams of research including: (a) studies focusing on factors that influence span of control and (b) studies examining the relationships between span of control and performance. The first stream of studies identified several factors influencing span of control; however, these factors were not included in the second stream with the exception of the study by McCutcheon (2003). Specifically, many studies used a numerical measure (i.e., the total number of staff reporting directly to the manager) to determine the size of the manager's span of control (Cogliser & Schriesheim 2000; Gittell, 2001; Green et al., 1996; Hechanova Alampay & Beehr, 2001; McCutcheon). In addition to the numerical measure, some of the factors influencing span of control were examined in a study by McCutcheon including number of staff categories reporting to the manager, number of units the manager is responsible for, unit unpredictability, type of unit, and number of staff providing support for the unit. The challenge lies in developing a tool to measure span of control based on all of these factors.

5.6.2 What Is the Desired Scope of the Measure of Span of Control?

As discussed above, the first stream of studies (Dewar & Simet, 1981; Stieglitz, 1962; Van Fleet, 1983; Van Fleet & Bedeian, 1977) identified several factors influencing span of control including similarity and complexity of the workers' functions; geographic proximity of the workers; direction, control, and coordination required; planning for future programs and objectives; and organizational assistance. The studies that examined the relationships between span of control and performance did not include these factors. Considering that span of control has been identified as a useful measure of the closeness of contact between a manager and staff (Ouchi & Dowling, 1974), there is a need to measure the factors that decrease or increase the manager's time spent with staff.

5.7   Evidence Concerning Approaches to Measuring Managers' Span of Control

The literature identified only one measure of the manager's span of control, that is, the total number of staff reporting directly to the manager, reported as a numerical measure. Factors in the work environment that influence span of control need to be examined and taken into consideration when determining span of control. Some of these factors include similarity and complexity of the workers' functions, unit unpredictability, and number of staff providing support for the unit. The challenge lies in developing a tool to measure span of control based on all of these factors.

5.8   Measures of Span of Control

As discussed, the measure used to determine the manager's span of control is the total number of staff reporting directly to the manager. Some studies used the number of full-time equivalents. Others used the total number of people (i.e., full-time, part-time, and casual), because full-time equivalent did not accurately reflect the number of people reporting directly to the manager. In some instances one full-time equivalent consisted of two part-time nurses, and in other cases one full-time equivalent consisted of one part-time and two casual nurses. No other published measures of span of control are available.

5.9   Implications and Future Directions

The results of the review of literature provide acknowledgment of the importance of the manager's span of control in creating a positive work environment. There is evidence of the need to develop a tool to measure span of control and to conduct studies that examine the relationships between span of control and patient outcomes.

Span of control matters. Span of control has a direct effect on performance measures that have been found to influence patient outcomes and a moderating effect on the relationship between leadership and performance. Specifically, wider spans of control are associated with lower levels of performance and higher unit turnover rate. As span of control increases, the relationships between managers and staff become less positive. Furthermore, the wider the span of control, the smaller the positive effect of supportive leadership styles on nurses' job satisfaction and the greater the negative effect of less supportive leadership styles on job satisfaction.

The research supports the need to develop guidelines regarding the number of staff a nurse manager may effectively support. It is very difficult, if not impossible, to consistently provide positive leadership to a large staff while at the same time ensuring the effective and efficient operation of a large unit on a daily basis.

The review of literature provides support for the need to develop a tool to measure span of control. The challenge is for researchers to develop a tool that includes the various factors influencing span of control.

There is a need to conduct studies to examine the relationships between span of control and patient outcomes.

5.10 References

Bakker, B., Killmer, C., Siegriest, J., & Schaufeli, W. (2000). Effort-reward imbalance and burnout between nurses. *Journal of Advanced Nursing, 31,* 884–891.

Bass, B. (1998). *Transformational leadership: Industrial, military, and educational impact.* Mahwah, NJ: Lawrence Erlbaum Associates, Inc.

Baumann, A., O'Brien-Pallas, L., Armstrong-Stassen, M., Blythe, J., Bourbonnais, R., Cameron, S. et al. (2001). *Commitment and care: The benefits of a healthy workplace for nurses, their patients and the system.* Retrieved October 10, 2001, from http://www.chsrf.ca

Blythe, J., Baumann, A., & Giovannetti, P. (2001). Nurses' experiences of restructuring in three Ontario hospitals. *Journal of Nursing Scholarship, 33,* 61–68.

Buchan, J. (1999). Still attractive after all these years? Magnet hospitals in a changing health care environment. *Journal of Advanced Nursing, 30,* 100–108.

Cogliser, C., & Shriesheim, C. (2000). Exploring work unit context and leader-member exchange: A multilevel perspective. *Journal of Organizational Behavior, 21,* 487–511.

Decker, F. (1997). Occupational and nonoccupational factors in job satisfaction and psychological distress between nurses. *Research in Nursing & Health, 20,* 453–464.

Dewar, R., & Simet, D. (1981). A level specific prediction of spans of control examining the effects of size, technology, and specialization. *Academy of Management Journal, 24,* 5–24.

Gittell, J. (2001). Supervisory span, relational coordination and flight departure performance: A reassessment of postbureaucracy theory. *Organization Science, 12,* 468–483.

Green, S., Anderson, S., & Shivers, S. (1996). Demographic and organizational influences on leader-member exchange and related work attitudes. *Organizational Behavior and Human Decision Processes, 66,* 203–214.

Gulick, L. (1937). Notes on the theory of organization. In L. Gulick & L. Urwick (Eds.), *Papers on the science of administration* (pp. 191–195). New York: Institute of Public Administration, Columbia University.

Hammond, T. (1990). In defence of Luther Gulick's "Notes on the theory of organizations." *Public Administration, 68,* 143–173.

Hattrup, G., & Kleiner, B. (1993). How to establish the proper span of control for managers. *Industrial Management, 35*(6), 28–30.

Hechanova Alampay, R., & Beehr, T. (2001). Empowerment, span of control, and safety performance in work teams after workforce reduction. *Journal of Occupational Health Psychology, 6,* 275–282.

Irvine, D., & Evans, M. (1995). Job satisfaction and turnover between nurses: Integrating research findings across studies. *Nursing Research, 44,* 246–253.

Loke, J. (2001). Leadership behaviors: Effects on job satisfaction, productivity and organizational commitment. *Journal of Nursing Management, 9,* 191–204.

Lucas, M. (1991). Management style and staff nurse job satisfaction. *Journal of Professional Nursing, 7,* 280–289.

McCutcheon, A. (2003). *The relationships between span of control, leadership and performance.* Unpublished doctoral dissertation. University of Toronto, Ontario.

McGillis Hall, L., Doran, D., Baker, G., Pink, F., Sidani, S., O'Brien-Pallas, L., et al. (2001). *A study of the impact of nursing staff mix models on patient outcomes.* Retrieved October 30, 2001, from http://www.nursing.utoronto.ca

McNeese-Smith, D. (1993). Leadership behavior and employee effectiveness. *Nursing Management, 28*(5), 38–39.

McNeese-Smith, D. (1995). Job satisfaction, productivity, and organizational commitment: The result of leadership. *Journal of Nursing Administration, 25*(9), 17–26.

Medley, F., & Larochelle, D. (1995). Transformational leadership and job satisfaction. *Nursing Management, 26*(9), 64JJ–LL.

Meier, K., & Bohte, J. (2000). Ode to Luther Gulick: Span of control and organizational performance. *Administration & Society, 32,* 115–137.

Ouchi, W., & Dowling, J. (1974). Defining the span of control. *Administrative Science Quarterly, 19,* 357–365.

Pillai, R., & Meindl, J. (1998). Context and charisma: A "meso" level examination of the relationship of organic structure, collectivism and crisis to charismatic leadership. *Journal of Management, 24,* 643–671.

Rodger, G. (2002). *Span of control decision making indicators with ranking.* Unpublished work. The Ottawa Hospital, Ontario.

Schriesheim, C., Castro, S., & Yammarino, F. (2000). Investigating contingencies: An examination of the impact of span of supervision and upward controllingness on leader–member exchange using traditional and multivariate within- and between-entities analysis. *Journal of Applied Psychology, 85,* 659–677.

Scott, J., Sochalski, J., & Aiken, L. (1999). Review of magnet hospital research: Findings and implications for professional nursing practice. *Journal of Nursing Administration, 29,* 9–19.

Simon, H. (1946). The proverbs of administration. *Public Administration Review, 4,* 16–30.

Spence Laschinger, H., Sabiston, J., Finegan, J., & Shamian, J. (2001). Voices from the trenches: Nurses' experiences of hospital restructuring in Ontario. *Canadian Journal of Nursing Leadership, 14*(10), 6–13.

Stieglitz, H. (1962). Optimizing span of control. *Management Record, 24,* 25–29.

Stordeur, S., D'Hoore, W., & Vandenberghe, C. (2001). Leadership, organizational stress, and emotional exhaustion between hospital nursing staff. *Journal of Advanced Nursing, 35,* 533–542.

Urwick, L. (1956). The manager's span of control. *Harvard Business Review, May-June,* 39–47.

Van Fleet, D. (1983). Span of management research and issues. *Academy of Management Journal, 26,* 546–552.

Van Fleet, D., & Bedeian, A. (1977). A history of the span of management. *Academy of Management Review, 2,* 356–372.

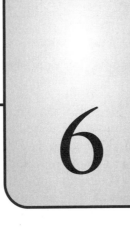

6

Workload and Productivity

Linda O'Brien-Pallas

Raquel Meyer

Donna Thomson

6.1 Introduction

Measuring nursing workload and using workload and staffing data to understand the productivity on nursing units are important management tools. However, the utility of these indicators is highly dependent on the quality of the data collected and the soundness of the analytic process used in understanding their relevance to the nursing work environment.

Workload measurement systems (WMS) have been in existence for over 60 years. Pioneering work by Connor (1961) identified that different patients required different amounts of care and that different staffing responses were needed to provide that care. The work measurement studies that formed the basis of Connor's research identified that nurses were spending significant amounts of their time in non-nursing activities such as housekeeping and dietary tray delivery. Numerous studies since then have demonstrated that nurses are still spending time completing non-nursing duties.

This review examined theoretical and empirical literature in the field of nursing workload measurement as well as productivity, using the methodology outlined in Chapter One. In total, over 1,000 relevant sources were identified, of which 93 met the criteria for inclusion in this chapter. Articles were selected that explored advances in the theoretical underpinnings of workload and productivity as well as research studies investigating these concepts in relation to patient, nurse, and system outcomes. This chapter focuses on the most common WMSs and productivity measures currently utilized.

In order to understand the scientific basis and application of workload measurement tools and measures of productivity, this chapter:

- Defines the concepts of nursing workload measurement and productivity in relation to the guidelines for Management Information Systems (MIS) in Canadian health service organizations (Canadian Institute for Health Information [CIHI], 1999)

- Presents the theoretical underpinnings of nursing workload and productivity

- Critically examines the factors that influence nursing workload and productivity

- Links nursing workload and productivity to outcome achievement

- Discusses specific issues in the assessment of nursing workload and productivity

- Suggests areas for future work based on the gaps identified in the literature

6.2 Definition of the Concepts of Workload and Productivity in Nursing

6.2.1 Nursing Workload

Nursing workload or nursing intensity is defined as the amount and type (i.e., direct and indirect) of nursing resources needed to care for an individual patient on a daily basis (O'Brien-Pallas & Giovannetti, 1992). The hours of nursing resources can be summed over the patient stay to provide an indication of the amount of nursing resources that were used over a patient's entire episode of care (O'Brien-Pallas & Giovannetti). Individual patient workload can be summed across all patients on a unit or a program to determine the total resources required on a daily basis. Consistent with the MIS guidelines, workload can be reported prospectively, as the amount of care the patient requires, and retrospectively, as the amount of care the patient received, and institutions must declare which format they report (CIHI, 1999). In Ontario and New Brunswick, nursing workload is tracked at the unit or functional center level of hospitals in the MIS reporting framework.

The terms patient classification system (PCS) and WMS have been used interchangeably in the literature. Patient classification is a generic term used to denote a methodology for grouping patients based on some explicit criteria (Thompson & Diers, 1988). When used in nursing, both PCSs and WMSs measure patient requirements for nursing care (i.e., nursing intensity) and estimate the number of nursing care hours (i.e., workload) required to meet those patients' needs (O'Brien-Pallas & Giovannetti, 1993). WMSs generally do not measure the complexity of nursing work or identify the skill and knowledge required to perform the work. They do, however, estimate the relative amount of nursing care one patient will require relative to another patient. Unless specifically stated, the term WMS will be used throughout this chapter to denote both concepts.

MIS guidelines were developed in Canada in the 1980s to serve as a standardized framework for the collection and reporting of financial and statistical data related to the day-to-day operations of health service organizations (CIHI, 1999). These guidelines allow for the integration of clinical, financial, and statistical information for service recipient costing. As defined by the MIS guidelines, a WMS is a time-based tool that measures the volume of activity provided by the Unit Producing Personnel (i.e., hands-on care providers) of a specific functional center (i.e., nursing unit or program) in terms of a standardized unit of time (CIHI).

6.2.2 Nursing Productivity

A variety of definitions of productivity exist in the literature. Holcomb, Hoffart, and Fox (2002) observed that authors frequently use, but do not define, the term productivity. In a concept analysis of productivity, Holcomb and colleagues noted that "When productivity was defined, it was either as the ratio of outputs to inputs (Benefield, 1996; Finkler & Kovner, 2000; Lengacher et al., 1996; McConnell, 1986; Scheffler, Waitzman, & Hillman, 1996) or as the relationship between inputs and outputs (Barron, 1994; Curtin, 1995; Griffith, 1995; Hilsenrath, Levey, & O'Neill, 1997; Jordan, 1994)" (p. 379). The focus has been on the physical units that workers shaped and assembled. This measure of productivity has dominated the minds of economists and business executives (Haas, 1984).

A lack of consistency in defining input and output measures has led to poor conceptual clarity as attempts are made to build a body of science in this area. Output in nursing is conditioned on predicated expectations of service from nurses and status changes in patients rather than absolute ones (Ruh, 1982). Dennis, Dunn, and Benson (1980) suggested that workload may capture the efficiency of the processes on nursing but fails to capture the effectiveness of the service provided. Productivity is defined as the relationship between the amount of acceptable output produced and the input required to produce the output. *Acceptable* presumes that commonly held and generally acceptable standards exist. Output infers that the result of the activity has some recognizable shape and the significance has some economic worth to the consumer. Acceptability can be constantly renegotiated and output can be intangible (Jelinek & Dennis, 1976; Thomson, 2003). Omachonu and Nanda (1989) argued that output expressed in terms of quantity of service rendered (i.e., hours of care) ignored the value of service provided, and that the comparison of actual nursing hours to required nursing hours constituted a definition of efficiency, not productivity. Efficiency is the ratio of actual output to a standard expected output. The most common definition of productivity is "nursing hours per patient day," but this considers only direct patient care. A definition of productivity is needed that considers the context in which nursing occurs and the effect of all resources consumed (Thomson).

Since the output of nursing is difficult to define and traditionally not well measured, CIHI (1999) proposed that the measure for nursing productivity be the relationship between nursing workload units and direct care worked hours (O'Brien-Pallas, Thomson, Alksnis, & Bruce, 2001). Under this definition, productivity measures the throughput of the nursing unit relative to the resources used to provide care. The CIHI formulas for productivity provide a framework for examining the relationship between the demands for service, as measured by the WMS, and the amount of resources used to provide that service, but do not consider the quality of the service provided. The CIHI formulas provide a limited measure of nursing productivity. Even when outcomes can be clearly defined, productivity reflects the joint influences of many factors including technology, capital investments, utilization of capacity, energy and materials, organization of production, and workforce characteristics including skill and organization (Dean & Harper, 1998; O'Brien-Pallas, Thomson, et al., 2001). Given all the influences that are not considered in the CIHI productivity measure, the formulas might well be considered a measure of "labor capacity" or "utilization," rather than "productivity" (O'Brien-Pallas, Thomson, et al., 2001; O'Brien-Pallas, Thomson, McGillis Hall, et al., 2003). O'Brien-Pallas and colleagues (2003) note that the maximum productivity (i.e., workload divided by worked hours) of any employee is 93%. Seven percent is allocated to paid breaks during which time no workload is contractually expected. At 93%, nurses are working flat out with no flexibility to meet unanticipated demands or rapidly changing patient acuity.

6.3 Theoretical Underpinnings of Nursing Workload and Productivity

Early nursing WMSs were developed using the industrial and management engineering approaches that have dominated industry with time and motion studies since the early twentieth century (O'Brien-Pallas, Giovanetti, Peereboom, &

Marton, 1995). Nursing time was calculated by determining the average time associated with each nursing task. Data were used primarily for staffing. The early conceptual underpinnings of WMS dichotomized nursing work into two broad categories of direct care and indirect care. Depending on which system was used to classify patients, direct care involved an assessment of some or many of the tasks that nurses did on behalf of patients or that required the presence of the patient or family. Indirect care encompassed all of the other activities that nurses completed for the patients, for maintenance of the unit, or for information exchange and training. From a theoretical perspective, some developers used nursing theorists such as Henderson, Orem, and Roy as the guiding framework to organize the listing of direct care activities included in the WMS (Auger & Dee, 1983; Thibault, David, O'Brien-Pallas, & Vinet, 1990).

Open systems theory, applied operations research methods, and econometric analysis were utilized by Jelinek (1967, 1969) to develop and test the Patient Care System Model for examining nursing work. This model consisted of *input* factors including personnel types and physical facilities; *throughput* factors including workload, organizational, and environmental factors; and *output* factors including patient care, patient satisfaction, and personnel satisfaction.

Expanding on the work of Halloran (1985) and Jelinek (1967, 1969), O'Brien-Pallas and colleagues developed, tested, and refined a care delivery model based on open systems theory (O'Brien-Pallas, Irvine, Peereboom, & Murray, 1997; O'Brien-Pallas et al., 1998). The model enables conceptual linking of resource utilization, nurse measures of quality, and client or patient outcomes. By moving beyond the traditional unidimensional approach of examining only direct and indirect care time, this model provides a framework for understanding the factors that cause patients with very similar medical conditions to have significantly different nurse resource requirements.

The model has been tested in the community as the Client Care Delivery Model (O'Brien-Pallas et al., 1998; O'Brien-Pallas, Irvine Doran, et al., 2001, 2002) and in the hospital sector as the Patient Care Delivery Model (O'Brien-Pallas, Thomson, McGillis Hall, et al., 2003). The model emphasizes that inputs from the care delivery system (e.g., characteristics of patients, nurses, and the system, as well as system behaviors) and throughput factors (e.g., communication and coordination, environmental complexity, and care delivery activities) cross the patient care subsystem boundaries. A transformation occurs as a consequence of interactions and processes among system substructures that result in outputs for the system (intermediate outputs include unit productivity and daily hours of care per patient; distal outputs include patient, nurse, and system outcomes) and provides feedback for the entire system. The model employs setting-specific variables and has effectively identified unique factors in both the community and hospital sectors that contribute to environmental complexity. O'Brien-Pallas and colleagues (2003) realized that multiple variables interact to influence the process of care delivery, the nursing time that patients need and receive, as well as patient, nurse, and system outcomes. The challenge in this work is to determine and routinely capture the most significant variables in settings where nursing care is delivered.

Concurrently, Prescott (1986) suggested that current approaches to workload measurement failed to adequately address patients' physiological instability and need for teaching and emotional support. The Patient Intensity for Nursing Index (PINI; Prescott & Phillips, 1988) addressed the amount of care, the complexity of care, and the clinical judgment necessary to care for patients in specific clinical settings. The four multidimensional but interrelated constructs that underpin the PINI are medical severity of illness, dependency, complexity, and time.

Donabedian's (1988) structure, process, and outcomes model forms the theoretical basis for many productivity studies. In this model, structure comprises the attributes of a setting where care occurs (i.e., material, human, and organizational structure); process denotes what was actually done; and outcome is the effect of care (Donabedian). Although Open Systems Theory and Donabedian's model offer theoretical frameworks to conceptualize the relationships between inputs/structure and outputs/outcomes, the operationalization of the concepts into measurable variables has not been fully articulated. Given the variability in definition and conceptualization, the dynamic interaction of these concepts is not yet fully understood. In advancing a theoretical framework of nursing productivity based on nursing intellectual capital, McGillis Hall (2003) has moved away from traditional economic models. This framework is currently being tested to investigate the contribution of nursing knowledge, which is measured as education, experience, career planning and development, autonomy, organizational trust and commitment, and job satisfaction, on nursing productivity indicators (e.g., nursing costs; turnover; absenteeism; costs for replacement, orientation, and education; nursing errors related to patient safety; and patient satisfaction).

Considerable progress has been made in advancing the science of workload measurement beyond a focus on nursing tasks and medical conditions. Nurse researchers and theorists recognize that provision of nursing services is influenced by a complex array of health care system inputs (e.g., patient, provider, and agency characteristics), throughputs (e.g., practice environment), and outputs (e.g., for patients, providers, and the system). To date, conceptualization of nursing productivity has been limited. Further work is needed to fully understand the interaction of the concepts that underpin current theoretical frameworks and to translate these into measurable variables that have utility for consumers of nursing workload and productivity measures.

6.4 Factors that Influence Nursing Workload and Productivity

A number of factors that influence nursing workload and productivity are identified in the literature. These factors include patient and care provider characteristics, staffing patterns, and the organization of patient care.

6.4.1 Patient Characteristics

In the hospital system, patient characteristics such as age and nursing and medical diagnoses have demonstrated different influences on nursing workload (Cohen et al., 1999; Halloran, 1985; O'Brien-Pallas, Irvine, Peereboom, & Murray, 1997). Halloran identified that as patient age increased, the average nursing workload increased as well. Nursing and medical diagnoses explained 60% of the variation in daily nursing workload, and nursing diagnoses explained twice the variation in nursing workload as did medical diagnoses (Halloran). In an acute care pediatric population (n = 1,435; patient days n = 9,102), O'Brien-Pallas and colleagues found an inverse relationship between age and nursing workload, with younger children generating greater nursing workload than older children. Nursing diagnoses were significant in explaining variation in hospital stay workload for pediatric patients, adding 21% to the explanatory power of the model (F overall = 18.49, df = 106:1312, p < .001, Adjusted R^2 = .57). The Project Research in Nursing (PRN) 80 was used to measure nursing workload in this study (O'Brien-Pallas et al.).

Mion, McLaren, and Frengley (1988) identified that patient age was modestly but positively correlated with four of the eight elements of a patient acuity system (PAS) that measures nursing workload. However, when nursing workload was correlated with severity of illness, moderately positive correlations were noted for all eight elements of the PAS. Prescott, Ryan et al. (1991) found that PINI correlated positively with the number of secondary medical diagnoses (r = .33, p < .001), medical consults (r = .17, p < .001), medical severity (r = .44, p < .001), and length of stay (r = .31, p < .001). Shorter lengths of stay have also been associated with increased daily nursing workload (O'Brien-Pallas et al., 1997; Shamian, Hagen, Hu, & Fogarty, 1992).

Cohen et al. (1999) used the Project Research in Nursing (PRN), a measure of nursing workload, to examine workload associated with adverse events in postanesthetic care patients (n = 2,031). Patients who required the lowest amount of nursing services were women, had an American Society of Anesthesiologists' (n.d.) physical status score of 1-2 (i.e., normal healthy patients or those with mild systemic disease), had surgeries that lasted less than 1 hour, and received neurolept anesthesia. Although patients with more postoperative events had higher workload scores, the relationship was not linear. For example, patients who had an unplanned intensive care unit (ICU) admission represented 0.5% of the sample and generated 1.6% of the total workload. In contrast, patients with nausea and vomiting and no other problems represented 6.0% of the patients and 6.1% of the workload costs. Patients with no adverse events comprised 60.1% of the sample and used 48.8% of the costs.

In the community sector, variation in average nurse visit time or the number of nurse visits have been associated with client age (Carr-Hill & Jenkins-Clarke, 1995; Marek, 1996; O'Brien-Pallas, Irvine Doran, et al., 2001; O'Brien-Pallas et al., 2002; Williams, Phillips, Torner, & Irvine, 1990), nursing diagnoses (Marek; O'Brien-Pallas, Irvine Doran, et al.; O'Brien-Pallas et al.), medical diagnoses (Carr-Hill & Jenkins-Clarke; Helberg, 1993; Marek; O'Brien-Pallas,

Irvine Doran, et al.; O'Brien-Pallas et al.; Williams et al.), number of comorbidities and complications (Helberg), instrumental activities of daily living (Helberg; Payne, Thomas, Fitzpatrick, Abdel-Rahman, & Kayne, 1998), clinical instability (Payne et al.), and income (Marek).

6.4.2 Care Provider Characteristics

The characteristics of the providers of nursing services constitute another factor that explains variation in nursing workload. In a study of community nursing workload in a metropolitan city in Ontario, clients ($n = 751$) cared for by baccalaureate-prepared Registered Nurses (RNs) had fewer visits than those cared for by non-baccalaureate-prepared nurses and Registered Practical Nurses, after controlling for patient complexity (O'Brien-Pallas, Irvine Doran, et al., 2001). Nurses with an RN designation and more years of community experience were less likely to report stress with amount of time available to complete their duties (Cockerill et al., 2002).

In a study of nursing performance and staffing in cardiac and cardiovascular units in six Canadian hospitals, O'Brien-Pallas, Thomson, McGillis Hall, et al. (2003) found that unit productivity (i.e., workload divided by worked hours) was influenced by nurse characteristics ($n = 727$). Productivity levels were more likely to be higher when nurse autonomy was higher and were more likely to be lower when a higher proportion of nurses on the unit were emotionally exhausted or mentally healthy. The authors suggested that emotionally exhausted nurses may not be able to work at the same level of productivity as when they are not emotionally exhausted, while mentally healthy nurses may be inclined to say no to unrealistic work expectations. For every 10% increase in the number of baccalaureate-prepared nurses on the unit, delayed interventions were 27% less likely and nurses were 40% more likely to report improved quality of care over the past year.

6.4.3 Staffing Patterns

Little is known about how management decisions regarding staffing, continuity of care providers, and caseload influence nursing workload. In the community setting, Payne et al. (1998) found that visit type, scheduled visits, caseload, and travel and case coordination time significantly influenced average visit time. O'Brien-Pallas, Irvine Doran, et al. (2001) observed that as the number of nurses visiting the client increased, so too did the average visit time and the number of visits. The greater the proportion of visits made by the primary nurse, the shorter the visit time and number of visits that were required. As would be expected, the greater the nurses' caseload on a particular day, the shorter the visit time per patient.

In the hospital sector, in a study of 24 cardiac and cardiovascular units, O'Brien-Pallas, Thomson, McGillis Hall, et al. (2003) demonstrated that nursing productivity (defined as unit workload divided by worked hours) is not linear, and although the goal is to maximize nurse activity, at productivity levels above 80%, negative outcomes emerge because nurse capacity is inadequate to meet demands. Significant benefits, both fiscal and human, could be achieved by moderating productivity levels within a range of 85% ± 5%. In terms of nurse staffing, the authors found that higher unit productivity levels were more likely when the proportion of Registered Nurse worked hours on the unit was greater, when higher nurse-to-patient ratios were reported, and when nurses required more time to complete the work as specified by the patient care plan. On 61.5% of the study days (n = 8113), productivity levels were higher than 85%. And although the maximum productivity of any employee is 93% (with the remaining 7% allocated to paid breaks), on 46.5% of the study days, productivity levels were higher than 93%.

In the Netherlands, Tummers, Landeweerd, and van Merode (2002) found that the number of staff nurses (r = -.65, p < .01), sufficient technical resources (r = -.33, p < .01), and predictable nursing care requirements (r = -.21, p < .01) were negatively associated with perceived nursing workload conditions (e.g., working under pressure, strenuous work) in general hospital settings. The availability of support staff also followed a similar pattern in an earlier study by Shamian et al. (1992).

Bloom, Alexander, and Nuchols (1997) examined the efficiency of patient care delivery of four nurse staffing patterns in a 20% random sample (n = 1,222) of U.S. hospitals. The ratio of an organization's output to input was used to measure efficiency, where output comprised hospital admissions and input consisted of both personnel and nonpersonnel operating costs. Using a transaction cost analysis, the researchers specified four regression models to examine the effects of staffing plans on personnel and benefit costs and nonpersonnel operating costs. Thirteen variables were used to control for the costs associated with the organizational and environmental determinants of costs. Use of part-time career RNs who worked exclusively at the hospital and experienced staff reduced the overall personnel and benefit and nonpersonnel operating costs. The use of agency staff increased the nonpersonnel operating costs. The use of an RN-intensive staff mix was not associated with either measure of hospital costs. This study suggested that the use of agency staff may reduce hospital productivity when defined as the ratio of outputs to inputs.

Eastaugh (2002) conducted a production function analysis of data from 1997 to 2000 from 37 U.S. hospitals to determine if the employment of Nurse Extender Technicians (NEs) increased the technical efficiency of nursing departments. The role of NEs, which evolved in response to shortages of RNs for primary nursing staff, consists of assisting RNs in completing non-nursing tasks including noninterpretive vital signs, tests, and paperwork (Eastaugh; Shukla cited in Eastaugh). The production function analysis led to the following conclusions: (a) primary care nursing could be either very productive or inefficient; (b) all-RN staffing resulted in the worst productivity performance; and (c) employment of NEs reduced waste labor and enhanced RN productivity.

6.4.4 Organization of Patient Care

In the community sector, variation in average nurse visit time or the number of nurse visits has been associated with agency characteristics such as type of visit (O'Brien-Pallas, Irvine Doran, et al., 2001; Payne et al., 1998), program of service (Payne et al.; Williams et al., 1990), type of insurance (Marek, 1996; Payne et al.), and type of agency providing the service (Payne et al.).

Several studies have hypothesized that the time nurses spend doing non-nursing tasks impinges on the time nurses perform direct care activities with patients and their families. Young, Daehn, and Busch (1990) examined the WMS and analyzed workflow in a Virginia medical center with 210 beds to evaluate the productivity of the nursing practice. Results revealed that nursing staff had assumed many non-nursing responsibilities in response to losses of full-time equivalents from support service departments. In a review of eight work sampling studies, Prescott, Phillips, Ryan, and Thompson (1991) reported that on average nurses spent only about 20% to 43% of their time completing direct care activities with patients and families. The remaining time was spent in combined indirect care and unit management activities, as well as personal time. Nurses continue to spend time portering, cleaning, restocking supplies, performing clerical duties, and delivering meal trays (Prescott, Phillips, et al.), activities that do not require the skills of RNs.

In long-term care environments, McGillis Hall and O'Brien-Pallas (2000) noted that RNs, despite their strong affinity for direct patient care activities, performed the lowest percentage of direct care (26% of their time), chiefly due to their accountability for planning and coordinating the care provided by others. The health care aides, who provided the bulk of direct patient care (35.5% of their time), found little gratification with this aspect of their role.

In a 235-bed hospital, Shukla (1990) evaluated how an admission, monitoring, and scheduling system designed to reduce fluctuations in workload on nursing units influenced productivity. The productivity of units was described as the ratio of staff cost outputs to staff full-time equivalents inputs. Streamlining the admission planning process and linking it to workload on the units actually improved productivity by 3% and reduced the number of days that nurses were sent home without pay on low census days by 40%. In an evidence-based nurse staffing study of cardiac and cardiovascular care units, O'Brien-Pallas, Thomson, McGillis Hall, et al. (2003) found that unit productivity was more likely to be lower when units were specialized (i.e., units that only service patients with cardiology conditions).

In the hospital sector, Helt and Jelinek (1988) examined the workload, productivity, and quality of care for four large urban teaching centers in the United States in four separate studies. Data were collected for admitted patients over a 3-month period. This descriptive study identified a decline in the ratio of actual hours of nursing care (i.e., inputs) to patient workload (i.e., outputs) during the years 1983 to 1985. Despite shorter average length of stay, actual quality of care as measured by the Medicus quality system (a process measure) improved in many hospitals. The major rationales given for this improvement were an increase in the number of RNs providing care and close monitoring of the process using the Medicus Nursing Quality and Productivity System.

In the Ontario hospital sector in Canada, Birch, O'Brien-Pallas, Alksnis, Tomblin Murphy, and Thomson (2003) used a production function analysis to examine changes in the inputs of nursing human resources and the acuity-adjusted flow of patients between the years 1994/95 to 1998/99. These years marked the most extreme health care restructuring years in Ontario. Productivity was described as the number of relative intensity weighted days to nursing worked hours. Using worked hours and patient acuity data from MIS and CIHI, a 20% reduction in beds per adjusted episode and a 3.7% reduction in nurses per adjusted episode were observed over the years of the data analysis. This suggests that decisions made in the 1990s to reduce the number of hospital beds in Ontario had major implications for nurse human resource requirements. In the absence of equiproportional reductions in the number of episodes of all levels of severity, additional nursing inputs per episode were required in order to support the technological innovations required to reduce hospital lengths of stay.

Numerous factors have been identified that influence nursing workload and productivity. These include characteristics of the patient (e.g., age, gender, acuity, complexity of nursing care, teaching and emotional support needs, medical condition, and adverse events), care provider (e.g., age, skills, clinical judgment, educational preparation, and employment status), organization (e.g., continuity of care, caseload, skill mix, and time spent on non-nursing tasks), and practice environment (e.g., competing demands, unanticipated case complexity and admissions). While the research to date has effectively identified factors that contribute to nursing workload, less attention has been directed towards linking these to outcomes.

6.5 Linking Nursing Workload and Productivity to Outcome Achievement

6.5.1 Nursing Workload and Productivity and Nurse Outcomes

Commonly, studies have related workload to adverse outcomes in nurses. Research indicates that heavy workloads contribute to job strain and suggests that short-term increases in productivity lead to long-term health costs (O'Brien-Pallas,

Thomson, et al., 2001). Nurses in most clinical units in Ontario hospitals, particularly nurses in emergency and medical surgical units, work at intensities that could harm their health. This study noted an almost perfect correlation between the hours of overtime worked and sick time claimed. Heavy workloads may also explain why full-time nurses have higher rates of absenteeism than part-time nurses (Burke & Greenglass, 2000). In U.S. hospitals, an increase of one patient per nurse was associated with a 23% increase in burnout and a 15% increase in job dissatisfaction (Aiken, Clarke, Sloane, Sochalski, & Silber, 2002).

Clarke, Rockett, Sloane, and Aiken (2002) examined the relationship between organizational climate as measured by the Nursing Work Index and workload (i.e., self-reported patient load) to needlestick injuries in nurses (n = 2,287) in 22 U.S. hospitals. Nurses who reported the lowest administrative support (i.e., Nursing Work Index scores less than 10) and the heaviest patient loads (i.e., more than six patients on an average day shift) were 50% more likely to sustain needlestick injuries. Near-miss incidents related to needlestick injuries were 40% more likely when nurses had the heaviest patient loads.

In cardiac and cardiovascular hospital units, improved nurse-physician relationships were associated with increases in Registered Nurse worked hours on the unit (O'Brien-Pallas, Thomson, McGillis Hall, et al., 2003). When unit productivity levels exceeded 85%, deterioration in nurse-physician relationships was observed, although nurses reported higher autonomy above this level. Higher nurse autonomy was also associated with higher nurse-patient ratios. Higher nurse job satisfaction was 57% less likely when unit productivity exceeded 80%. Reduced absenteeism rates were observed when unit productivity remained below 80%, and intent to leave increased as unit productivity levels exceeded 83% (O'Brien-Pallas, Thomson, McGillis Hall, et al.).

6.5.2 Nursing Workload and Productivity and Patient Outcomes

Few studies have linked nursing workload and patient outcome achievement. High percentages of nurses in Canada, the United States, the United Kingdom, and Sweden have reported work pressures severe enough to affect patient care (Nolan, Lundh, & Brown, 1999; Shindul-Rothschild & Duffy, 1996; Shullanberger, 2000; White, 1997), and there is evidence that lower nurse-to-patient ratios lead to complications and poorer patient outcomes (Kovner & Gergen, 1998; Lancaster, 1997; Shullanberger). Conversely, higher staffing levels are linked to better outcomes (Aiken, Sloane, & Sochalski, 1998; Lancaster).

In a study of 232,342 medical and surgical patients from 168 hospitals in Pennsylvania, for every additional patient in an average nursing workload Aiken et al. (2002) identified a 7% increase in both the odds of patient mortality within 30 days of admission and the odds of failure to rescue. Therefore, if a nurse's workload increases from four to six patients, the odds of patient mortality would increase by 14%. Rohrer, Momany, and Chang (1993) analyzed physical function as an outcome measure for nursing home residents ($n = 827$) and found that fewer heavy care residents resulted in better resident functioning. The relationship between mortality rates in very low birthweight infants ($n = 692$) and nursing staff levels in an Australian neonatal intensive care unit was examined between 1996 and 1999 (Callaghan, Cartwright, O'Rourke, & Davies, 2003). The study found that the odds of risk-adjusted mortality improved by 82% when infant staff ratios were greater than 1.71.

Kovner and Gergen (1998) examined the relationship between nurse staffing levels (number of full-time equivalent RNs working per adjusted patient day) and adverse patient outcomes after major surgery including venous thrombosis or pulmonary embolism, urinary tract infection (UTI), and pneumonia. An increase of 0.5 RN hours per day was associated with a 4.5% decrease in UTIs, a 4.2% decrease in pneumonia, a 2.6% decrease in thrombosis, and a 1.8% decrease in pulmonary complications. Sovie and Jawad (2001) studied the impact of restructuring as a cost containment exercise in 29 U.S. teaching hospitals. An increase in the number of hours worked per patient per day by registered nurses was associated with fewer patient falls ($F = 11.73$, $p = .002$) and higher levels of satisfaction regarding pain management by patients ($F = 15.05$, $p = .0007$).

In a study of 1997 data from 799 U.S. hospitals, Needleman, Buerhaus, Mattke, Stewart, and Zelevinsky (2002) reported that greater absolute hours of care provided by RNs among medical patients ($n = 5,075,969$) were associated with shorter lengths of stay ($p < .001$) and lower rates of urinary tract infections ($p = .003$) and upper gastrointestinal bleeding ($p = .007$), and among surgical patients ($n = 1,104,659$) were related to lower rates of failure to rescue ($p = .008$). In an examination of total hours of care worked by all nursing personnel (i.e., workload), Blegen, Goode, and Reed (1998) found a direct association with complaints, decubiti, and mortality. Tarnow-Mordi, Hau, Warden, and Shearer (2000) identified that variations in adjusted ICU mortality may be partially explained by excess ICU workloads. The excess workload could include an inadequate number of nursing staff, medical staff, training, supervision, and equipment.

In an evidence-based nurse staffing study of cardiac and cardiovascular care units, O'Brien-Pallas, Thomson, McGillis Hall, et al. (2003) determined that improvements in patient SF-12 physical scores at discharge were 45% less likely when unit productivity surpassed 80% and 7% less likely for each additional hour of nurse overtime. Patient behavior scores were more likely to decrease when unit productivity exceeded 88%. Improved patient knowledge scores at discharge were 74% more likely for every 10% increase in RN worked hours on the unit. Patient knowledge scores were 44% less likely to improve for every 10% increase in nurses on the unit with more than one shift change during the past two weeks. When unit productivity exceeded 91%, patients were more likely to have longer than expected lengths of stay.

By conceptually linking inputs with outputs, O'Brien-Pallas et al. (2002) found that average visit time was negatively associated with knowledge and behavior outcomes as measured by the OMAHA Problem Rating Scale for Outcomes developed by the Omaha Visiting Nurses Association (Martin & Scheet, 1992) and with social functioning outcomes as measured by the SF-36 Health Status Survey (Acute) Form (Ware, Snow, Kosinski, & Gandek, 1993) in community home nursing. These findings were consistent with the trend noted by Fortinsky and Madigan (1997). This finding warrants careful interpretation as it may be reflective of clients with more complex health needs (e.g., long-term or palliative clients) who may have less potential for improved outcomes, and thus may require more nursing resources.

6.5.3 *Nursing Workload and Productivity and Organizational Outcomes*

Rohrer, Momany, and Chang (1993) analyzed physical function as a measure of nursing home resident outcomes in ten nursing homes and found that organizational design variables were important. Results were consistent with contingency theory, which posits that to maximize performance, organizational structure should be adjusted to variations in task difficulty and variability. This study revealed that better resident outcomes could be achieved in faster paced nursing homes when employees were less closely supervised and the basis for job assignment was clear and consistent. A more hierarchical structure may be effective when workload is heavy; however, when workload and pace are held constant, better outcomes are associated with smaller hierarchies and nonspecific job assignment (Rohrer, Momany, & Chang). In a study of cardiac and cardiovascular hospital units, lower costs per Resource Intensity Weight were more likely when unit productivity levels remained below 90% and actual patient care hours declined as unit productivity exceeded 90% (O'Brien-Pallas, Thomson, McGillis Hall, et al., 2003).

6.6 Issues in the Assessment of Nursing Workload and Productivity

If WMSs are to provide the basis for resource intensity monitoring in nursing, then the reliability and validity of these data are a function of (a) the initial reliability and validity of the tools used to measure workload, (b) continued validity and reliability monitoring over time once a system is implemented, and (c) comparability of results between WMSs. The various systems differ in the way in which they measure nursing workload and the ease with which they can be modified. In turn, this may have an impact on efforts to effectively measure nursing productivity.

6.6.1 Establishing the Reliability and Validity of Measures

At best, most of the tools used to measure workload rely on a simple evaluation of face and content validity and interrater reliability. Task-based systems such as GRASP have had extensive attention placed on the face and content validity of the measure because the WMSs are usually built to reflect practice in each unit when implemented. Since its inception in the early seventies, the PRN system has maintained face and content validity by holding regular meetings where experts in nursing complete a nominal group process to validate the content of the PRN workload measurement system (Chagnon, Audette, Lebrun, & Tilquin, 1978a; Thibault et al., 1990). Each revision of the PRN measure has resulted in the identification of additional nursing interventions for inclusion in the measurement model. System developers and vendors have argued that if the WMS estimates closely correlate with the care provided, then this serves as an indication of predictive validity. However, researchers suggested that the care provided may not represent the amount or quality of care that patients require, and therefore, cannot be utilized as a gold standard criterion (Alward, 1983; Chagnon, Audette, Lebrun, & Tilquin, 1978b; Hernandez & O'Brien-Pallas, 1996; O'Brien-Pallas, Cockerill, & Leatt, 1992; Thibault et al.).

With a WMS, determination of construct validity focuses on the abstract concept or construct underlying the instrument (e.g., the need for nursing care) and assesses its relationship to one or more hypothetically related concepts. The least amount of work has been done in the area of construct validity of WMSs (Hernandez & O'Brien-Pallas, 1996). Chagnon and colleagues (1978b) evaluated and published the construct validity of the PRN PCS. They examined the relationship between the supply of nursing personnel and the demand for nursing services. At nonpeak times in the nursing shifts, the nurses' degree of occupation or busyness was observed and compared to the staffing estimates derived from the PCS. A high positive and significant correlation was observed between the two variables ($r = .91$, $p = .02$). The degree of occupation explained 80% of the variation in the staff working on the unit.

6.6.2 Maintaining Reliability and Validity of Measures

Maintaining the integrity of a measure once it is developed and implemented is equally as important as establishing the initial reliability and validity. For example, since the mid-1980s infection control practices have needed to keep pace with such phenomena as AIDS, nosocomial multiresistant bacteria, and Sudden Acute Respiratory Syndrome (SARS). Accordingly, WMSs must be updated regularly to ensure they have the ability to capture the nursing workload implications of evolving clinical practices including new infection control measures (Saulnier et al., 2001). For example, in a study conducted during 1995 and 1996, using the third version of PRN 87, nursing workload was found to be underestimated in association with infection control practices for multiresistant nosocomial bacteria (Saulnier et al.). Ongoing validation of the tool is necessary. As of 2003, a newer version of PRN is available (C. Tilquin, personal communication, September 12, 2003).

In the practice setting, the face and content validity of WMSs must be updated at least annually or more often if the case mix on a unit changes and agencies must demonstrate that the quantification coefficients (i.e., the time weighting associated with each category) have been evaluated annually. For example, with the Medicus system the target hours assigned to a unit must be reevaluated to determine if changes in patient mix, care practices, or staff mix have occurred and whether these changes affect the target hours selected for the unit. Task-based systems (e.g., GRASP) need to be evaluated to determine if the items included on the patient care hours chart reflect the majority of the patient care activities that constitute the greatest amount of nursing time (O'Brien-Pallas & Giovannetti, 1992). Ongoing monitoring of reliability is a prerequisite for maintaining validity. It is recommended that interrater reliability monitoring be carried out on 10% of the cases classified annually and that checks should be completed at regular intervals throughout the year. For systems where patients are placed in categories of care prior to assigning an hours estimate, agreement between raters should be at least 95%. Category of care approaches need to be more stringent because incorrect categorization of a patient may result in a difference of hours, rather than minutes, being assigned to the patient.

6.6.3 Issues in the Equivalence of Measures

Studies have demonstrated that when different WMSs were applied to the same patient, significantly different hours of care estimates were generated (Carr-Hill & Jenkins-Clarke, 1995; O'Brien-Pallas et al., 1992; O'Brien-Pallas, Leatt, Deber, & Till, 1989; Phillips, Castorr, Prescott, & Soeken, 1992; Thompson & Diers, 1988). Low to moderate correlations have been observed between WMSs, which suggests that the systems are measuring similar phenomena. To date, none of the systems has been declared the "gold standard." However, since the PRN system has demonstrated construct validity (Chagnon et al., 1978b), one could argue that it most closely approximates a gold standard. In one study, the PRN system estimated on average 4.53 more hours of care per day than did Medicus, GRASP, or the Nursing Information System for Saskatchewan (NISS; O'Brien-Pallas et al., 1992). In another study, O'Brien-Pallas et al. (1989) found that PRN estimated an average of 2.43 and 2.49 more hours of care per patient day than Medicus and GRASP, respectively. When the hour estimates were converted to costs, each WMS provided different cost estimates for the same patient stay (Cockerill, O'Brien-Pallas, Bolley, & Pink, 1993). These findings suggest that comparison of case costs across settings is difficult because of the different WMSs utilized. In a purposive sample of 24 clinical units in four United States hospitals, Phillips et al. (1992) concurrently rated patients using PINI and Medicus ($n = 1,829$), and PINI and GRASP ($n = 1,117$). In terms of hours of care, the amount of shared variability between PINI and the other two WMSs was low at 34%. The researchers suggested that this may be accounted for by differing measurement techniques (i.e., estimates derived from time and motion studies for Medicus and GRASP versus nurse-assessed hours of care for PINI). Further, since 50% of the variability in the Medicus and GRASP scores was not accounted for by the PINI tool, these WMSs may have measured different phenomena than PINI.

6.6.4 *Effectively Capturing Productivity*

The key issue in measuring productivity is to move beyond the econometric model of outputs, such as cost, being analyzed relative to personnel inputs. Studies examining the most effective and efficient number and mix of nursing personnel and the appropriate methods of care delivery required to improve productivity and patient outcomes have yet to be identified. Recent studies suggest that nurses in Ontario hospitals are working beyond capacity with over 25% of units reporting productivity standards of greater than 93% (O'Brien-Pallas, Thomson, Alksnis, et al., 2003; O'Brien-Pallas, Thomson, McGillis Hall, et al., 2003). Although evidence suggests that work overload is associated with nurse burnout and lost day injury rates (Aiken et al., 2002; Shamian et al., 2001), the impact of these unrealistic productivity levels on patient outcomes has been emerging (O'Brien-Pallas, Thomson, McGillis Hall et al.). In order to understand the work capacity of nurses, several forces over and above the product mix need to be considered and quantified. These include the work environment of the nurse, the complexity of cases, scheduling issues, and quality of care (O'Brien-Pallas, Thomson, McGillis Hall, et al.). The target for effective capacity is expected to vary by nursing unit and agency size and type, given the variation in ability to anticipate demand, the roles of different organizations in the health care system, and economies of scale related to size. These variations in effective capacity have yet to be defined, but ongoing research is addressing important considerations in this process. However, when actual capacity exceeds the target for effective capacity, consequences in cost and quality arise (O'Brien-Pallas, Thomson, et al., 2001). For example, in situations where overtime is increased to meet workload demands, the odds of having a lost day claim for a musculoskeletal injury increase by 70% for each quartile increase in overtime hours worked (Shamian et al.). At this time, a methodology to measure the difference between design and effective capacity has not been developed.

6.7 Evidence Concerning Approaches to Measuring Nursing Workload and Productivity

Although a great deal of anecdotal evidence exists in the literature about WMSs and productivity, few studies provide direction for future development. While WMSs have been in place for over 50 years in North American hospitals, little innovation is found in the approaches used or in the applications to nonhospital sectors. Recent literature suggests that conceptualizations of nursing and patient care need to move beyond counting nursing tasks to a systems perspective for understanding the unique characteristics of the client, those who provide care, the environment in which care is delivered (in particular the management decisions and behaviors), the factors that influence the care delivery process, and the impact of the interactions of these on patient, nurse, and system outcomes including productivity (O'Brien-Pallas et al., 1997, 2002; O'Brien-Pallas, Irvine Doran, et al., 2001; O'Brien-Pallas, Thomson, McGillis Hall, et al., 2003; Prescott & Phillips, 1988). In order to achieve this broader conceptualization, the influences of multiple measures of workload and productivity need to be examined. To date, not all of these data are routinely collected. There is an urgent need to define concepts, develop and validate measures, and ensure routine collection of data elements to inform analysis.

6.7.1 Measures of Nursing Workload

Several reports in the literature describe the development of WMSs for nursing. Many reflect a single hospital's efforts to develop a WMS. The following descriptions focus on the most commonly used measures that have displayed good evidence of reliability and validity testing. These include GRASP, PINI, Medicus, PRN, and the Environmental Complexity Scale (ECS) (see Table 6.1, page 124). In addition, the potential usefulness of MIS data as a source of nursing workload data is examined.

6.7.1.1 GRASP

The GRASP methodology studies the tasks nurses complete on behalf of patients. Tasks are divided into the following categories: nursing process, direct nursing care, indirect nursing care, teaching and emotional support, and transportation activities. The tasks relative to teaching and emotional support are considered but are less detailed. Tasks can easily be measured per shift and per category of personnel to capture the number of patient care hours and nursing care hours. GRASP's methodology takes into account variables such as the effect of fatigue, slowing down due to the time of the day or due to other phenomena, and the importance of personnel participation, but these variables are not determined. The tasks studied were deduced from the application of Pareto's law (i.e., 15% of the activities in which nurses are involved take up 85% of their time). Emotional support needs are not derived from the application of Pareto's law, rather, these items are included as a separate category in the system application. Additional items that are relevant to a particular unit are added based on group process and work measurement on the unit. The GRASP database held by the vendors holds extensive task listings and time associated with tasks from the numerous studies completed in the system implementations over time.

6.7.1.2 *Patient Intensity for Nursing Index (PINI)*

PINI was developed as a measure of nursing intensity for examining nursing care costs (Prescott & Phillips, 1988; Prescott, Ryan, et al., 1991). Intended for use by RNs caring for hospital patients in medical, surgical, and intensive care settings (Prescott, Soeken, & Ryan, 1989), PINI attempts to incorporate factors such as the patient's physiological instability and need for teaching and emotional support into PCSs.

Nursing intensity, as defined by the PINI model, includes the amount of care, the complexity of care, and the clinical judgment necessary to care for patients in specific clinical settings. PINI comprises four multidimensional but related constructs: medical severity of illness, dependency, complexity, and time (Prescott, Ryan, et al., 1991). As a medical construct, severity of illness refers to the gravity of the patient's condition. Dependency, or the patient's need for nursing, includes items found in traditional WMSs, such as the need for assistance with activities of daily living. Items related to teaching and psychosocial support are also included. Complexity, the third dimension, encompasses the knowledge, skill, and experience related to the nursing interventions required by the patient. As well, it includes the problem-solving dimension of the nursing process, during which a nurse applies his or her knowledge and skill to the clinical decision-making associated with the nursing care. Time, the final component of the PINI, refers to the hours of care provided within a specified time frame.

The PINI was not originally intended as a staffing system. It is completed at the end of a work shift to estimate the actual time spent on different aspects of patient care during the shift. It produces an estimate of total nursing care delivered rather than an estimate of the care needed (Prescott, Ryan, et al., 1991).

6.7.1.3 *Medicus*

The Rush Medicus system for classifying patients was originally developed by Jelinek and Dennis (1976) from the Medicus Corporation. Medicus differs from the task-based systems because it purports to measure the dependency on nursing created by different patient conditions. The current 37-item measure was derived from extensive research that examined patients' conditions, the interventions that nurses complete for patients, and the time involved in providing care. Initial unpublished studies identified that the 37 items included in the generic Medicus

Table 6.1 Nursing Measures of Workload and Productivity

Instrument Author/Date of Publication	Target Population	Domains	Method of Administration	Reliability	Validity	Sensitivity to Nursing
Patient Intensity for Nursing Index (PINI)	Hospital settings; measures intensity of nursing care as a combination of the complexity and the quantity of care needed within a defined amount of time (Prescott & Phillips, 1988).	Four components: severity of illness; complexity; patient need for nursing; and time (Prescott & Phillips, 1988); the initial 12 items were later reduced to 10.	Nurses assign a rating to patients based on the amount of care they actually provide versus an estimate of the care the patient needs (Prescott & Phillips, 1988).	Internal consistency, $\alpha = 0.85$; interrater reliability, $\alpha = 0.62$ based on 408 paired ratings; (Prescott & Phillips, 1988); internal consistency (Prescott, Ryan, Soeken, Castorr, Thompson & Phillips, 1991).	Validity was demonstrated through rigorous testing. (Prescott, Ryan, Soeken, Castorr, Thompson & Phillips, 1991).	The time nurses spent in providing patient care was significantly correlated with the estimates of nursing time reflected on the PINI. (Prescott, Ryan, Soeken, Castorr, Thompson & Phillips, 1991).
Project Research in Nursing (PRN) (1974; 1980; 1987; 2002)	Hospital sector; prospective and retrospective use of tool in the following types of units: medicine, surgery, nursery, postpartum, pediatrics, psychiatry, geriatrics, rehabilitation, and long-term care; retrospective use in: emergency (Thibault et al, 1990).	PRN 1974: 129 nursing interventions (Chagnon et al, 1978a); PRN 1974 – 1987: 214-259 primary indicators of bedside care (Thibault et al, 1990). Records the estimate of time versus the real time required to complete specific patient care activities.	Staff nurse administered.	Reliability is user dependent (Chagnon et al, 1978a); no data on interrater reliability.	Construct validity (Chagnon et al, 1978b); face, content, and predictive validity (Thibault et al, 1990).	Indicators based on Henderson's 14 basic nursing needs that are integrated into Orem's categories of self-care; exhaustive list of indicators will be sensitive to very small changes in patient requirements for nursing care (Thibault et al, 1990).
GRASP (1976)	Nursing, allied health and support departments in hospitals, nursing homes and home health care; suggests prospective and retrospective use of tool in the following types of units: medicine, surgery,	Task categories: nursing process, direct nursing care, indirect nursing care, teaching and emotional support, and transportation. Productivity indicators: optimal, good, and essential care.	Data entered by staff nurse each shift.		Internal validity; some questions exist regarding external validity; much of the scientific basis is unpublished; content validity is user dependent; face validity is adequate; concept validity; no evidence to support.	The nursing process is the organizing framework and concern has been expressed that it may be weak in its ability to determine the items (i.e. interventions) that are captured (Thibault et al, 1990).

α = Cronbach's alpha coefficient
p = probability
r = Pearson's product-moment correlation coefficient
α = Cohen's weighted kappa

Table 6.1 (continued)

Instrument Author/Date of Publication	Target Population	Domains	Method of Administration	Reliability	Validity	Sensitivity to Nursing
GRASP (continued)	out-patient clinic, nursery, postpartum, psychiatry, geriatrics, hemodialysis, rehabilitation, and long-term care; retrospective use in: emergency, obstetrics and delivery room (Thibault et al, 1990).				development of productivity indicators (Thibault et al, 1990).	
The MEDICUS Nursing Management Information System (Medicus Corporation)	Hospital sector; prospective and retrospective use of tool in the following types of units: medicine, surgery, nursery, postpartum, psychiatry, geriatrics, rehabilitation, and long-term care; retrospective use in: emergency, out patient clinic, obstetrics, delivery room, and hemodialysis (Thibault et al, 1990).	Four patient types: type two signifies the average patient; a set of 32 (later 37) indicators within three categories (patient condition, basic care, and therapeutic intervention); one productivity indicator; tool intended to capture "visible and invisible nursing work."	Staff nurse administered; to be completed on any shift.	The system is described as enabling interrater reliability of 95%. (Thibault et al, 1990).	External validity is supported by user satisfaction and replication of the patient groupings; nominal face validity; unable to evaluate content validity due to unavailability of original research (Thibault et al, 1990); r (101) = .920, p < .01; r (76) = .853, p < .01 (Halloran 1981 cited in Halloran, 1985).	Conceptual basis is the nursing process that is described as weak because it does not "create a unique link between dependency and workload" (Thibault et al, 1990).

α = Cronbach's alpha coefficient
p = probability
r = Pearson's product-moment correlation coefficient
α = Cohen's weighted kappa

tool were significant, and the greatest amount of variation was in patients' dependence on nursing, measured in time spent with patients (Thibault et al., 1990). Initially, patients were placed in one of four levels of dependency, and each level had a relative value assigned that reflected the amount of resources required by each level relative to the other levels. For example, in the early Medicus system, the average or standard patient was a type 2 patient and was assigned a relative value of 1. A type 1 patient had a relative value of 0.5 and therefore was half as dependent on nursing as a type 2 patient. A type 4 patient with a relative value of 4 was 2.3 times as dependent as a type 2 patient using the six-type Medicus system of patients in recognition of the increasing complexity of patients admitted to hospitals (Thibault et al.; N. Hilborn, personal communication, July 23, 2003).

Through a process of workflow analysis and work measurement, target hours for standard type 2 patients are determined for each nursing unit. Medicus, like other vendors, has an extensive database that reflects the target hours of different types of units in numerous hospitals. Once target hours are established, the relative value for each patient type on the unit is multiplied by the target hours for the unit, then summed to determine the workload on the unit. The workload index is used to compare the unit's relative dependency on nursing. Usual staffing on the unit is developed through consultation with the unit managers and an analysis of the mix of patients on the unit. Medicus introduced the notion of variable staffing in its early system implementations. Units were staffed according to the normal workload, then, based on daily variations from the norm, staffing was adjusted through the use of float pools or agency staff to meet the needs on a day to day basis.

According to Thibault et al. (1990), although Medicus representatives assert that the level of reliability of the instrument is high based on its ease of use, the methods that were originally used to establish the reliability of the instrument remain unknown. The vendor states that his classification system permits interrater reliability of 95%. While not explicitly stated in formal publications, the content validity of the levels of care can be assumed because of the early work measurement studies that were done including validation of the categories by nurse experts during system development (M. Hundert, personal communication, 1990). Since that time, additional indicators and categories have been developed to ensure system integrity (N. Hilborn, personal communication, July 23, 2003). The link between patient dependence and workload has not been validated, and the clinical reality is that the semiautonomous patient may entail a larger workload than the totally dependent patient. The variables used are very limited and reflect the more easily observed and measurable aspects of the workload, but do not always capture the most important specific or burdensome aspects of nursing.

A quality of care measure (Jelinek, Haussman, Hegyvary, & Newman, 1975) is often applied with each Medicus implementation in order to understand the relationship between staffing and quality of care. While the Medicus system has been used extensively in Canada and the United States, primarily in large teaching hospitals, use has declined in Canada for two reasons: (a) nursing staff do not always understand the principles of patient dependency and become frustrated when the tasks they complete do not appear on the classification instrument; and (b) a financial investment is required to make the system MIS compatible.

6.7.1.4 Project Research in Nursing (PRN)

The PRN methodology has had extensive testing (Chagnon et al., 1978a, 1978b), and has gone through several iterations since it was first developed in 1972. To begin the project, a list of activities of required care for certain classes of patients was developed. Over time, diverse methods were employed to validate the tasks that were inscribed with the aid of (a) real nursing care plans and standard nursing care plans, (b) the times estimated by the nurses with the help of precise timing studies, and (c) the required care compared to the given care. The first research goal was to develop a classification of patients, and eventually, one measure of time required by patients was identified.

The nursing framework for the system was based on Virginia Henderson's definition of nursing, and later, the work of Orem (Thibault et al., 1990). The activities of required care were listed from the 14 basic nursing needs described by Henderson, then integrated into Orem's categories of self-care. One strength of this approach is that it is derived from an analysis over a long period of time of the care patients required based on a theoretical view of man and nursing. Another strength of this approach is the application of this view through the use of care plans reflecting the elements of the nursing process to treat usual patients in each hospital area. This application was systematic and rigorous. The strength of this system is that the approach is dynamic and can continue to evolve as the process of nursing evolves. The second version published, the PRN 80 (Tilquin, Carle, Saulnier, & Lambert, 1981) gives more extensive treatment to psychosocial aspects of nursing. The units of analysis for the initial development and the subsequent revisions were the nursing care plan and the activities performed by the nursing staff to care for patients with a given standard/individual care plan. Over 2,000 care plans formed the basis of this analysis (Thibault et al., 1990). The next version of the tool, the PRN 6.0, is currently available in French and Spanish (C. Tilquin, personal communication, September 12, 2003).

This instrument lists 214 indicators or tasks that nurses complete over a 24-hour period. Each indicator has a standard point value that reflects the time involved to complete tasks for patients; each point represents 5 minutes. A higher point value indicates that greater amounts of nursing care are required. The system is based on the measurement of the activities that nurses complete for patients' care. The system measures the time required to complete the task rather than the actual completion time. A focus on the care required allows for staffing decisions that are based on need, not just the amount of time available or the status quo, which may reflect an understaffed situation.

The internal validity of the project appeared excellent; it was developed utilizing the Delphi and nominal group methods successively. The system was revised four times and was published in a fifth version. Internal validity for this system was further strengthened by the evaluation that was conducted by peers on two occasions. Face validity was adequate, and content validity was established by nurse experts during a series of meetings held over time (Thibault et al., 1990). Chagnon et al. (1978a, 1978b) established the construct and predictive validity of the tool. Time studies of nurses at nonpeak work periods demonstrated that the time estimates predicted by the PRN tool corresponded with the degree of busyness of nurses and work actually done at the nonpeak times (Chagnon et al., 1978b). Interrater reliability was user dependent.

The PRN system may be used for budgeting, adjusting the workload of each team member on each shift, simulation of a unit before its opening, addressing skill mix issues, admitting patients to the unit, evaluating issues of professional development, evaluating the impact of certain types of professional practice, and identifying comparisons across units. While the system may be used to consider productivity issues, it does not permit the verification of the productivity of personnel; this was not one of its goals. The system measures visible work (direct clinical activities), indirect clinical activities, non-nursing activities, and nonclinical activities.

6.7.1.5 *Environmental Complexity Scale (ECS)*

Developed by O'Brien-Pallas et al. (1997), the ECS examines the push and pull that nurses experience while delivering patient care on a day to day basis. Factor analyses in a number of preliminary studies have revealed that the ECS taps three main domains including unanticipated delays and resequencing of work in response to others, unanticipated delays due to changes in patient acuity, and characteristics and composition of the caregivers (O'Brien-Pallas et al.). Both exploratory and confirmatory factor analysis have supported these domains in two studies that examined over 2,000 patient days of data (Estabrooks et al., 2003; O'Brien-Pallas, Thomson, McGillis Hall, et al., 2003).

In the hospital sector, both exploratory and confirmatory factor analyses were completed on the 22-item scale (O'Brien-Pallas, Thomson, McGillis Hall, et al., 2003). Three identical factor solutions were obtained and explained 60.31% of the variance. The first subscale, explaining 49.8% of the variance, measures delays associated with resequencing work in response to others including the following variables: doctors not answering pages, keys missing, clarifying doctors' orders, multiple delays, more than the usual number of calls to the doctors, language barriers with the patients and families, teams not pulling together, completing the work of others, and participating in nursing research. The second subscale included extra charting and paperwork, psychosocial support for patients, psychosocial support for families, extra vital signs, more than the usual amount of teaching, interruptions that increased time with families, increased patient acuity, rushing to complete work, and stat blood work; this subscale accounted for 5.78% of the variance explained in the factor analysis. The final subscale, which addressed characteristics and composition of the caregiving team, comprised three items including: (a) students requiring assistance, supervision, and access to charts; (b) equipment and supplies; and (c) absence of unit staff. This subscale added 4.74% to the explanatory power of the model. The alpha reliabilities for the three subscales were .87, .90, and .77 respectively (O'Brien-Pallas, Thomson, McGillis Hall, et al.).

In the earliest studies, the environmental complexity items explained a small but significant amount of variation in both daily and hospital stay workload after considering patient characteristics. Characteristics and composition of the caregiving team were negatively related to average hospital stay workload and added an additional 3% to the explanatory power of the model (O'Brien-Pallas et al., 1997). Whereas in the community sector, shifting case complexity and the number of new admissions to the caseload explained 20.5% of the variation observed in average visit time after controlling for patient, geographical, and provider characteristics (O'Brien-Pallas, Irvine Doran, et al., 2001). In this setting, environmental complexity was associated with longer visit times, the number of visits, and patient outcomes (O'Brien-Pallas, Irvine, et al.; O'Brien-Pallas et al., 2002).

6.7.1.6 MIS Data

In Ontario and New Brunswick, nursing workload data are part of routine reporting of hospitals through the MIS system. Hospitals are required to report both service recipient workload (i.e., activities directed toward the care of a patient or group of patients) and nonservice recipient workload (i.e., activities not directly related to an individual patient but critical to the care delivery process). Reported under the assessment, therapeutic interventions, and consultation categories, service recipient workload is derived primarily from WMSs. Nonservice recipient workload is reported under four ledgers including functional center activities, organizational professional activities/facility and community professional activities, teaching and in-service, and lastly, research.

One of the difficulties in using the workload measurement data reported in the MIS system for research purposes centers on the reliability of the data. While hospitals are required to monitor and maintain acceptable levels of interrater reliability of the WMS used in the facility, this is not always achieved. Another reliability issue stems from the fact that hospitals that do not have a WMS have been known to create a workload value for the various reporting centers in the hospital and report this value to the Ministry of Health and Long-Term Care in Ontario (D. Thomson, personal communication, May, 2003). The Ontario government has developed guidelines for auditing and compliance with reference to workload and these should improve the consistency of the results (D. Thomson, personal communication, May, 2003). Currently, when hospitals do not submit workload, the Ontario Ministry of Health and Long-Term Care assigns a default value of 1 hour (D. Thomson, personal communication, May, 2003). Unless researchers understand the particularities of the MIS system, this can lead to erroneous conclusions.

6.7.2 Measures of Nursing Productivity

In production lines where an operator is working at a single task, the workload is usually measured through time studies and is defined as the time involved in completing an entire task from start to finish. A standard time per task allows the managers to understand how many units of work can be completed in a work shift after factoring a time for fatigue and delay and the productivity of an individual worker or group of workers in a specified period of time.

The measure purported by CIHI (1999) involves examining the following ratio: *Unit productivity = (workload hours/worked hours) × 100*. Hospitals do not always report workload data reliably, if at all. Therefore, estimates of productivity using the CIHI method may be very unreliable. Researchers need to examine the productivity data carefully and delete extreme values that are most likely reporting errors from the analysis.

6.8   Implications and Future Directions

Nursing workload and productivity are important concepts relative to patient outcomes, quality of care, nurse outcomes, and health system costs. This literature review identifies that although WMSs have been in use for a number of years in the acute care sector, the conceptual adequacy of these measures and their psychometric properties have been relatively unexplored until the last two decades. Currently in Canada, the CIHI measure of productivity is consistent with the world view that the "amount of nursing care" is the key indicator of productivity; however, this measure does not contribute to developing potential improvements in the cost and quality of the care delivered. Furthermore, a paucity of research exists in measuring nursing workload and productivity in nonacute care sectors including community, long-term, and chronic care.

Further research is needed to define a gold standard for measuring nursing workload. Once a gold standard is achieved, all acute care institutions should use the same measure to facilitate comparisons across settings and jurisdictions. At present, both the PRN WMS and the ECS could be used for this purpose because good reliability and validity have been achieved and the authors have made the methodology transparent. The PINI measure also has adequate reliability and validity; however, the methodology is not published in the public domain. In the interim, hospitals should report their workload using existing tools but ensure the quality of the data submitted for MIS reporting is reliable.

Any workload system developed should involve multiple measures that capture the complexity of patient conditions, the decisions that providers make, environmental complexity, as well as the factors that influence processes and patient, nurse, and system outcomes. From a theoretical perspective these variables could be specified by using broad frameworks that link inputs to outputs such as the Patient Care Delivery Model (O'Brien-Pallas, Irvine Doran, et al., 2001; O'Brien-Pallas et al., 2002; O'Brien-Pallas, Thomson, McGillis Hall, et al., 2003) or the Nursing Role Effectiveness Model (Irvine, Sidani, & McGillis Hall, 1998).

Further work is required to enable the development of quality-adjusted measures of productivity that are sensitive to the multiple factors that influence inputs, throughputs, and outputs of the system.

In the community sector, the collection of data elements related to number, type, and length of visits, as well as characteristics of and outcomes for clients, providers, and agencies should be standardized. In community and hospital sectors, the ECS can be used to capture unique environmental complexity factors that explain variation in workload. Future studies to examine the constraints on nurse productivity and the impact of client-controlled care settings and to refine existing models are recommended.

6.9 References

Aiken, L. H., Clarke, S. P., Sloane, D. M., Sochalski, J., & Silber, J. H. (2002). Hospital nurse staffing and patient mortality, nurse burnout, and job dissatisfaction. *Journal of the American Medical Association, 288*, 1987–1993.

Aiken, L. H., Sloane, D. M., & Sochalski, J. (1998). Hospital organisation and outcomes. *Quality in Health Care, 7*(4), 222–226.

Alward, R. R. (1983). Patient classification systems: The ideal vs. reality. *Journal of Nursing Administration, 13*(2), 14–19.

American Society of Anesthesiologists. (n.d.). *ASA physical status classification system.* Retrieved September 9, 2003, from http://www.asahq.org/clinical/physicalstatus.htm.

Auger, J., & Dee., V. (1983). A patient classification system based on the behavioral system model of nursing: Part 2. *Journal of Nursing Administration, 13*(4), 38–43.

Barron, J. (1994). Productivity and cost per unit of service. In R. Spitzer-Lehman (Ed.), *Nursing management desk reference: Concepts, skills and strategies* (pp. 260–277). Philadelphia: W. B. Saunders.

Benefield, L. E. (1996). Component analysis of productivity in home care RNs. *Public Health Nursing, 13*, 233–243.

Birch, S., O'Brien-Pallas, L., Alksnis, C., Tomblin Murphy, G., & Thomson, D. (2003). Beyond demographic change in health human resources planning: An extended framework and application to nursing. *Journal of Health Services Research and Policy, 8*(4), 225–229.

Blegen, M., Goode, C., & Reed, L. (1998). Nurse staffing and patient outcomes. *Nursing Research, 47*(1), 43–50.

Bloom, J. R., Alexander, J. A., & Nuchols, B. A. (1997). Nurse staffing patterns and hospital efficiency in the United States. *Social Science & Medicine, 44,* 147–155.

Burke, R. J., & Greenglass, E. R. (2000). Effects of hospital restructuring on full time and part time nursing staff in Ontario. *International Journal of Nursing Studies, 37*(2), 163–171.

Callaghan, L. A., Cartwright, D. W., O'Rourke, P., & Davies, M. W. (2003). Infant to staff ratios and risk of mortality in very low birthweight infants. *Archives of Disease in Childhood Fetal and Neonatal Edition, 88,* F94–F97.

Canadian Institute for Health Information (1999). *MIS Guidelines for Canadian Health Care Facilities.* Ottawa, Canada: Author.

Carr-Hill, R., & Jenkins-Clarke, S. (1995). Measurement systems in principle and in practice: The example of nursing workload. *Journal of Advanced Nursing, 22,* 221–225.

Chagnon, M., Audette, L., Lebrun, L., & Tilquin, C. (1978a). A patient classification system by level of nursing care requirements. *Nursing Research, 27,* 107–113.

Chagnon, M., Audette, L. M., Lebrun, L., & Tilquin, C. (1978b). Validation of a patient classification through evaluation of the nursing staff degree of occupation. *Medical Care, 16,* 465–475.

Clarke, S. P., Rockett, J. L., Sloane, D. M., & Aiken, L. H. (2002). Organizational climate, staffing, and safety equipment as predictors of needlestick injuries and near-misses in hospital nurses. *American Journal of Infection Control, 30*(4), 207–216.

Cockerill, R., O'Brien-Pallas, L. L., Bolley, H., & Pink, G. (1993). Measuring nursing workload for case costing. *Nursing Economic$, 11,* 342–349.

Cockerill, R., O'Brien-Pallas, L. L., Murray, M., Doran, D., Sidani, S., Laurie-Shaw, B., et al. (2002). Adequacy of time per visit in community nursing. *Research and Theory in Nursing Practice, 16*(1), 43–51.

Cohen, M., O'Brien-Pallas, L., Copplestone, C., Wall, R., Porter, J., & Rose, K. (1999). Nursing workload associated with adverse events in the postanesthesia care unit. *Anaesthesiology, 91,* 1882–1890.

Connor, R. J. (1961). A work sampling study of variations in nursing work load. *Hospitals, 35,* 40–41.

Curtin, L. L. (1995). Nursing productivity from data to definition. *Nursing Management, 26,* 25, 28–29, 32–36.

Dean, E., & Harper, M. (1998). The BLS Productivity Measurement Program. Bureau of Labor Statistics presentation at the Conference on Research in Income and Wealth—New Directions in Productivity Analysis.

Dennis, L., Dunn, M., & Benson, G. (1980). *An empirical model for measuring nursing in acute care hospitals.* Chicago: Medicus Systems Corporation.

Donabedian, A. (1988). The quality of care: How can it be assessed? *Journal of the American Medical Association, 260,* 1743–8.

Eastaugh, S. R. (2002). Hospital nurse productivity. *Journal of Health Care Finance, 29*(1), 14–22.

Estabrooks, C. A., Lander, J., Norris, J., Boschma, G., Lau, F., Watt-Watson, J., et al. (2003). *The determinants of research utilization in an acute clinical setting.* Toronto, Canada: Nursing Effectiveness, Utilization and Outcomes Research Unit, University of Toronto. Manuscript in preparation.

Finkler, S. A., & Kovner, C. T. (2000). Determining health care costs and rates. In *Financial management for nurse managers and executives* (2nd ed., pp. 153–202). Philadelphia: W. B. Saunders.

Fortinsky, R. H., & Madigan, E. A. (1997). Home care resource consumption and patient outcomes: What are the relationships? *Home Health Care Services Quarterly, 16*(3), 55–73.

Griffith, J. R. (1995). *The well-managed healthcare organization* (3rd ed.). Ann Arbor, MI: AUPHA Press/Health Administration Press.

Haas, S. A. W. (1984). Sorting out nursing productivity. *Nursing Management, 15,* 37–40.

Halloran, E. (1985). Nursing workload, medical diagnosis related groups and nursing diagnosis. *Research in Nursing and Health, 8,* 421–433.

Helberg, J. L. (1993). Factors influencing home care nursing problems and nursing care. *Research in Nursing, 16,* 363–370.

Helt, E. H, & Jelinek, R. C. (1988). In the wake of cost cutting, nursing productivity and quality improve. *Nursing Management, 19*(6), 36–38.

Hernandez, C. A., & O' Brien-Pallas, L. L. (1996). Validity and reliability of nursing workload measurement systems: Strategies for nursing administrators. *Canadian Journal of Nursing Administration, 9*(4), 33–52.

Hilsenrath, P., Levey, S., & O'Neill, L. (1997). Management and economic perspectives on efficiency. *Best Practices and Benchmarking in Healthcare, 2,* 208–213.

Holcomb, B. R., Hoffart, N., & Fox, M. H. (2002). Defining and measuring nursing productivity: A concept analysis and pilot study. *Journal of Advanced Nursing, 38,* 378–386.

Irvine, D. M., Sidani, S., & McGillis Hall, L. (1998). Linking outcomes to nurses' roles in health care. *Nursing Economic$, 16,* 58–64.

Jelinek, R. (1967). A structural model for the patient care operation. *Health Services Research, (Fall-Winter),* 226–242.

Jelinek, R. C. (1969). An operational analysis of the patient care function. *Inquiry, 6*(2), 53–58.

Jelinek, R. C., & Dennis, L. C. (1976). *A review and evaluation of nursing productivity.* (DHEW Publication No. HRA 77-15). Bethesda, MD: U.S. Department of Health, Education, and Welfare.

Jelinek, R. C., Haussman, R. K. D., Hegyvary, S. T., & Newman, J. F. Jr. (1975). *A methodology for monitoring quality of nursing care* (DHEW Publication No. HRA 76-25). Bethesda, MD: U.S. Department of Health, Education, and Welfare.

Jordan, S. D. (1994). Nursing productivity in rural hospitals. *Nursing Management, 25,* 58–62.

Kovner, C., & Gergen, P. J. (1998). Nurse staffing levels and adverse events following surgery in U.S. hospitals. *Image: Journal of Nursing Scholarship, 30*(4), 315–321.

Lancaster, A. D. (1997). Consult stat: Understaffing can increase infection rates. *RN, 60*(10), 79.

Lengacher, C. A., Mabe, P. R., Heinemann, D., VanCott, M. L., Swymer, S., & Kent, K. (1996). Effects of the PIPC model on outcome measures of productivity and costs. *Nursing Economic$, 14,* 205–212, 238.

Marek, K. (1996). Nursing diagnoses and home care nursing utilization. *Public Health Nursing, 13,* 195–200.

Martin, K., & Scheet, N. (1992). The OMAHA system: Applications for community health nursing. Philadelphia: W.B. Saunders.

McConnell, C. R. (1986). *The Health Care Supervisor's Guide to Cost Control and Productivity Improvement.* Rockfield, MD: Aspen.

McGillis Hall, L. (2003). Nursing intellectual capital: A theoretical approach for analyzing nursing productivity. *Nursing Economic$, 21*(1), 14–19.

McGillis Hall, L., & O'Brien-Pallas, L. L. (2000). Redesigning nursing work in long-term care environments. *Nursing Economic$, 18*(2), 79–87.

Mion, L. C., McLaren, C. E., & Frengley, J. D. (1988). The impact of patients' severity of illness and age on nursing workload. *Nursing Management, 19*(12), 26–34.

Needleman, J., Buerhaus, P., Mattke, S., Stewart, M., & Zelevinsky, K. (2002). Nurse-staffing levels and the quality of care in hospitals. *New England Journal of Medicine, 346,* 1715–1722.

Nolan, M., Lundh, U., & Brown, J. (1999). Changing aspects of nurses' work environments: A comparison of perceptions in two hospitals in Sweden and the UK and implications for recruitment and retention of staff. *NT Research, 4*(3), 221–234.

O'Brien-Pallas, L. L., Cockerill, R., & Leatt, P. (1992). Different systems, different costs: An examination of the comparability of workload measurement systems. *Journal of Nursing Administration, 22*(12), 17–22.

O'Brien-Pallas, L. L., & Giovannetti, P. (1992). Nursing intensity. *Papers from the Nursing Minimum Data Set Conference,* 68–76.

O'Brien-Pallas, L. L., & Giovannetti, P. (1993). *Nursing case costing: Directions for the future.* Paper presented at the International Scientific Conference on Nursing Economics, May 13–14, 1993. Winnipeg, Canada.

O'Brien-Pallas, L., Giovannetti, P., Peereboom, E., & Marton, C. (1995). *Case costing and nursing workload: Past, present, and future.* Working Paper Series, 95-1. University of Toronto, Quality of Nursing Worklife Research Unit.

O'Brien-Pallas, L. L., Irvine, D., Peereboom, E., & Murray, M. (1997). Measuring nursing workload: Understanding variability. *Nursing Economic$, 15,* 172–182.

O'Brien-Pallas, L. L., Irvine Doran, D., Murray, M., Cockerill, R., Sidani, S., Laurie-Shaw, B., et al. (2001). Evaluation of a client care delivery model, Part 1: Variability in nursing utilization in community home nursing. *Nursing Economic$, 19*(6), 267–276.

O'Brien-Pallas, L., Irvine Doran, D., Murray, M., Cockerill, R., Sidani, S., Laurie-Shaw, B., et al (2002). Evaluation of a client care delivery model, Part 2: Variability in client outcomes in community home nursing. *Nursing Economic$, 20,* 13–36.

O'Brien-Pallas, L. L., Leatt, P., Deber, R., & Till, J. (1989). A comparison of workload estimates using three methods of patient classification. *Canadian Journal of Nursing Administration, 2*(3), 16–23.

O'Brien-Pallas, L., Murray, M., Irvine, D., Cockerill, R., Sidani, S., Laurie-Shaw, B., et al. (1998). *Factors that influence variability in nursing workload and outcomes of care in community nursing.* Working Paper 98-1. Hamilton, Canada: Nursing Effectiveness, Utilization, and Outcomes Research Unit.

O'Brien-Pallas, L., Thomson, D., Alksnis, C., Baumann, A. O., Luba, M., Pagniello, A., et al. (2003). Health human resources: An analysis of nursing personnel in Ontario. Toronto, Canada: Nursing Effectiveness, Utilization and Outcomes Research Unit, University of Toronto. Manuscript in preparation.

O'Brien-Pallas, L. L., Thomson, D., Alksnis, C., & Bruce, S. (2001). The economic impact of nurse staffing decisions: Time to turn down another road. *Hospital Quarterly, 4*(3), 42–50.

O'Brien-Pallas, L., Thomson, D., McGillis Hall, L., Pink, G., Kerr, M., Wang, S. (2003). *Evidence based standards for measuring nurse staffing and performance* (Project RC1-0621-06). Final report submitted to the Canadian Health Services Research Foundation, Ottawa, Ontario.

Omachonu, V. K., & Nanda, R. (1989). Measuring productivity: Outcome vs. output. *Nursing Management, 20*(4), 35–38, 40.

Payne, S. M., Thomas, C. P., Fitzpatrick, T., Abdel-Rahman, M., & Kayne, H. L. (1998). Determinants of home health visit length: Results of a multisite prospective study. *Medical Care, 36*(10), 1500–1514.

Phillips, C. Y., Castorr, A., Prescott, P. A., & Soeken, K. (1992). Nursing intensity: Going beyond patient classification. *Journal of Nursing Administration, 22*(4), 46–52.

Prescott, P. A. (1986). DRG prospective reimbursement: The nursing intensity factor. *Nursing Management, 17*(1), 43–48.

Prescott, P. A., & Phillips, C. Y. (1988). Gauging nursing intensity to bring costs to light. *Nursing & Health Care, 9*(1), 17–22.

Prescott, P. A., Phillips, C. Y., Ryan, J. W., & Thompson, K. O. (1991). Changing how nurses spend their time. *Image: Journal of Nursing Scholarship, 23*(1), 23–28.

Prescott, P. A., Ryan, J. W., Soeken, K. L., Castorr, A. H., Thompson, K. O., & Phillips, C. Y. (1991). The patient intensity for nursing index: A validity assessment. *Research in Nursing & Health, 14,* 213–221.

Prescott, P. A., Soeken K. L., & Ryan, J. W. (1989). Measuring patient intensity: A reliability study. *Evaluation & the Health Professions, 12,* 255–69.

PRN 87. (1987). PRN 87: The measurement of the level of nursing care required. Montreal, Canada: Département d'administration de la santé, Faculté de médecine, Université de Montréal.

Rohrer, J. E., Momany, E. T., & Chang, W. (1993). Organizational predictors of outcomes of long-stay nursing home residents. *Social Science & Medicine, 37,* 549–54.

Ruch, W. A. (1982). The measurement of white collar productivity. *National Productivity Review, Autumn, 1,* 416–426.

Saulnier, F. F., Hubert, H., Onimus, T. M., Beague, S., Nseir, S., Grandbastien, B. et al. (2001). Assessing excess nurse work load generated by multiresistant nosocomial bacteria in intensive care. *Infection Control and Hospital Epidemiology, 22*(5), 273–278.

Scheffler, R. M., Waitzman, N. J., & Hillman, J. M. (1996). The productivity of physician assistants and nurse practitioners and health work force policy in the era of managed care. *Journal of Allied Health, 25,* 207–217.

Shamian, J., Hagen, B., Hu, T-W., & Fogarty, T. (1992). Nursing resource requirement and support services. *Nursing Economic$, 10,* 110–115.

Shamian, J., O'Brien-Pallas, L., Kerr, M., Koehoorn, M., Thomson, D., & Alksnis, A. (2001). Effects of job strain, hospital organizational factors and individual characteristics on work-related disability among nurses. Toronto, Canada: Workplace Safety and Insurance Board.

Shindul-Rothschild, J., & Duffy, M. (1996). The impact of restructuring and work design on nursing practice and patient care. *Best Practices and Benchmarking in Healthcare: A Practical Journal for Clinical and Management Applications, 1*(6), 271–282.

Shukla, R. K. (1990). Effect of an admission monitoring and scheduling system on productivity and employee satisfaction. *Hospital & Health Services Administration, 35*(3), 429–441.

Shullanberger, G. (2000). Nurse staffing decisions: An integrative review of the literature. *Nursing Economic$, 18*(3), 124–132, 146–148.

Sovie, M. D., & Jawad, A. F. (2001). Hospital restructuring and its impact on outcomes: Nursing staff regulations are premature. *Journal of Nursing Administration, 31*(12), 588–600.

Tarnow-Mordi, W. O., Hau, C., Warden, A., & Shearer, A. J. (2000). Hospital mortality in relation to staff workload: A 4-year study in an adult intensive-care unit. *The Lancet, 356,* 185–189.

Thibault, C., David, N., O'Brien-Pallas, L. L., & Vinet, A. (1990). *Workload measurement systems in nursing.* Montreal, Canada: Quebec Hospital Association.

Thomson, D. (2003). Untitled. Unpublished doctoral thesis proposal, University of Toronto, Canada.

Thompson, J. D., & Diers, D. (1988). Management of nursing intensity. *Nursing Clinics of North America, 23*(3), 473–492.

Tilquin, C., Carle, J., Saulnier, D., & Lambert, P. (1981). *PRN 80. Measuring the level of nursing care required.* Montreal, Canada: Equipe de Recherche Operationnelle en Santé, Institut National de Systématique Appliquée, & Department of Health Administration, Université de Montréal.

Tummers, G. E., Landeweerd, J. A., & van Merode, G. G. (2002). Organization, work and work reactions: A study of the relationships between organizational aspects of nursing and nurses' work characteristics and work reactions. *Scandinavian Journal of Caring Science, 16*, 52–58.

Ware, J. E., Snow, K. K., Kosinski, M., & Gandek, B. (1993). *SF-36 Health Survey. Manual and Interpretation Guide.* Boston: The Health Institute, New England Medical Center.

White, J. P. (1997). Health care, hospitals, and reengineering: The nightingales sing the blues. In A. Duffy, D. Glenday, & N. Pupo (Eds.), *Good jobs, bad jobs, no jobs: The transformation of work in the 21st century.* Toronto, Canada: Harcourt & Brace.

Williams, B. C., Phillips, E., Torner, J. C., & Irvine, A. A. (1990). Predicting utilization of home health resources: Important data from routinely collected information. *Medical Care, 28* (5), 379–391.

Young, S. W., Daehn, L. M., & Busch, C. M. (1990). Managing nursing staff productivity through reallocation of nursing resources. *Nursing Administration Quarterly, 14*(3), 24–30.

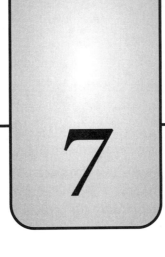

7

Autonomy and Decision-Making in Nursing

Joan Tranmer

7.1 Introduction

Although the importance of professional nurse autonomy is extensively addressed in the literature as a key indicator of quality work environments, definition, measurement, and interpretation of research findings have complicated the effective integration and promotion of this key indicator into nursing work environments.

In this chapter:

- The concept of professional nurse autonomy is examined.

- A conceptual definition of professional nurse autonomy is proposed.

- The empirical evidence linking professional nurse autonomy to quality work environments and to patient outcomes is critically examined.

- The measurement tools and methods are reviewed in regard to their psychometric soundness (i.e., reliability, validity, and sensitivity) and their appropriateness as a measure for professional nurse autonomy.

- Recommendations are proposed based on the strength and availability of the evidence concerning the relationship between professional nurse autonomy and nursing and patient outcomes, and approaches to measurement.

- Conclusions and future directions are suggested.

A detailed literature review identified articles or references that included the theoretical construct of autonomy or a discussion or presentation of the conceptual underpinnings of autonomy—definitions and domains, characteristics and attributes, impact, and outcomes. A second review identified articles that reported assessment of the psychometric measurement of autonomy, descriptive correlational or experimental studies, or evaluation of interventions to enhance professional autonomy. The search yielded a large number of references, of which 65 met the criteria for inclusion in this chapter. Only literature published within the past 10 years, unless a seminal work, was included.

7.2 Definition of Professional Nurse Autonomy

The concept of professional nurse autonomy has been visible and replete in the nursing literature for many years. Maas and Jacox (1977), in their seminal work, solicited from nurses their definition and meaning of professional autonomy and laid the groundwork for defining the importance between autonomous nursing practice and patient welfare. The prevailing assumption and belief is that autonomous practice is desired and of benefit to nurses, patients, employers, and the discipline. Despite this longstanding belief, autonomy has been poorly defined, operationalized, and measured.

Autonomy is a complex, multidimensional phenomenon, an interactive, relational process that occurs within the context of one's being and work. Wade (1999), in her concept analysis of professional nurse autonomy, distinguished between: (a) structural and work autonomy as the worker's freedom to make decisions based upon job requirements; (b) attitudinal autonomy as the belief in one's freedom to exercise judgment in decision-making; and (c) aggregate autonomy, which encompasses attitudinal and structural dimensions, the socially and legally granted freedom of self-governance and control of the profession without influence from external sources. Wade defined professional nurse autonomy as a "belief in the centrality of the client when making responsible decisions both independently and interdependently, that reflect advocacy for the client" (p. 3). This definition builds upon historical definitions in which autonomy was defined as the freedom to make decisions consistent with one's scope of practice and the evolving trend of shared control and interdependence in health care freedom to act upon these decisions (Batey & Lewis, 1982); the practice of one's occupation in accordance with one's education with members of that occupation governing, defining, and controlling their own activities in the absence of external controls (Schutzenhofer, 1987).

There are two basic dimensions of nurses' work autonomy: organizational and clinical practice (Keenan, 1999; Scott, Sochalski, & Aiken, 1999). Organizational autonomy refers to the capacity of nurses to be involved as participants in the decision-making process that guides the work of their unit or organization. Clinical practice autonomy occurs within the scope and milieu of clinical practice. Autonomy does not imply independence (Mitchinson, 1996). Professional nurse autonomy implies the right to exercise clinical and organizational judgment within the context of an interdependent health care team and in accordance with the socially and legally granted freedom of the discipline (MacDonald, 2002). The outcome of autonomy is accountable practice and practice decisions (Holden, 1991), and ultimately, improved patient care and nursing work.

7.3 Theoretical Underpinnings of Autonomy

Autonomy has been explored from a philosophical, moral, ethical, social, and feminist perspective (Ballou, 1998; Batey & Lewis, 1982; de Casterle, Roelens, & Gastmans, 1998; Keenan, 1999; MacDonald, 2002; Mundinger, 1980; Scott, 1998; Wilkinson, 1997). Ballou identified several recurring themes in her conceptual analysis of autonomy. These were themes related to self-governance within a system of principles, competence or capacity, decision-making, critical reflection, freedom, and self-control (Ballou). Autonomy is contingent upon personal factors:

- Inherent intellectual capacity
- Morality
- Exposure to a system of beliefs, laws, standards and principles
- Knowledge sufficient to develop competence
- Knowledge of personal values and beliefs
- Ability to reason
- Ability to control self

Critical attributes of autonomy include:

- Professional knowledge and skill

- Defined area of practice

- Desire for autonomy

- Responsibility and authority to make decisions based on professional knowledge and skill and the ability to execute these in practice

- An environment that supports professional nursing practice and respects nurses' individual and collective right to challenge circumstances and decisions (Batey & Lewis; Wilkinson)

7.4 Factors that Influence Nurse Autonomy

7.4.1 Personal versus Professional Autonomy

Autonomy is a multidimensional concept with many layers of interaction. There is a continuous interdependent interaction between personal and professional autonomy, which at times presents challenges for nurses and employers (Kennerly, 2000). For example, nurses who have lower personal and professional autonomy needs may work best and feel more satisfied when they have concrete direction from other professionals and work within practice models, such as case management models, that allow for interprofessional direction. Nurses with higher autonomy needs may be more productive in practice models where direction is less (Dwyer, Schwartz, & Fox, 1992). Variation in levels of personal and professional autonomy should be expected and supported. However, clarity of roles and expectations with respect to levels of autonomous decision-making is essential when establishing the domains of nursing responsibility. This particularly applies to nursing where diverse preparation, education, and orientation, along with increasing complexity of the work environment present unique challenges. Nurses have the authority to provide care within their scope of practice in accordance with their professional standards. Thus, in order to provide competent care they must possess the required levels of personal and professional autonomy to ensure competent decision-making and behaviors (College of Nurses of Ontario, 2003).

7.4.2 Education, Professional Development, and Professional Autonomy

It is unclear whether advanced education and positions enhance autonomy or if autonomous nurses seek higher levels of education and more decisional responsibility (Schutzenhofer & Musser, 1994). Basic and graduate educational curriculums should increase students' knowledge, understanding, and skill of autonomous practices, particularly decision-making processes, and foster inquiry (Wade, 1999). Clearly, nursing work environments that support and reward lifelong learning are more likely to have more autonomous nurses. Nursing work environments must promote and encourage the development of nursing autonomy, especially within the context of the therapeutic nurse–patient relationship. Factors such as the rules and policies of the organization, the expectations of other health professionals and coworkers, and the expectations of patients and family, influence and provide the context for the development of autonomous nursing practice (de Casterle et al., 1998; Singleton & Nail, 1984). The attainment of clinical autonomy, regardless of nursing position or scope, should be a priority. Decentralization, increasing educational level or knowledge capacity, role modeling, role taking, peer review, and peer consultation foster clinical autonomy. Kramer and Schmalenberg (1988a) stated that nurses at all levels need to learn to tolerate more uncertainty and chaos and to work with nonstandardization even when the regulations and demands of external agencies become more prevalent and demanding. Learning about and continual development of the knowledge and skill related to autonomous nursing practice should position nurses well to meet these challenges.

7.4.3 Critical Reflection and Decision-Making

Autonomous decision-making occurs when nurses deliberatively and critically analyze a practice or organizational issue, and when nurses make a judgment about plans of action and ensure the plans are carried out as planned (Erlen & Sereika, 1997). A comprehensive knowledge base and critical thinking is integral to decision-making and includes activities such as the organization of necessary background and assessment information and the recognition of patterns and evidence to support analysis and conclusions. Teamwork and autonomous decision-making are synergistic to each other (Rafferty, Ball, & Aiken, 2001). Decision-making is facilitated with decentralization of control and nonhierarchical organizational structures that support nurses to think and act (Kramer & Schmalenberg, 1988a, 1988b; Ritter-Teitel, 2002). Staff nurses desire individual authority and accountability for patient care decisions, whereas for unit-based decisions, group participation is preferred (Blegen et al., 1993). Nursing experience along with experiential knowledge enhances confidence and the individualization of decision-making for patients as previous patient experiences can be applied in subsequent patient care situations (Radwin, 1998). Autonomous decision-making is the capacity and the freedom to make sound decisions consistent with one's scope of practice and professional standards.

7.4.4 Professional Practice Environments

The importance of the professional practice environment to autonomous practice cannot be overstated. Practice models provide an organizing framework for the creation of structure and processes to facilitate autonomous practice and decision-making at patient and unit-levels. In fact, Porter-O'Grady (1996) postulated that 90% of the decisions of an organization should be made by staff if their work outcomes are ever to be sustained. Staff have the right and the obligation to make decisions that affect what they do and how they do it. Practice models should be accountability- and community-focused. They should provide the framework to support professional development from novice to expert and to help sustain and develop professional practice. Traditional systems- and department-oriented structures support a provider-focused orientation and do not support the development of point-of-care-focused roles and functions (Comack, Brady, & Porter-O'Grady, 1997; Wolf, Boland, & Aukerman, 1994). An effective professional practice environment that supports autonomous practice increases nurses' job satisfaction (Upenieks, 2000, 2002, 2003a).

7.4.5 Job Satisfaction

Much has been written about the positive relationship between nurse autonomy and job satisfaction and retention, particularly in the early 1980s, and more recently in the early 2000s (Blanchfield & Biordi, 1996; Mark, Salyer, & Wan, 2003; McCloskey, 1990; Mrayyan, 2003; O'Brien-Pallas, Thomson, Alksnis, & Bruce, 2001; Scott et al., 1999). The cyclic reemergence of job satisfaction and nurse autonomy in the literature has paralleled changes in health care systems and nursing shortages. In the early 1990s, there was ongoing restructuring and redesign of hospital settings that led to less integration among nurses, competitiveness for scarce jobs, dissipated professional leadership, uncertainty, unfamiliar work environments, and deskilling—all changes that contributed to less autonomy in the workplace and increased job dissatisfaction (Blythe, Baumann, & Giovannetti, 2001). Efforts to enhance job satisfaction, and corollary nurse retention and recruitment, have looked carefully at the magnet hospital research. This research has clearly shown that autonomy and staff involvement in decision-making were significant predictors of job satisfaction (Laschinger, Finegan, Shamian, & Almost, 2001; Scott et al., 1999). Optimum employee autonomy along with the existence of firm central direction, an attribute labeled "simultaneous loose–tight property" has allowed nurses to have full command of expert knowledge and control over decision-making within the context of shared key values (Kramer & Schmalenberg, 1988a, 1988b) and contributes to quality health care environments. As a large cohort of the nursing workforce reaches retirement age and the younger generation of baccalaureate-prepared nurses enters employment, job satisfaction and work autonomy will become major workplace issues.

7.5 Linking Nurse Autonomy to Outcome Achievement

Twenty studies were identified and reviewed. All of these studies empirically measured aspects of nurse autonomy.

No empirical studies were found that examined primarily the relationships between nurse autonomy and patient outcomes. However, magnet hospital research, in which autonomous practice is alluded to, has explored the effect of nurse staffing, nursing work, and nurse satisfaction on patient outcomes including mortality (Aiken, Clarke, & Sloane, 2002; Aiken, Clarke, Sloane, & Sochalski, 2001; Aiken, Clarke, Sloane, Sochalski, & Silber, 2002). Doran, Sidani, Keatings, and Doidge (2002) examined the impact of role performance including job autonomy on selected patient outcomes for medical-surgical patients. Using a cross sectional design, a total of 372 patients self-reported on their perception of the quality of nursing care, self-care ability, functional status, and mood at time of discharge; 254 nurses from 26 general medical-surgical units rated the quality of nurse communication and coordination of care, adequacy of time to provide care, role tension, and autonomy. Job autonomy, measured with the Hackman and Oldhan's Job Diagnostic Survey (Hackman & Oldham, 1980) was positively associated with quality of nurse communication and negatively associated with coordination of care and the quality of nurses' independent role performance. There was no direct association between autonomy and patient outcomes, supporting the investigators' hypothesis that the effect of autonomy is mediated by the nurses' role performance. The findings from this study are important, especially for future research, as they provide beginning empirical evidence for an organizing framework for the study of nurse autonomy on patient outcomes. The majority of the studies reviewed focused on individual or organizational factors related to the development of professional nurse autonomy.

7.5.1 Nurse Autonomy

One of the first known studies of nurse autonomy found that higher autonomy scores were associated with education, leadership, academic setting, and nontraditional social climates (Pankratz & Pankratz, 1974). Fifteen years later, when 368 registered nurses (RNs) in a 520-bed hospital completed the same Nursing Autonomy/Patients Rights Questionnaire, perceptions of autonomy remained relatively similar (Collins & Henderson, 1991). Respondents ($n = 208$, 56.5%) reported that they were expected to practice autonomously, but the majority felt little support to do so in their hospital work environment. Nurses who scored highest on the autonomy scale were more likely to be female with postgraduate education and in an administrative role or a specialty clinical area (e.g., emergency). Other studies have shown similar relationships between personal and professional variables and autonomy (Schutzenhofer & Musser, 1994; Weisman,

Alexander, & Chase, 1980). In a large survey of 2,000 RNs from four states in the United States, respondents ($n = 542$, 27.1%) completed a questionnaire containing the Nursing Activity Scale (NAS; Schutzenhofer, 1987) and a measure of personal attributes and other demographic information (Schutzenhofer & Musser). Significant relationships were noted among autonomy and nursing education, practice setting, clinical specialty, functional role, membership in professional organizations, and gender stereotyped personality traits. Public health nurses reported higher levels of autonomy than hospital-based nurses, with no significant differences between type of hospital or type of nursing model (i.e., primary care, team, or functional) noted. Nurses who identified themselves as clinical specialists or practitioners reported higher autonomy than nurse managers and staff nurses. Membership in a professional organization and male personality traits were positively correlated with autonomy.

Blegen et al. (1993) explored the preferences for decision-making between staff nurses ($n = 356$) and head nurses ($n = 130$) from 16 hospitals. Staff nurses, in general, preferred independent decision-making for patient care decisions and shared decision-making for unit operations. Nursing managers indicated that staff nurses should have a higher level of autonomy than the staff nurses indicated for themselves. Differences existed between staff nurses' and nurse leaders' desired level of authority and autonomy for more than half of the decisions, suggesting there is a need to ensure a better fit between desired and actual level of decisional involvement.

The links between authority and autonomy and the importance of both adds complexity to the measurement of autonomy. Blanchfield and Biordi (1996) distributed a questionnaire containing the Nursing Authority and Autonomy Scale (NAAS), a scale designed specifically for this study, to 1,048 nurses from four Midwestern hospitals. The purpose of the study was to determine the level of agreement between staff nurses and nurse leaders about desired and importance of autonomy to deliver patient care. Significant and moderately positive correlations were found between authority and autonomy. Nurses correlated authority with autonomy and highly valued both. Staff nurses reported a significantly higher perception of autonomy to enact patient care in comparison to the nurse leaders, indicating a potential area for conflict. Nurse leaders who worked nights and staff nurses from specialized units and smaller hospitals reported higher levels of authority and work autonomy in comparison to nurses from larger hospitals or more general units. It would seem that the bureaucratic management structures created in larger hospitals or during the regular business day hours undermine nurses' authority and autonomy. The ability to practice autonomously should not change from shift to shift. Schutzenhofer and Musser (1994) recommended collaboration between nurse leaders and staff nurses to ensure autonomy and authority, "Without authority, autonomy is lacking a vital element of empowerment: sanctioned power" (p. 48).

Foley, Kee, Minick, Harvey, and Jennings (2002) explored the differences between autonomy, control over practice, and nurse–physician collaboration between civilian and military nurses who worked in two military hospitals. Military RNs in comparison to civilian RNs were likely to be male, educated at the baccalaureate level, younger, and more apt to be European American. Scores on autonomy, control over practice, and nurse–physician relationships were indicative of positive work environments in both military hospitals. The status of nurses in military hospitals, the high proportion of male nurses, and the high education level of military nurses seemed to contribute to an environment that promoted high job satisfaction and collegial relationships. It was suggested that the more homogeneous military culture and the high visibility and rank of nursing within the hospital promoted autonomy—factors that perhaps civilian hospitals should consider.

An international study of 225 registered nurses in a general hospital in New Zealand examined the effect of the work environment (i.e., autonomy, control, and nurse–physician relationships) on the health status of nurses (Budge, Carryer, & Wood, 2003). Less autonomy and control and better nurse–physician relations were reported in the New Zealand hospital in comparison to similar hospitals in the United States. Of importance were the findings that quality-of-life scores for nurses were on the average lower than those of comparable national groups. Lower quality-of-life was associated with lower scores in the three workplace attributes studied. A workplace composed of workers reporting low levels of physical and emotional well-being should be a major concern for organizations, especially in relation to the aging nursing workforce, and the impact and costs associated with high levels of sick time.

Finally, when examining the development of professional autonomy, consideration needs to be given to the level of autonomy on entry into the profession. Boughn (1992) compared levels of individual autonomy in nursing students to women students in other traditional female occupations (e.g., education) and nontraditional occupations (e.g., business, technology, and arts and sciences). Scores on autonomy were not different between graduating nursing students and women students in other disciplines. However, nursing students scored significantly higher on questions concerning advocacy and activism, specifically as it related to patients' rights to be informed to choose and to refuse treatments. Nursing students were more inclined to correct injustices and to fight for employment rights. Nursing students, in this study, possessed individual autonomy, implying that poor development of professional autonomy is likely related to the work environments and organizations in which nurses work.

Professional autonomy builds upon individual autonomy. In an earlier study, Pinch (1985) explored decision-making and attitudes toward professional autonomy in freshman students ($n = 109$), senior students ($n = 103$) and graduates ($n = 84$). Participants completed a three-part questionnaire containing: (a) situation specific case studies that explored types of nurse–patient relationship models, risk taking, perceived work restrictions, and perceived anxiety; (b) a shortened form of the Pankratz Nursing Autonomy and Patients' Rights Scale (Pankratz & Pankratz, 1974); and (c) a section on demographics. Freshman nursing students were less likely to take risks and to select the patient advocate model as their choice of interaction, and they perceived higher levels of work restriction and anxiety in relation to the specific dilemmas. Freshman students reported lower levels of nurse autonomy, promotion of patients' rights and rejection of the traditional nursing role in comparison to seniors and graduates. These results suggest that educational processes impact the development of autonomy, and graduate nurses enter the work setting with relatively high levels of professional autonomy, at least when faced with theoretical, ethical, or work dilemmas. Further exploration of the development of professional autonomy within the context of real clinical dilemmas is warranted.

7.5.2 *Autonomy and Organizational Attributes*

Studies have revealed a positive relationship between workplace attributes and autonomy. Upenieks (2002) surveyed 700 clinical nurses at designated magnet and nonmagnet hospitals, along with 16 nurse leaders from the same hospitals, to determine if there was a difference in job satisfaction among clinical nurses employed in diverse hospital settings. Magnet hospital work satisfaction scores, as measured with the Revised Nurses Work Index (NWI-R; Kramer & Hafner, 1989), were higher than those reported by nurses employed at nonmagnet hospitals. Nurses in magnet hospitals reported better physician–nurse relationships and greater autonomy and control over practice. Nurse leaders in magnet hospitals reported that clinical nurses were the most essential component of a successful professional organization and reflected this belief in their actions, such as assurance of adequate staffing levels. Nurse leaders were able to articulate and reinforce the importance of autonomy and accountability for nurses' clinical practice. Differences in autonomy scores were potentially linked to the different professional practice environments—the magnet environment that supported risk and assumption of responsibility and the nonmagnet environment that tended to use a more top-down style of management (Upenieks).

It was somewhat surprising, then, to find that when Kramer and Schmalenberg (2003) interviewed 20 staff nurses from 14 magnet hospitals they found that 26% of nurses working in these hospitals reported situations of unsupported or no autonomy. Poor levels of autonomy were reported in hospitals where the nurses felt they were no longer magnet hospitals. Autonomy was negatively affected by mergers and changes, poor relationships with the physicians, and no control over practice. Staff nurses perceived clinical autonomy to be an action beyond the usual standard of practice and felt that nurse leaders needed to support and reward their clinical autonomy.

Autonomy has been explored within the context of different types of nursing professional practice models. Rafferty et al. (2001) surveyed 10,022 staff nurses in 32 hospitals in England to explore the relationship between interdisciplinary teamwork and nurse autonomy on hospital care. Nurse autonomy was positively correlated with better perceptions of quality of care and higher job satisfaction. Nurses with higher teamwork scores reported higher levels of autonomy and more involvement in decision-making; a finding that suggests autonomy and teamwork are synergistic and not in conflict with one another. Kangas, Kee, and McKee-Waddle (1999) surveyed 92 nurses in three different hospitals representing three different nursing care delivery models (i.e., team, case management, and primary) to identify differences and relationships among nurse job satisfaction, patient satisfaction, nursing care delivery models, and organizational attributes. The type of nursing care delivery model had no impact on levels of nursing job satisfaction. Perceiving the environment as supportive and working in a critical care environment were significant predictors of nurses' job satisfaction (i.e., autonomy) scores (Kangas et al.).

In a quasi-experimental study, Kennerly (2000) conducted a before and after evaluation of a shared governance implementation. Nurse and nonnurse perceptions of their work and work environment were examined at 6, 18, and 36 months. Job satisfaction, role conflict, and peer leadership emerged as the best predictors of worker perceptions of autonomy on units implementing shared governance. Kennerly reported that fluctuations across time in worker perceptions of autonomy were unexpected and of significance. Workers perceived moderate to high levels of autonomy prior to implementation of shared governance with levels increasing slightly 6 months post implementation and returning to preproject levels by 18 months. The author suggested that moderate to high levels of autonomy may be a prerequisite for effective implementation of professional practice models such as shared governance, and not an outcome.

Nursing leadership is an influential workplace attribute. Ferguson-Paré (1998) conducted a triangulated ethnographic study using a quantitative survey to describe nurses' perceptions of leadership attributes and autonomy. Twelve patient-care managers formed the sample for the ethnographic study. The findings showed that nursing managers most successful in promoting autonomous professional practice of registered nurses in a team-based environment provided necessary structures to assure the achievement of quality and the maintenance of standards. They provided policy and individual direction of staff where needed, and did so in a supportive manner. They focused on building and recognizing strengths and commitment of staff. Recruitment and development of managers in nursing who exhibit these human, professional, and leadership qualities will contribute to the supports necessary to provide autonomous professional practice of nurses (Ferguson-Paré).

McCloskey (1990) explored the links between autonomy and social integration for newly employed nurses who joined a large Midwestern hospital. Nurses ($n = 150$) completed questionnaires during the first month of employment, at the end of approximately 6 months, and after a year of employment. This study found that autonomy and social integration are important job concepts for nurses. When both autonomy and social integration were perceived to be low, nurses reported low job satisfaction and work motivation, poor commitment to the organization, and less intent to stay on the job. Higher levels of social integration seemed to buffer the bad effects of lower autonomy. Nurses with the lowest autonomy and social integration scores were more likely to be from medical units, in comparison to intensive care or obstetrical units. Nurses seem to desire autonomy and feelings of connectedness (McCloskey).

7.5.3 Summary

In summary, much of the empirical work has defined the important relational and contextual factors for nurse autonomy. In several of the studies, nurses or nursing students have completed questionnaires designed specifically to measure nurses' or nursing students' autonomy. These instruments included the Pankratz and Pankratz Nursing Autonomy Scale (Pankratz & Pankratz, 1974; Pinch, 1985), the Nursing Authority and Autonomy Scale (Blanchfield & Biordi, 1996), the Kurtines' Autonomy Scale (Boughn, 1992, 1995), the Nursing Activity Scale (Blegen et al., 1993; Schutzenhofer, 1987; Schutzenhofer & Musser, 1994), and a ranked category scale (Kramer & Schmalenberg, 2003). Other studies used questionnaires that included measures of autonomy in subscales or specific questions. These instruments included the Nursing Workload Index (Rafferty et al., 2001), the Revised Nursing Work Index (NWI-R); Aiken, Clarke, & Sloane, 2002; Aiken et al., 2001; Aiken, Clarke, Sloane, Sochalski, et al., 2002; Aiken, Havens, & Sloane, 2000; Budge et al., 2003; Foley et al., 2002; Upenieks, 2000, 2002, 2003a), the Job Diagnostic Survey (Doran et al., 2002), the Nursing Job Satisfaction Scale (Kangas et al., 1999), the Job Characteristics Inventory (McCloskey, 1990), and specially designed instruments for individual studies (Kennerly, 2000). Manojlovich and Spence Laschinger (2002) looked at autonomy as a component of psychological empowerment and used Spreitzer's Psychological Empowerment Tool in which autonomy was one of four attributes measured. Most of the studies were targeted at nurses working in hospital environments including general and specialized units. A number of studies were conducted with staff from hospitals designated as magnet hospitals. Sample sizes ranged from 185 to more than 10,000. Where reported, response rates were varied and ranged from a low of 27.1% (Schutzenhofer & Musser) to a high of 86% (Aiken & Patrician, 2000). On the whole, response rates were below 60% and some studies reported differences in response rates for staff nurses, managers, and patients.

7.6 Issues in the Assessment of Nurses' Autonomy

There are two major issues associated with the empirical assessment of autonomy: (a) lack of a standardized conceptualization of professional nurse autonomy, and (b) inability to isolate autonomy and autonomous behaviors from other influential and confounding personal and contextual factors.

7.6.1 Standardized Conceptualization of Professional Nurse Autonomy

Concepts such as control over work; control of nursing practice; and clinical, individual, practice, and professional autonomy have all been labeled *autonomy* and have been used interchangeably and measured with the same tools. Notwithstanding this confusion and lack of definitional precision, high levels of nurse autonomy have been reported in magnet hospitals, and autonomy is considered to be essential to the productivity of quality care and nurse job satisfaction (Kramer & Hafner, 1989; Kramer & Schmalenberg, 1988a, 1988b, 1993, 2003). If autonomy is a highly desirable behavior related to nurse effectiveness, job satisfaction, and retention, a clear and standardized concept is needed in order to develop tools to measure it and conduct research to identify the factors leading to and supporting it. Moreover, there is a need to clearly define autonomous behaviors that are measurable and of relevance to nursing practice and the care of patients.

7.6.2 Understanding Autonomy Within Personal and Organizational Contexts

Personal autonomy and work-related autonomy have been strongly related to professional nurse autonomy. Any direct relationship between these variables may have been obscured by the fact that individuals with high needs for achievement and autonomy tended to seek higher education and environments that were conducive to using their knowledge and skills. Autonomous nurses have been a positive attribute of quality work environments, and quality work environments support and develop autonomous nurses. Thus, it is difficult to isolate and measure autonomy when it is embedded within the being and work of nurses and measured as a component of larger measures of personal being or workplace attributes (i.e., job satisfaction and nursing work). No instruments directly assessed the nature and extent of autonomous clinical nursing patient care behaviors. Thus, it is difficult to determine the impact of nursing autonomy on patient outcomes.

7.7 Evidence Concerning Approaches to Measuring Nurses' Autonomy

The literature identified a number of scales, questionnaires, or measures that have attempted to quantify aspects of professional nurse autonomy. Many of the constructs and items on these scales may be of relevance in the measure of autonomy, but most require further testing and evaluation in both hospital and community settings to determine their validity and sensitivity for nursing work and patient outcomes. Eight measures of nursing autonomy were reviewed; six were reviewed in detail (see Table 7.1). Four measures of nurses' work that included a measure of autonomy were also reviewed with one reviewed in detail.

7.8 Nursing Measures of Autonomy

7.8.1 Nursing Authority and Autonomy Scale (NAAS)

The NAAS, is a three part instrument developed by Blanchfield and Biordi (1996). The first part consists of 28 items that measure nurses' perceptions of their authority and autonomy; the second part measures nurses' perceptions of the importance of their authority and autonomy; and the third part contains demographic information. The scale was derived from Katzman's Authority and Nursing Roles Instrument (Katzman, 1989) and the autonomy subscale of Stamps and Piedmonte's Job Satisfaction Index (Stamps, 1986). This instrument was used in one study to determine the extent of agreement between nurse managers and staff nurses with respect to staff nurses' authority and autonomy (Blanchfield & Biordi). This measure quantifies two important concepts: autonomy and authority.

7.8.2 Staff Nurse Autonomy Questionnaire

The Staff Nurse Autonomy Questionnaire consists of 42 decisions—21 patient care and 21 unit operations—developed by 15 nurse experts. It is derived from the experience of the team members, the nursing administration literature, and specific items included in the work of Schutzenhofer (1987) and Katzman (1989). Desired level of involvement in decision-making was determined for the 42 activities on a 5-point response level, ranging from 1 (assuming no authority and accountability) to 5 (having full authority and accountability). The questionnaire also asks respondents to indicate in general their current authority for patient care and unit decisions and the extent to which they desired more authority. This questionnaire was used in Blegen et al.'s (1993) study of 600 nurses from all general hospitals in one American state. This tool does not empirically quantify aspects of autonomy. It allows for categorization of levels of decision-making for patient care and unit operation activities.

7.8.3 Nursing Attitude Scale

Pankratz and Pankratz (1974) developed a 69-item questionnaire—27 items related to patient rights, 29 items related to nurse autonomy, and 13 items related to elements of both. The original measure was tested in a sample of 702 nurses and nurse administrators from a variety of hospital settings. Three subscales emerged:

Table 7.1 Nursing Measures of Autonomy

Instrument Author/Date of Publication	Target Population	Domains	Method of Administration	Reliability	Validity	Sensitivity to Nursing
Nursing Authority and Autonomy Scale (NAAS) (Blanchfield & Biordi, 1996)	Nurses.	Three-part instrument: first part (28 items) measured nurses' perceptions of staff nurses' authority; second part (10 items) measured nurses' perceptions of the importance of staff nurses' authority and autonomy; third section (12 items) asked demographic information.	Self-administered questionnaire.	Part 1: authority (α = .86); autonomy (α = .72) Part 2: importance of authority items (α = .84); importance of autonomy items (α = .78).	Content validity.	
Staff Nurse Autonomy Questionnaire (Blegen, et al., 1993)	Staff nurses in hospitals.	42-item; 5-point Likert scale; measures autonomy in patient care decisions and unit operations.	Self-administered questionnaire.		Questions were derived from nursing literature and specific items in Schutzenhofer (1987) and Katzman (1989).	
Autonomy: the Care Perspective (ACP) Instrument (Boughn, 1995)	Nursing students.	Designed specifically to measure the attitudes and behaviors of nursing students based on the caring perspective; 50 items designed to relate to four concepts: regard for self, regard for others, advocacy and activism for self, and activism for others.	Self-administered questionnaire.	Stability reliability (r = .90); internal consistency (α = .84).	Content validity index of .76; construct validity.	

α = Cronbach's alpha coefficient

154

Table 7.1 (continued)

Instrument Author/Date of Publication	Target Population	Domains	Method of Administration	Reliability	Validity	Sensitivity to Nursing
Authority in Nursing Roles Inventory (ANRI) (Katzman, 1989)	Registered nurses (RNs) and licensed practical nurses (LPNs) in any setting.	25-item scale asking about current and ideal conditions of autonomy or authority.	Self-administered questionnaire.	High rating on psychometric soundness (Huber et al., 2000).	High rating on psychometric soundness (Huber et al., 2000).	
Clinical Autonomy Ranked Category Scale (Kramer and Schmalenberg, 2003)	Registered nurses (RNs).	Five-category ranked scale: autonomous patient care action, autonomous nursing care action, limited autonomy, unsanctioned autonomy, no autonomous practice.	Qualitative interviews.	Scale requires more psychometric validation.	Scale requires more psychometric validation.	
Kurtines Autonomy Scale (Kurtines, 1978)	All workers.	Short, easy to administer scale based on the California Psychological Inventory (CPI).	Self-administered.	Several analyses conducted to determine reliability.	Content validity; construct validity.	
Maas and Jacox Semantic Differential (Maas, 1977)	Registered nurses (RNs).	Twenty bipolar adjectives with a 7-point Likert scale identifying the meaning of the concept of professional autonomy.	Self-administered questionnaire.			

α = Cronbach's alpha coefficient

Table 7.1 (continued)

Instrument Author/Date of Publication	Target Population	Domains	Method of Administration	Reliability	Validity	Sensitivity to Nursing
Maas and Jacox Concept interview (1977)	Registered nurses (RNs).	Eleven open-ended questions soliciting perceptions about the definition and meaning of professional autonomy in nursing.	Self-administered.			
Nursing Attitude Scale (PNAS) (Pankratz, 1974)	Measures autonomy of hospital nurses; used with student and community nurse populations.	69 items; three subscales: a) nurse autonomy and patient advocacy; b) patient's rights, and c) rejection of nurses' traditional role limitations.	Self-administered.		Content and construct validity questionable because the tool may be outdated (Wade, 1999).	
Nursing Activity Scale (NAS) (Schutzenhofer, 1987)	Registered nurses (RNs) in clinical settings; used to measure professional nursing practice autonomy.	30-item scale with five unscored items that serve to measure internal consistency; the items on the NAS describe clinical nursing situations, applicable to a variety of clinical specialties, in which a nurse must exercise some degree of professional nursing autonomy.	Self-administered questionnaire.	Published internal consistency reliability estimates were .91; ($r = .79$).	Content validity based on a review of current nursing literature and a survey of nursing leaders.	

α = Cronbach's alpha coefficient

nurse autonomy and advocacy, patients' rights, and rejection of traditional role limitations. This scale was more recently used by Collins and Henderson (1991) in their descriptive study of hospital nurses. They found that nursing autonomy had not substantially changed over the years. This scale has been criticized for its methodological weaknesses (Wade, 1999). Wade commented that the wording in the items is ambiguous and open to interpretation by the respondents and suggested that the content and construct validity of these instrument is questionable and dated.

7.8.4 Professional Nursing Autonomy Scale (PNAS)

The Professional Nursing Autonomy Scale (PNAS) is a 30-item scale developed from nursing literature and a survey of nursing deans, nursing directors of clinical services, and nursing specialists (Schutzenhofer, 1987). Items describe situations where nurses must act autonomously, for example, "refuse to administer a contraindicated drug despite the physician's insistence that the drug be given." Blegen et al. (1993) adapted this scale, as previously described, for use in their Staff Nurse Autonomy Questionnaire. Schutzenhofer and Musser (1994) later used this tool to measure the relationships between nurses' personal and professional characteristics and autonomy.

7.8.5 Autonomy, the Caring Perspective Instrument (ACP)

Autonomy, the Caring Perspective (ACP) Instrument was designed to measure autonomy-related attitudes and behaviors, specifically for nursing students (Boughn, 1992, 1995). Each of the 50 items relates to four concepts: regard for self, regard for others, advocacy and activism for self, and advocacy and activism for others. Items were designed to contrast respondents' attitudes and behaviors pertaining to self and with those pertaining to others, for example, "I would jeopardize my job for patients' rights." The reliability and validity of the ACP was tested over a 3-year period through application to a population of 400 students at various levels in a baccalaureate program. Seven factors were identified: regard for self, regard for women, regard for nurses, advocacy and activism for self, advocacy and activism for women, advocacy and activism for nurses, and advocacy and activism for patients. Stability reliability, internal consistency, and content and construct validity were established. The tool is an important measure of the socialization process—the development of self and patient, activism, and advocacy during nursing education.

7.8.6 Kurtines' Autonomy Scale

Kurtines' Autonomy Scale was developed within the framework of a multidimensional model of moral development (Kurtines, 1978). Content, criterion-related, and construct validity were determined in a sample of students and military officers. The purpose of the scale is to measure autonomous rule compliance as a dimension of moral conduct. Boughn (1992) used this tool to measure the characteristics of autonomy in female students enrolled in nursing, business, and arts programs.

7.9   General Measures that Include Autonomy

7.9.1 Revised Nursing Work Index (NWI-R)

The Revised Nursing Work Index (Aiken et al., 2000; Kramer & Hafner, 1989) is the instrument most commonly used to measure organizational attributes of professional practice environments and has been used extensively internationally, predominantly in the magnet hospital research (Aiken et al.; Rafferty et al., 2001; Upenieks, 2000, 2002, 2003a, 2003b). Nurses report on the presence or absence of factors that contribute to a professional practice environment. The original NWI was developed directly from the early research on magnet hospitals (Kramer & Hafner) in which nurses identified 65 traits as important to their satisfaction, useful to their ability to provide quality care, and present in their current work environment. The instrument was intended to measure individual values related to job satisfaction, ability to provide care, and the presence of professional organizational attributes. To better measure the characteristics of a unit or organization, the NWI was modified. Fifty-five of the original 65 items were retained. Three subscales were conceptually derived: autonomy, control over work environment, and relationships with physicians. The autonomy subscale contains five items: "A supervisory staff that is supportive of nurses"; "Nursing controls its own practice"; "Freedom to make important patient care and work decisions"; "Not being placed in a position of having to do things that are against my judgment"; and "A nursing manager backs up the nursing staff in decision-making even if there is conflict with a physician." Aiken and Patrician (2000) were able to demonstrate that nurse autonomy, as measured with the NWI-R significantly varied between magnet hospital units and nonmagnet hospital units, and specialized units and nonmagnet general units. The NWI-R is a promising tool to measure organizational attributes of a hospital–unit from the nurses' perspective; however, it is a relatively limited measure of professional nurse autonomy and autonomous behaviors that directly impact patient care.

7.9.2 Other Measures that Include Autonomy

Many nursing job satisfaction measures include a subscale of autonomy and the reader is referred to the chapter on Nurses' Job Satisfaction prepared by L. McGillis Hall in the *Nursing Sensitive Outcomes: State of the Science* book (McGillis Hall, 2003). Other scales that measure aspects of autonomy include: The Decisional Involvement Scale (DCI), formally the Distribution of Authority Scale; the Job Diagnostic Survey (JDS); and the Spreitzer Empowerment Scale.

7.10   Implications and Future Directions

The reviewed literature and studies suggest that nurses and nursing units who practice (i.e., think and act) autonomously should affect the quality of care and outcomes for patients. However, there is no empirical evidence to support this claim. As described in this chapter, most of the studies reviewed are descriptive examinations of the relationships between the concept and personal- or work-related characteristics of students and nurses. There are no rigorous trials that have specifically examined the impact of autonomous behaviors on patient outcomes. Despite this gap, there is an opportunity to build upon the detailed descriptive work completed and instruments developed to meet this gap.

There is a desperate need for a unifying concept and measure of the different aspects of professional nurse autonomy. There is sufficient evidence about the important personal, social, and workplace factors that are antecedents to and consequences of autonomy, and the instruments reviewed have addressed many of these factors. To build upon this important work, the future measures of autonomy need to be of relevance within the various domains in nursing (i.e., practice, leadership, and education) and across various roles. Autonomous practice needs to be explored within the context of the nurses' work environments. Professional nurse autonomy should be reflected in professional nursing behaviors and actions and tools developed to measure such. For example, a nurse who feels that professional autonomy has been attained should demonstrate behaviors that reflect sound knowledge, critical thinking, independent–interdependent provision of care, professional consultation, professional communication, patient activism and advocacy, and peer leadership in a self-directed, self-controlled and self-regulated manner. Nursing units or communities that function autonomously should demonstrate the same behaviors at the unit level. No measures have thoroughly assessed nurse autonomous behaviors or actions in relation to nurses' work, and thus, there has been little, if any, assessment of autonomous nursing practice on important patient outcomes.

Based on the instruments reviewed, the NWI-R (Aiken et al., 2000) along with the ranking of the autonomous clinical behavior scale tested by Kramer and Schmalenberg (2003) should be used and tested in future research studies. The NWI-R has demonstrated good psychometric properties in a number of studies and examines autonomy within the context of the work environment. The ranking scale requires further development and validation in other sites and settings, but this scale has the potential to specifically and empirically measure autonomous clinical practice behaviors.

Understanding and measuring professional nurse autonomy from an organizational perspective in relation to patient outcomes should be a priority research agenda. There is an urgent need to measure and define the characteristics of organizations (and units) that demonstrate autonomous nursing practice and the impact of autonomous nursing practice on patient outcomes. If we cannot design and test interventions through rigorously designed trials, then we are poorly positioned to recommend autonomous nursing practice as a standard of professional nursing care.

Acknowledgements:

The author of this chapter gratefully acknowledges the scholarly work of A. Heino and C. Bolton in the preparation of this chapter.

7.11   References

Aiken, L. H., Clarke, S. P., & Sloane, D. M. (2002). Hospital staffing, organization, and quality of care: Cross-national findings. *Nursing Outlook, 50,* 187–194.

Aiken, L. H., Clarke, S. P., Sloane, D. M., & Sochalski, J. (2001). Cause for concern: Nurses' reports of hospital care in five countries. *LDI Issue Brief, 6,* 1–4.

Aiken, L. H., Clarke, S. P., Sloane, D. M., Sochalski, J., & Silber, J. H. (2002). Hospital nurse staffing and patient mortality, nurse burnout, and job dissatisfaction. *Journal of American Medical Association, 288,* 1987–1993.

Aiken, L. H., Havens, D. S., & Sloane, D. M. (2000). The Magnet Nursing Services Recognition Program: A Comparison of Two Groups of Magnet Hospitals. *American Journal of Nursing, 100,* 26–36.

Aiken, L. H. & Patrician, P. A. (2000). Measuring organizational traits of hospitals: the Revised Nursing Work Index. *Nursing Research, 49,* 146–153.

Ballou, K. A. (1998). A concept analysis of autonomy. *Journal of Professional Nursing, 14,* 102–110.

Batey, M. V. & Lewis, F. M. (1982). Clarifying autonomy and accountability in nursing service, part 1. *Journal of Nursing Administration, 8,* 1213–1218.

Blanchfield, K. C. & Biordi, D. L. (1996). Power in practice: A study of nursing authority and autonomy. *Nursing Administration Quarterly, 20,* 42–49.

Blegen, M. A., Goode, C., Johnson, M., Maas, M., Chen, L., & Moorhead, S. (1993). Preferences for decision-making autonomy. *Image: the Journal of Nursing Scholarship, 25,* 339–344.

Blythe, J., Baumann, A., & Giovannetti, P. (2001). Health policy and systems. Nurses' experiences of restructuring in three Ontario hospitals. *Journal of Nursing Scholarship, 33,* 61–68.

Boughn, S. (1992). Nursing students rank high in autonomy at the exit level. *Journal of Nursing Education, 31,* 58–64.

Boughn, S. (1995). An instrument for measuring autonomy-related attitudes and behaviors in women nursing students. *Journal of Nursing Education, 34,* 106–113.

Budge, C., Carryer, J., & Wood, S. (2003). Health correlates of autonomy, control and professional relationships in the nursing work environment. *Journal of Advanced Nursing, 42,* 260–268.

College of Nurses of Ontario. (2003). *Entry to practice competencies: For Ontario registered nurses as of January 1, 2005.* Toronto, ON: College of Nurses of Ontario.

Collins, S. S., & Henderson, M. C. (1991). Autonomy: Part of the nursing role? *Nursing Forum, 26,* 23–29.

Comack, M., Brady, J., & Porter-O'Grady, T. (1997). Professional practice: A framework for transition to a new culture... Essential Elements Model. *Journal of Nursing Administration, 27,* 32–41.

de Casterle, B. D., Roelens, A., & Gastmans, C. (1998). An adjusted version of Kohlberg's moral theory: Discussion of its validity for research in nursing ethics. *Journal of Advanced Nursing, 27,* 829–835.

Doran, D. I., Sidani, S., Keatings, M., & Doidge, D. (2002). An empirical test of the Nursing Role Effectiveness Model. *Journal of Advanced Nursing, 38,* 29–39.

Dwyer, D. J., Schwartz, R. H., & Fox, M. L. (1992). Decision-making autonomy in nursing. *Journal of Nursing Administration, 22,* 17–23.

Erlen, J. A., & Sereika, S. M. (1997). Critical care nurses, ethical decision-making and stress. *Journal of Advanced Nursing, 26,* 953–961.

Ferguson-Paré, M. (1998). Nursing leadership and autonomous professional practice of registered nurses. *Canadian Journal of Nursing Administration, 11,* 7–30.

Foley, B. J., Kee, C. C., Minick, P., Harvey, S. S., & Jennings, B. M. (2002). Characteristics of nurses and hospital work environments that foster satisfaction and clinical expertise. *Journal of Nursing Administration, 32,* 273–282.

Hackman, J. R., & Oldham, G. R. (1980). *Work redesign.* Reading, MA: Addison-Wesley.

Holden, R. J. (1991). Responsibility and autonomous nursing practice. *Journal of Advanced Nursing, 16,* 398–403.

Huber, D., Maas, M., McCloskey, J., Scherb, C., Goode, C., & Watson, C. (2002). Evaluating nursing administration instruments. *Journal of Nursing Administration, 30*(5), 251–272.

Kangas, S., Kee, C. C., & McKee-Waddle, R. (1999). Organizational factors, nurses' job satisfaction, and patient satisfaction with nursing care. *Journal of Nursing Administration, 29,* 32–42.

Katzman, E. M. (1989). Nurses' and physicians' perceptions of nursing authority. *Journal of Professional Nursing, 5,* 208–214.

Keenan, J. (1999). A concept analysis of autonomy. *Journal of Advanced Nursing, 29,* 556–562.

Kennerly, S. (2000). Perceived worker autonomy: The foundation for shared governance. *Journal of Nursing Administration, 30,* 611–617.

Kramer, M., & Hafner, L. P. (1989). Shared values: Impact on staff nurse job satisfaction and perceived productivity. *Nursing Research, 38,* 172–177.

Kramer, M., & Schmalenberg, C. (1988a). Magnet hospitals: Institutions of excellence, part 1. *Journal of Nursing Administration, 18,* 13–24.

Kramer, M., & Schmalenberg, C. (1988b). Magnet hospitals: Institutions of excellence, part 2. *Journal of Nursing Administration, 18,* 11–19.

Kramer, M., & Schmalenberg, C. (1993). Learning from success: Autonomy and empowerment. *Nursing Management, 24,* 58–59.

Kramer, M., & Schmalenberg, C. E. (2003). Magnet hospital staff nurses describe clinical autonomy. *Nursing Outlook, 51,* 13–19.

Kurtines, W. M. (1978). A measure of autonomy. *Journal of Personality Assessment, 42,* 253–257.

Laschinger, H. K. S., Finegan, J., Shamian, J., & Almost, J. (2001). Testing Karasek's Demands–Control Model in restructured healthcare settings: Effects of job strain on staff nurses' quality of worklife. *Journal of Nursing Administration, 31,* 233–243.

Maas, M. J. A., & Jacox, A. K. (1977). *Guidelines for Nurse Autonomy/Patient Welfare.* New York: Appleton-Century Crofts.

MacDonald, C. (2002). Nurse autonomy as relational. *Nursing Ethics, 9,* 194–201.

Manojlovich, M. & Spence Laschinger, H. (2002). The relationship of empowerment and selected personality characteristics to nursing job satisfaction. *Journal of Nursing Administration, 32,* 586–595.

Mark, B. A., Salyer, J., & Wan, T. T. (2003). Professional nursing practice: Impact on organizational and patient outcomes. *Journal of Nursing Administration, 33,* 224–234.

McCloskey, J. C. (1990). Two requirements for job contentment: Autonomy and social integration. *Image: the Journal of Nursing Scholarship, 22,* 140–143.

McGillis Hall, L. (2003). Nursing Outcome: Nurses' Job Satisfaction. In D. Doran (Ed.), *Nursing-Sensitive Outcomes: State of the Science* (pp. 283–318). Boston: Jones and Bartlett Publishers.

Mitchinson, S. (1996). Are nurses independent and autonomous practitioners? *Nursing Standard, 10,* 34–38.

Mrayyan, M. (2003). Nurse autonomy, nurse job satisfaction and client satisfaction with nursing care: Their place in nursing data sets. *Canadian Journal of Nursing Leadership, 16,* 74–82.

Mundinger, M. O. (1980). *Autonomy in Nursing.* Germantown, MD: Aspen Systems Corporation.

O'Brien-Pallas, L., Thomson, D., Alksnis, C., & Bruce, S. (2001). The economic impact of nurse staffing decisions: Time to turn down another road? *Hospital Quarterly, 4,* 42–50.

Pankratz, L., & Pankratz, D. (1974). Nursing autonomy and patients' rights: Development of a nursing attitude scale. *Journal of Health and Social Behaviour, 15,* 211–216.

Pinch, W. J. (1985). Ethical dilemmas in nursing: The role of the nurse and perceptions of autonomy. *Journal of Nursing Education, 24,* 372–376.

Porter-O'Grady, T. (1996). Multidisciplinary shared governance: The next step. *Seminars for Nurse Managers, 4,* 43–48.

Radwin, L. E. (1998). Empirically generated attributes of experience in nursing. *Journal of Advanced Nursing, 27,* 590–595.

Rafferty, A. M., Ball, J., & Aiken, L. H. (2001). Are teamwork and professional autonomy compatible, and do they result in improved hospital care? *Quality Health Care, 10,* ii32–ii37.

Ritter-Teitel, J. (2002). The impact of restructuring on professional nursing practice. *Journal of Nursing Administration, 32,* 31–41.

Schutzenhofer, K. K. (1987). The measurement of professional autonomy. *Journal of Professional Nursing, 3,* 278–283.

Schutzenhofer, K. K., & Musser, D. B. (1994). Nurse characteristics and professional autonomy. *Image: the Journal of Nursing Scholarship, 26,* 201–205.

Scott, J. G., Sochalski, J., & Aiken, L. (1999). Review of magnet hospital research: Findings and implications for professional nursing practice. *Journal of Nursing Administration, 29,* 9–19.

Scott, P. A. P. (1998). Morally autonomous practice? *Advances in Nursing Science, 21,* 69–79.

Singleton, E. K., & Nail, F. C. (1984). Role clarification: A prerequisite to autonomy... in nursing practice. *Journal of Nursing Administration, 14,* 17–22.

Stamps, P. P. E. (1986). *Nurses and Work Satisfaction.* Ann Arbor, MI: Michigan Health Administration Press.

Upenieks, V. (2000). The relationship of nursing practice models and job satisfaction outcomes. *Journal of Nursing Administration, 30,* 330–335.

Upenieks, V. V. (2002). Assessing differences in job satisfaction of nurses in magnet and nonmagnet hospitals. *Journal of Nursing Administration, 32,* 564–576.

Upenieks, V. V. (2003a). The interrelationship of organizational characteristics of magnet hospitals, nursing leadership, and nursing job satisfaction. *Health Care Management (Frederick), 22,* 83–98.

Upenieks, V. V. (2003b). What's the attraction to magnet hospitals? Unlimited opportunity, resources, and autonomy draw nurses to these empowering facilities. *Nursing Management, 34,* 43–44.

Wade, G. H. M. R. (1999). Professional nurse autonomy: Concept analysis and application to nursing education. *Journal of Advanced Nursing, 30,* 310–318.

Weisman, C. S., Alexander, C. S., & Chase, G. A. (1980). Job satisfaction among hospital nurses: A longitudinal study. *Health Services Research, 15,* 341–364.

Wilkinson, J. (1997). Professional issues: Developing a concept analysis of autonomy in nursing practice. *British Journal of Nursing, 6,* 703–707.

Wolf, G. A., Boland, S., & Aukerman, M. (1994). A transformational model for the practice of professional nursing: the model, part 1. *Journal of Nursing Administration, 24,* 51–57.

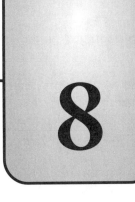

8

Professional Development Opportunities

Ellen Rukholm

8.1 Introduction

Professional development is a term that covers a wide variety of educational activities ranging from formal professional requirements to informal, individual actions (Lawton & Wimpenny, 2003). Sadler-Smith, Allinson, and Hayes (2000) further characterize that professional development has three key roles or functions: maintenance, survival, and mobility (as cited in Lawton & Wimpenny, p. 42). The maintenance role refers to lifelong learning; the survival role refers to competence; while mobility refers to employment capacity. Generally, most models of professional development focus on the survival role or competency. Regulatory bodies whose purpose is to protect the public tend to focus predominantly on competency. Workplace settings whose mandate is to provide efficient care tend to focus on employment capacity, while learners themselves may be more likely to see themselves as lifelong learners in ever-changing work environments (Lawton & Wimpenny). These three roles are compatible and may co-exist; the challenge lies in the measurement of professional development opportunities and their connection to nursing-sensitive outcomes.

This chapter:

- Proposes a conceptual definition of professional development based on the literature

- Presents the theoretical underpinnings of nursing professional development

- Identifies factors that influence nurses' professional development opportunities

- Critically examines the empirical evidence linking nursing professional development opportunities to studies relating professional development to patient outcome achievement

- Discusses issues in the assessment of professional development opportunities

- Reviews approaches to measuring nurses' professional development

- Identifies implications and directions for the future

This review examined literature relating to theoretical and empirical work in the area of professional development opportunities for nurses. The search of this body of literature—using the keywords *nursing professional development, practice, patient outcomes*, and *measurement*—yielded more than 200 sources from the Ebsco Research Databases, Ovid, Proquest, and Ontario Scholars Portal. These online library databases allow access through the Ebsco "host" to more than 5 million articles in 3,304 text journals published by Academic Press, Elsevier Science, Hartcourt Health Sciences, and John Wiley & Sons. Many of the sources were anecdotal or conceptual in nature and tended to focus predominantly on nurse learner self-reports of learning, knowledge, and satisfaction as outcomes of continuing a professional development program or activity being evaluated. Very few studies that measured the effectiveness of continuing professional development on practice or patient outcomes from the perspective of patients were found. The literature reviewed in this chapter includes both comprehensive literature reviews and studies. The total number of relevant literature sources found was 200; 63 of these met the criteria for inclusion in this chapter.

8.2 Definitions of the Concept of Professional Development

Over the past 10 years there has been a movement away from using the term *continuing professional education* toward using the broader term of *professional development* (Lawton & Wimpenny, 2003). This shift acknowledges the wider range of activities that may be encompassed by professional development (Furze & Pearcey, 1999); however, both of these terms are still seen in the literature and are often used interchangeably. Consequently, this chapter draws on studies and reviews that use either terminology.

There has been considerable variation in the understanding and use of the term *professional development*, ranging from formal professional requirements to informal individualized activities. Lawton and Wimpenny (2003) suggested a definition of professional development that emerged from the architecture and construction industry: "the systematic maintenance, improvement and broadening of knowledge and skills, and the development of personal qualities necessary for execution of professional and technical duties throughout the individual's working life" (Friedman et al.'s study, as cited in Lawton & Wimpenny, p. 42). This definition implied lifelong learning, competence, and personal development; concepts that have been raised repeatedly throughout the literature on this topic (Barriball, While, & Norman, 1992; Lawton & Wimpenny; Nolan, Owen, Curran, & Venables, 2000; Perry, 1995).

A number of different functions for professional development have been reported in the literature. Miller (as cited in Adams, Miller, & Beck, 1996) included continuing education as an element of the broader concept of professionalism, and similar to the regulatory bodies, equated continuing education with competence. Beeler, Young, and Dull (1990) defined professional development as a process involving four developmental levels and five dimensions of professional nursing practice. The four developmental levels were professional awareness (level 1), professional identification (level 2), professional maturation (level 3), and professional mastery (level 4). The five dimensions of professional nursing practice included: nursing practice–process, communication–collaboration, leadership, professional integration, and research–evaluation. Bignell and Crotty (as cited in Perry, 1995) defined continuing professional education for nurses as "planned education activities intended to build upon the educational and experiential bases of the professional nurse for the enhancement of practice, education, administration, research or theory development to the end of improving the health of the public" (p. 766). Sadler-Smith et al. (2000) provided perhaps the most comprehensive way of viewing professional development by describing several different elements of professional development. These authors identified three key roles of continuing professional education including the maintenance role or lifelong learning, the survival role or competence, and the mobility role or employability.

The shift to using the term *professional development* rather than *continuing education* broadens its scope and incorporates notions of lifelong learning, competence, and employability. It has been suggested that professional development involves learning whereas continuing education implies the provision of learning experiences (Perry, 1995). Perry further differentiated that learning was not dependent upon the provision of educational opportunities and concurred with Illich (as cited in Perry) that, "most learning is not the result of instruction; it is rather the result of unhampered participation in a meaningful setting" (p. 767). Others have confirmed the contribution of peers to continuing professional development (Eisen, 2001; Francke, Garssen, & Abu-Saad, 1995; Hart, Clinton, Edwards, & Evans, 2000). Learning has been characterized as occurrences in real life situations with actual people and problems. Perry has linked learning to the development of critical thinking and reflection skills to deal with information and to augment knowledge through experience. She stressed the use of reflection, not only to modify existing knowledge, but also to keep the mind open to new ways of knowing. Hence, critical thinking and reflection grounded in *real life* experiences are also part of what defines professional development.

In summary, professional continuing education is in the process of evolving to a broader conceptualization called professional development. Both terms continue to appear in the literature and are often used interchangeably. However, professional development seems to be more comprehensive and is becoming the more prevalent term being used. Professional development ranges from informal to highly formal activities. The literature emphasizes that meaningful professional development opportunities involve critical thinking skills and reflection grounded in real life experiences. Although each of the defining characteristics of professional development opportunities (i.e., lifelong learning, competence, and employment) are important to each stakeholder (i.e., the nurse, the regulatory body, and the employer), the priority and meaning of these characteristics may vary in degree of importance for each stakeholder. Regulatory bodies tend to accentuate competence of the nurse, while employers emphasize employment flexibility and competence, and learners concentrate on lifelong learning, competence, and employability. Hence, it would seem that a definition that incorporates all of these functions and ideas might be the most helpful in looking at the impact of professional development opportunities on nurse-sensitive outcomes.

8.3 Theoretical Underpinnings of Nursing Professional Development

Currently, the dominant theoretical perspective underlying nursing professional development focuses on reflective practice and experiential or transformative adult learning (Benner, 1984; Dewey, 1933; Kolb, 1984; Kolb and Fry, 1975; Mezirow, 1991; Schon, 1983). Reflective practice is emphasized in undergraduate nursing education and is also a requirement of nursing regulatory bodies in Canada, the United States, and the United Kingdom. In the context of regulatory bodies, reflective practice is linked to competence. Reflective practice is defined by the Alberta Association of Registered Nurses (AARN; 2000) in the *Continuing Competence Handbook* as "the review of one's own nursing practice to determine learning needs and incorporate learning to improve one's own practice" and central to this process is "reflection on your practice against the

Nursing Practice Standards" (p. 8). In other words, nurses are required to assess the degree to which their practice meets these standards and then undertake activities to better their practice. Similar requirements exist across Canada, the United States, and the United Kingdom; some require specific numbers of hours of professional development while others do not. Thus, regulatory bodies link practice to professional development through reflection and competence.

According to Wilkinson (1999), there have been many attempts to define reflective practice and some would argue that it has been ill defined. Boud, Keogh, and Walker (1985) defined reflection as the learner's reaction to an experience. Others have defined reflective practice as "a means by which practitioners can develop a greater level of self-awareness about the nature and impact of their performance" (Osterman & Kottkamp, 1993, p. 19), and as an approach in which "actions are carefully planned in relation to the theory known to the professional and consciously monitored, so that outcomes of the action will be beneficial to the patient" (Jarvis, 1992, p. 177). Schon (1983) defined reflective practice as "a dialogue of thinking and doing through which I become more skillful" (p. 31), and later Schon (1987) described reflective techniques including reflection-in-action and reflection-on-action, both of which link reflection to experience. The former means to think about what one is doing while doing it, whereas the latter refers to retrospective exploration of an experience.

Although the popular use of reflection in nursing is a relatively recent phenomenon, the combined value of experiential learning and reflection has been widely acknowledged in the general literature on professional development and thinking since the 1930s (Benner, 1984; Dewey, 1933; Kolb, 1984; Kolb & Fry, 1975; Schon, 1983). These theorists have identified experiential learning as a valuable tool for improving professional practice and lifelong learning. In summary, reflection can be a process that formalizes the combination of experience and theory and the transition from novice to expert, thereby increasing opportunity for professional development (Ellis, 1999).

8.4 Factors that Influence Nurses' Professional Development Opportunities

The factors influencing nurses' professional development opportunities are examined from the perspective of the workplace and nurses themselves.

8.4.1 Professional Development from the Perspective of the Employer

Factors influencing professional development opportunities from the view of the employer include organization-defined needs related to competence, flexibility, cost of provision, and cost effectiveness as an outcome (Altimier, 1995; Altimier

& Sanders, 1999; Lyons, 1992). A great deal of emphasis is placed on patient-focused care, cross-training, and the orientation provided by employers as professional development opportunities (Bumgarner & Biggerstaff, 2000; Burchell & Jenner, 1996). More recently, the employers' perspective also seems to be driven by the impact of restructuring on staffing and the recruitment and retention of nurses (Eisen, 2001; Nolan et al., 2000; Stark, Warne, & Street, 2001). Yuen (as cited in Perry, 1995) identified a number of factors that serve as barriers to professional development opportunities including:

> Inability to convince nurse managers that staff development is of vital importance for the services, failure to encourage qualified nurses to value their own continuing personal and professional development, failure to recognize that the training personnel also need help, lack of appropriate criteria for nurse managers to select staff for continuing education programs, ineffective methods of publicizing programs, little systematic attention to identifying educational and training needs, inadequate evaluation of effectiveness of staff development programs, lack of coherent staff development programs, and inadequate funding of staff development. (p. 768)

Many of these obstacles identified by Yuen persist today (Jenner, 1998; Nolan et al.).

For cross-training and/or orientation, with the aims of increasing the cost effectiveness of care and ensuring nurse competence, continuing education programs may have been driven more by the needs of the workplace rather than by the individual professional development needs of nurses (Altimier, 1995; Altimier & Sanders, 1999; Bumgarner & Biggerstaff, 2000; Burchell & Jenner, 1996). Indeed, several authors have referred to tension existing between professional development needs at the organizational level and the personal and professional development needs of individuals (Furze & Pearcey, 1999; Lawton & Wimpenny, 2003; Nolan et al., 2000).

Cross-training refers to providing nurses with required education opportunities that allow nurses to be more flexible and competent to work in more areas within the system, for example, within a practice setting such as Maternal Child Health (Komara & Stefaniak, 1998). In this situation, a nurse may be educated to be able to work in labor and delivery, in an intensive care nursery, on the floor with new mothers, and with children. The advantage to the institution revolves around flexibility of staffing and the consequent cost savings of being able to move trained staff to several service areas according to demand. Proponents of this approach to continuing professional development cite the cost savings to the institution and emphasize nurse competence (Altimier, 1995; Altimier, & Sanders, 1999; Crompton, Roth, Eppley, & Phillips, 1999; Kozlowski, 1996). Those who oppose it argue that the individual nurse has no sense of control over her practice as a professional and there is no commitment to lifelong learning or personal development (Furze & Pearcey, 1999; Nolan et al., 2000). In many of these studies, learner needs are either not considered or considered only in the context of cross-training and orientation. However, several studies were identified where the learning needs of nurses were assessed and continuing education programs were identified in relation to those needs (Alexander, Chadwick, Slay, Petersen, & Pass, 2002; Bibb, Malebranche, Crowell, & Altman, 2003; Ozcan & Shukla, 1993; Werrett, Helm, & Carnwell, 2001). The reports of employer-provider approaches to professional development focused on assessment of nurse learner needs or on cross-training and orientation specific to organizational needs for flexibility, competence, and cost effectiveness.

8.4.2 *Professional Development from the Perspective of the Individual*

Factors influencing professional development from the perspective of the individual include learner motivation; learner defined needs; financial support—tuition and travel reimbursement; employer support—release time from work with pay and space; support—physician, workplace superior, peer, and family support; the shift worked; and availability and accessibility of programs (Ayer & Smith, 1998; Dowswell, Hewison, & Hinds, 1998; Francke et al., 1995; Glass & Todd-Atkinson, 1999; Rukholm, Carter, Bakker, & Viverais-Dresler, 2002; Waddell, 1993).

Perry (1995) hypothesized that failure of nurses to participate in educational development opportunities could also be attributed to resistance to change; a phenomenon she saw as being related to the reluctance of nurses to relinquish existing cultural nursing norms. As well, she suggested that little is known about what nurses expect to get from professional development opportunities.

Glass and Todd-Atkinson (1999) conducted a cross-sectional study of the continuing education needs of registered nurses and licensed practical nurses employed in randomly selected nursing homes in North Carolina. Sample selection excluded homes for the aged and hospital facilities because each of these settings required a different skill mix. One hundred and forty-one facilities met study criteria and a 10% sample was selected resulting in a sample of 14 facilities. Response rate from the 319 nurses employed in these facilities was 164 (51%). The questionnaire was a revised and extended version of a questionnaire developed by Bye (1988) and has been used with other gerontology study populations. The questionnaire contained six major categories of learning needs including the aging process, nursing interactions, nursing process, nursing management of elderly individuals with specific clinical problems, professional issues, and managerial and supervisory skills. Learning needs included 59 questions using a 5-point Likert scale. Nurses were asked to rate their knowledge, skills, or attitudes of the 59 learning needs. Independent variables, including age, education, experience, shift worked, and facility size, were also determined. The nurses identified many continuing education needs, but management skills, drug therapy–interactions, and behavioral problems were particularly important to them. Night shift workers and nurse educators had different learning needs. Factors facilitating or deterring attainment of continuing education were also investigated. In order of priority, facilitating factors were: (a) readily available programs, (b) supervisor and peer encouragement, (c) release time from work with pay and travel expenses reimbursed, and (d) tuition reimbursement. Deterrents included: (a) lack of information about programs, (b) family responsibilities, (c) tuition costs, (d) responsibilities at work, (e) lack of employment cooperation, and (f) peer opinions and attitudes. The greatest deterrent reported by the nurses was lack of tuition reimbursement.

The findings of the study *"Cardiac Care on the Web,"* which examined the online learning environment for registered nurses enrolled in a professional development university credit course in cardiovascular nursing, yielded information about the barriers and facilitators of online learning (Rukholm et al., 2002). The main reasons for withdrawal from the course, cited by *"Cardiac Care on the Web"* participants, included difficulties with scheduling, managing the time commitment required for a formal professional development course, and balancing course work with family and work responsibilities (Rukholm et al.). These reasons were similar to those cited in early studies of attrition in continuing education programs for nurses (Cookson, 1990; Kennedy & Powell, 1976; O'Kell, 1986; Phythian & Clements, 1980; Rekkedal, 1983; Woodley & McIntosh, 1977). In the rapidly evolving practice settings of our times, nurses' learning needs are constantly changing so that assessment of learner needs is a fundamental step required in order to provide relevant continuing professional development opportunities.

8.5 Linking Nurses' Professional Development to Patient Outcome Achievement

There is limited understanding of the impact of professional development opportunities on patient outcome achievement (Barriball et al., 1992; Lawton & Wimpenny, 2003; Waddell, 1993). Waddell's meta-analysis of 34 studies revealed that continuing professional education had a positive impact on practice, but did not explain why this happened. Lawton and Wimpenny agreed with Waddell's assertion that challenges with measuring effectiveness included the lack of experimental control and the multifactorial nature of continuing professional development. The vast majority of studies found were concerned with assessment of learner continuing professional development needs; some of these were very context-specific to learner needs in relation to industry driven organization goals while others were assessments of learner needs in relation to practice in general or to specific areas of practice such as medical surgical and intensive care (Synder & Nethersole-Chong, 1999), primary care (Stark et al., 2001; Werrett et al., 2001), or maternal and child health (Alexander et al., 2002).

Only two studies were found that linked continuing professional development to practice and patient outcomes (Dufault & Sullivan, 2000; Hart et al., 2000). Outcome measurement of continuing professional development opportunities in relation to nursing practice and nurse-sensitive outcomes grounded in best practice guidelines such as pain management was addressed in one of the studies reviewed (Dufault & Sullivan).

In a two-group, pre-test–intervention–post-test, quasi-experimental clinical trial composed of 173 surgical and oncology subjects with a history of pain, Dufault and Sullivan (2000) studied whether clinician participation in a collaborative research utilization model to generate and evaluate a research-based pain management standard resulted in changes in practice and improved outcomes in patients. Study assumptions included the beliefs that the complex nature of pain management and the difficulty in transferring–translating research evidence (i.e., knowledge) into practice required the participation of the multiple disciplines providing direct patient care. Practitioners and students from medicine, nursing, pastoral care, physical therapy, and pharmacy were linked in a partnership with the goal of examining the U.S. Agency for Health Care Policy and Research clinical practice guidelines for pain management and more recent pain management research evidence, generating a standard of care grounded in research, and testing the impact of the standard on patient outcomes. Continuing professional development in this study was multifaceted—it involved participants from multiple disciplines, engaged the learner in developing and testing the standard, and looked at the impact on patient outcomes. Furthermore, once the standard was developed, medical and nursing staff received "no pain" cue cards containing key elements of the new standard. As well, inservices on the standard were held on each unit on all shifts. Significant differences between control and treatment groups were found related to pain intensity.

Turnbull and Holt (1993) examined various frameworks for evaluating continuing education programs for health professionals and found that most evaluations focused on attendance, participant satisfaction, and change in knowledge and skills. These authors asserted that little or no evaluation research has measured the impact of professional development opportunities on patient outcomes. The conceptual framework developed by Donabedian (1966) for the evaluation of health care systems, which looks at structure, process, and outcome, could be helpful in guiding evaluation of professional development opportunities. Such a framework could provide insight into the linkage between professional development opportunities and patient outcomes.

8.6 Issues in the Assessment of Nurses' Professional Development Opportunities

Tension exists regarding who decides what professional development (i.e., continuing professional education) opportunities are priorities (Furze & Pearcey, 1999; Lawton & Wimpenny, 2003; Nolan et al., 2000; Rukholm et al., 2001). The issue may be a critical consideration in examining how learning can have an impact on practice and patient outcomes. If the major concern of nurses in the workplace is coping with stress, then perhaps a course on relaxation techniques that assists nurses in handling stress, and therefore, in functioning more effectively at work is an appropriate and important professional development activity. It may well be that the workplace institution and/or the professional regulatory body may question such an activity as an appropriate professional activity that would be acceptable in a professional portfolio or worthy of release time or workplace support. On the other hand, when the learning is formalized and has a direct link to practice, the workplace and regulatory bodies might view participation in a formal clinical course, where nothing new is learned but an obvious link to practice exists, as an appropriate professional development activity. Often, even in a formal course, the most meaningful learning occurs informally through interactions with colleagues.

Is professional development driven by the learner, employer, or regulatory body, or a combination of all three? What then are the implications for the measurement of continuing professional development? How can local context—local knowledge and general knowledge—be reconciled such that findings are meaningful beyond the situation being studied (Clarke & Wilcockson, 2002)? The work of Dufault and Sullivan (2000) illustrated an attempt to reconcile local and general knowledge through learner involvement in creating and testing a local standard grounded in best practice guidelines and then tested the impact of that standard on patient outcomes. A complex study by Hart et al. (2000) took a slightly different approach that illustrated an attempt to evaluate the impact of a continuing professional development program on a specific area of practice (i.e., mental health nursing) that incorporated learner involvement and professional development characteristics (i.e., reflection and critical thinking) and measured the impact on aspects peculiar to the specific practice (i.e., hope and empathy) and work performance. The researchers described the aim of the professional development program as "to improve the knowledge and skills of the participants, enhance the work environment and improve work performance" (Hart et al., p. 28). A combined quantitative and qualitative approach was used to measure critical thinking skills. The qualitative data regarding critical thinking and reflection was more useful in terms of understanding workplace performance, empathy, and critical thinking.

The Watson-Glaser Critical Thinking Appraisal (Watson & Glaser, 1980) used to measure critical thinking did not result in a significant difference between the two groups of accelerated professional development and peer consultation. Hart et al. (2000) raised concerns about the ability of this standard measurement to measure critical thinking in specific nursing contexts. Furthermore, the instrument was not adapted to the local context. Finally, the instrument was lengthy and respondent fatigue may have been a limitation.

Issues concerning the assessment of continuing professional development center on the lack of consensus on a definition of professional development, questions about whether critical thinking and reflection skills are outcomes of professional development or processes by which professional development is achieved, and questions about how best to measure critical thinking. If competence, lifelong learning, and employability are aspects of professional development, then it is critical to determine how these best be evaluated.

8.7 Evidence Concerning Approaches to Measuring Nurses' Professional Development

Measurement of nurses' professional development has been primarily focused on assessing the components of the learning opportunities such as the learners' critical thinking and reflection skills and self-reported responses concerning satisfaction or usefulness of programs (Postler-Slattery & Foley, 2003; Rukholm et al., 2002), rather than the effectiveness of programs in terms of their impact on practice and patient outcomes. There does seem to be consensus in the literature that continuing professional development is important (Lawton & Wimpenny, 2003); however, these authors contend that the actual measurement of the effectiveness of professional development opportunities is fraught with difficulties. It is easier to measure numbers of participants and participant satisfaction with learning than it is to actually try to measure the impact on practice and patients (see Table 8.1).

Approaches to evaluation have been both quantitative and qualitative. Quantitative studies that attempt to assess the impact of continuing professional development programs on practice and/or patient outcomes have been criticized for failure to report validity and reliability of the instruments used to measure the effects of education on practice. As well, lack of control of variables in relation to individual nurses, their practice, the number of patients they cared for, and the continuing professional development activity they received are but a few of the concerns that were identified by Wood (1998). Scheller (1993), in a qualitative study, identified three problems when attempting to measure the impact of continuing professional education on practice. These included: (a) the difficulty of measuring the impact of continuing professional education on nursing practice and the quality of care, (b) the lack of consensus on what comprises use of nursing knowledge, and (c) the use of knowledge gained from professional education programs is influenced by many different factors that interact to affect nursing practice. Waddell (2001), in a critical review of the literature related to the measurement of competence—an element of professional development—concluded that there is a need for educators and nurse managers to link national professional association practice standards with essential context-specific competencies. She further recommended the development of appropriate ways to measure these competencies and that regulatory bodies should then recognize successful outcomes of such activities as evidence of continued competence (Waddell).

Table 8.1 Nursing Measures of Professional Development

Instrument Author/Date of Publication	Target Population	Domains	Method of Administration	Reliability	Validity	Sensitivity to Nursing
Professional Development Self-Assessment Matrix (PDSAM) (Beeler et al., 1990)	Predominantly hospital staff registered nurses (RNs) attending baccalaureate nursing program.	Professional development is a process consisting of four developmental levels subdivided into five dimensions of professional nursing practice; professional awareness (level 1), professional identification (level 2), professional maturation (level 3), and professional mastery (level 4); the five dimensions are nursing practice–process, communication–collaboration, leadership, professional integration, and research–evaluation. Individuals rate themselves as being at one of the four levels on each of these five dimensions. Scores in each dimension are 1 to 4, with 1 representing beginning professional awareness, 4 representing professional mastery.	Self-report.	Analysis of students' scores on the PDSAM in 1995 were $\alpha = .8990$, for internal consistency. Data analysis in 1999 indicated $\alpha = .9193$ on the pre-test, $\alpha = .8788$ on the post-test. (Phillips, Palmer, Zimmerman & Mayfield, 2002)	Content validity.	

α = Cronbach's alpha coefficient

Table 8.1 (continued)

Instrument Author/Date Publication	Target Population	Domains	Method of Administration	Reliability	Validity	Sensitivity to Nursing
Professionalism inventory (Miller, Adams, & Beck, 1993)	Nurse executives and middle managers.	Professionalism based on the Miller et al. (1993) wheel of professionalism; tool measures degrees of professionalism, dichotomous responses to 48 items representing categories of educational preparation, autonomy, theory, and adherence to the American Nursing Association code of ethics, as well as participation in publication, research, professional organizations, community service and maintaining competence. Continuing education (professional development) is defined in terms of competence.	Questionnaire self-report.	Values of reliability ranged from α = .64 to α = .87. Adams, Miller and Beck (1996), α = .69.	Content validity was established by nurses in education and service settings.	Designed by nurse researchers for nursing.

α = Cronbach's alpha coefficient

Equally challenging is the evolving definition of professional development and the divergent functions (i.e., competence, employability, and lifelong learning) valued by the stakeholders (i.e., regulatory bodies, employers, and nurses). In the acute care hospital literature, much emphasis has been placed on the employability aspect of professional development opportunities (Lyons, 1992; Synder & Nethersole-Chong, 1999; Wheaton, 1996). Here, the employer's emphasis is on competence and employability, and professional development opportunities involve cross-training. The goal is the employer's need for a more cost effective use of nurses rather than on commitment to lifelong learning. Professional development opportunities may be directly linked to cost effectiveness and competence with little or no regard for nurse identification of learning needs or nurse commitment to lifelong learning. Such an approach to continuing professional development has potentially deleterious effects on learning and practice since learner motivation facilitates individual learner participation in continuing professional development activities.

In summary, the evaluation of continuing professional education opportunities has focused heavily on elements of learning rather than on practice and patient outcomes. Much of the literature has focused on nurses' self-reports of the effectiveness of learning and impact on practice. Critical thinking skills and reflection have been assessed as outcomes in formal programs while actual impact on practice has received little or no attention.

8.8 Implications and Future Directions

Continuing professional development is a complex multifaceted concept whose definition and measurement should incorporate stakeholder perspectives (i.e., employer, regulatory body, and individual) in relation to specific learning contexts. Attributes of the professional identified in the literature include knowledge, critical thinking ability, communication skills, leadership ability, participation and use of research in practice, involvement in professional nursing organizations, and reflection skills. Professional development may be general or context-specific.

Factors influencing professional development from the perspective of the individual include learner motivation, learner defined needs, financial support, time, space, and peer and family support. Factors influencing professional development from the view of the employer include organization defined needs related to competence, flexibility, cost of provision, and cost effectiveness as an outcome related to patient-focused care and cross-training. More recently, the employers' perspective seems to be driven in part by the impact of restructuring on staffing—recruitment and retention of nurses. Regulatory bodies, whose purpose is to protect the public, focus on competence and many emphasize mandatory hours of continuing education. Comprehensive understanding of professional development should incorporate the perspectives of all three stakeholders.

Further research is required that draws on the perspectives of all three stakeholders, is set in specific contexts, considers structured and unstructured professional development, and examines the impact of professional development on practice and nurse-sensitive patient outcomes.

Experimental designs, examination of the relationship between nursing professional development opportunities and patient outcomes, development of ways to measure contextualized professional development opportunities, further identification of factors influencing professional development opportunities, and examination of the relationship between individual organizational and regulatory definitions of *priority* professional development opportunities are among the areas requiring further research.

8.9   References

Adams, D., Miller, B., & Beck, L. (1996). Professionalism behaviors of hospital nurse executives and middle managers in 10 western states. *Western Journal of Nursing Research, 18,* 77–88.

Alberta Association of Registered Nurses. (2000). *Nursing Practice Standards: Standards for a New Millenium Canadian Nurses Association: Code of Ethics for Registered Nurses.* Edmonton, Canada: Alberta Association of Registered Nurses.

Alexander, G., Chadwick, C., Slay, M., Petersen, D., & Pass, M. A. (2002). Maternal and child health graduate and continuing education needs: A national assessment. *Maternal and Child Health Journal, 6*(3), 141–149.

Altimier, L. (1995). A perinatal cross-training program. *Nursing Management, 26*(11), 48–53.

Altimier, L., & Sanders, J. (1999). Cross-training in 3-D. *Nursing Management, 30*(11), 59–62.

Ayer, S., & Smith, C. (1998). Planning flexible learning to match the needs of consumers: A national survey. *Journal of Advanced Nursing, 27,* 1034–1047.

Barriball, K. L., While, A. E., & Norman, I. J. (1992). Continuing professional education for qualified nurses: A review of the literature. *Journal of Advanced Nursing, 17,* 1120–1140.

Beeler, J. L., Young, P. A., & Dull, S. M. (1990). Professional development framework: Pathway to the future. *Journal of Nursing Staff Development, 6,* 296–301.

Benner, P. (1984). *From novice to expert.* Menlo Park, CA: Addison Wesley.

Bibb, S., Malebranche, M., Crowell, D., & Altman, C. (2003). Professional development needs of RNs practicing at a military community hospital. *The Journal of Continuing Education in Nursing, 34,* 39–45.

Bignell, A., & Crotty, M. (1988). Continuing education: Does it enhance patient care? *Senior Nurse, 8*(4), 26–29.

Boud, D., Keogh, R., & Walker, D. (1985). *Reflection: Turning experience into learning.* London: Kogan Page.

Bumgarner, S., & Biggerstaff, S. (2000). A patient-centered approach to nurse orientation. *Journal of Nurses in Staff Development, 16*(6), 249–256.

Burchell, H., & Jenner, E. (1996). The role of the nurse in patient-focused care: Models of competence and implications for education and training. *International Journal of Nursing Studies, 33*(1), 67–75.

Bye, M. G. (1988). An analysis of the continuing education needs of nurses in nursing homes. *The Journal of Continuing Education in Nursing, 19*, 174–177.

Clarke, C., & Wilcockson, J. (2002). Seeing need and developing care: Exploring knowledge for and from practice. *International Journal of Nursing Studies, 39*, 397–406.

Cookson, P. (1990). Persistence in distance education. In M. G. Moore (Ed.) *Contemporary Issues in American Distance Education*. Oxford: Pergamon Press.

Crompton, D. A., Roth, R. M., Eppley, G. Y., & Phillips, C. R. (1999). Follow family-focused care principles. *Nursing Management, 30*(2), 47–50.

Dewey, J. (1933). *How we think*. New York: D. C. Health.

Donabedian, A. (1966). Evaluating the quality of medical care. *Millbank Memorial Fund Quarterly, 44* (Part 2), 166–206.

Dowswell, C., Hewison, J., & Hinds, M. (1998). Motivational forces affecting participation in post-registration degree courses and effects on home and work-life: A qualitative study. *Journal of Advanced Nursing, 28*, 1326–1333.

Dufault, M. A., & Sullivan, M. (2000). A collaborative research utilization approach to evaluate the effects of pain management standards on patient outcomes. *Journal of Professional Nursing, 16*(4), 240–250.

Eisen, M. J. (2001). Peer-based professional development viewed through the lens of transformative learning. *Holistic Nursing Practice, 16*(1), 30–42.

Ellis, S. (1999). The patient-centred care model: Holistic/multiprofessional/reflective. *British Journal of Nursing, 8*(5), 296–313.

Francke, A. L., Garssen, B., & Abu-Saad, H. H. (1995). Determinants of changes in nurses' behaviour after continuing education: A literature review. *Journal of Advanced Nursing, 21*, 371–377.

Furze, G., & Pearcey, P. (1999). Continuing education in nursing: A review of the literature. *Journal of Advanced Nursing, 29*, 355–363.

Glass, J. C., & Todd-Atkinson, S. (1999). Continuing education needs of nurses employed in nursing facilities. *The Journal of Continuing Education in Nursing, 30*(5), 219–225.

Hart, G., Clinton, M., Edwards, H., & Evans, K. (2000). Accelerated professional development and peer consultation: Two strategies for continuing professional education for nurses. *The Journal of Continuing Education in Nursing, 31*, 28–42.

Jarvis, R. (1992). Reflective practice and nursing. *Nurse Education Today, 12*, 174–181.

Jenner, E. (1998). A case study analysis of nurses' roles, education and training needs associated with patient-focused care. *Journal of Advanced Nursing, 27*, 1087–1095.

Kennedy, D., & Powell, R. (1976). Student progress and withdrawal in the Open University. *Teaching at a Distance, 7*, 61–75.

Kolb, D. A. (1984). *Experiential learning: Experience in the source of learning and development*. Englewood Cliffs, NJ: Prentice Hall.

Kolb, D., & Fry, F. (1975). *Towards an applied theory of experiential learning: Theories of group processes.* London: John Wiley.

Komara, C., & Stefaniak, K. (1998). Cross-training for obstetrics using an internship program. *Journal for Nurses in Staff Development, 14*(3), 154–158.

Kozlowski, S. (1996). Cross-training: Concepts, considerations and challenges. *Medical Laboratory Observer, February,* 50–54.

Lawton, S., & Wimpenny, P. (2003). Continuing professional development: A review. *Nursing Standard, 17*(24), 41–44.

Lyons, R. (1992). Cross-training: A richer staff for leaner budgets. *Nursing Management, 23*(1), 43–44.

Mezirow, J. (1991). *Transformative dimensions of adult learning.* San Francisco: Jossey-Bass.

Miller, B., Adams, D., & Beck, L. (1993). A behavioral inventory for professionalism in nursing. *Journal of Professional Nursing, 9*(5), 290–295.

Nolan, M., Owen, R., Curran, M., & Venables, A. (2000). Reconceptualising the outcomes of continuing professional development. *International Journal of Nursing Studies, 37,* 457–467.

O'Kell, S. P. (1986). A literature search into the continuing education undertaken in nursing. *Nurse Education Today, 6,* 152–57.

Osterman, K., & Kottkamp, R. (1993). *Reflective practice for educators: Improving schooling through professional development.* Newbury Park, CA: Corwin Press.

Ozcan, Y. A., & Shukla, R. K. (1993). The effect of a competency-based targeted staff development program on nursing productivity. *Journal of Nursing Staff Development, 9*(2), 78–84.

Perry, L. (1995). Continuing professional education: Luxury or necessity? *Journal of Advanced Nursing,* 21, 766–771.

Phillips, C. Y., Palmer, C. V., Zimmerman, B. J., & Mayfield, M. (2002). Professional development: Assuring growth of RN-to-BSN students. *Journal of Nursing Education, 41*(6), 282–284.

Phythian, T., & Clements, M. (1980). Post-foundation tutorial planning. *Teaching at a Distance, 18*(Winter), 38–43.

Postler-Slattery, D., & Foley, K. (2003). The fruits of lifelong learning. *Nursing Management, 34*(2), 34–37.

Rekkedal, T. (1983). Enhancing student progress in Norway. *Teaching at a Distance, 23* (Summer), 19–24.

Rukholm, E., Carter, L., Bakker, D., & Viverais-Dresler, G. (2002). *Cardiac Care on the Web: Final Report.* Sudbury, ON: School of Nursing and Centre for Continuing Education, Laurentian University.

Rukholm, E., Lemonde, M., Bailey, P., McGirr, M., Pong, R., Kaminski, V., et al. (2001). *System assessment and redesign for a new millennium. The Canadian Health Services Research Foundation; Interim Report, Case Study #1.* Sudbury, ON: School of Nursing, Laurentian University.

Sadler-Smith, E., Allinson, C. W., & Hayes, J. (2000). Learning preferences and cognitive style: Some implications for CPD. *Management Learning, 8*(4), 66–75.

Scheller, M. (1993). A qualitative analysis of factors in the work environment that influence nurses' use of knowledge gained from CE programmes. *Journal of Continuing Education in Nursing, 24,* 114–122.

Schon, D. (1983). *The reflective practitioner: How professionals think in action.* New York: Basic Books.

Schon, D. (1987). *Educating the reflective practitioner.* San Francisco: Jossey-Bass.

Stark, S., Warne, T., & Street, C. (2001). Practice nursing: An evaluation of a training practice initiative. *Nurse Education Today, 21*(4), 287–296.

Synder, J., & Nethersole-Chong, D. (1999). Is cross-training medical/surgical RNs to ICU the answer? *Nursing Management, 30*(2), 58–60.

Turnbull, D. C., & Holt, M. E. (1993). Conceptual frameworks for evaluating continuing education in allied health. *Journal of Continuing Education in the Health Professions, 13,* 177–186.

Waddell, D. (1993). The effects of continuing education on nursing practice: A meta-analysis. *Journal of Continuing Education in Nursing, 23*(4), 164–168.

Waddell, D. L. (2001). Measurement issues in promoting continued competence. *Journal of Continuing Education in Nursing, 32*(3), 102–106.

Watson, G.B., & Glaser, E.M. (1980). *Watson-Glaser critical thinking appraisal.* New York: Psychological Corporation.

Werrett, J., Helm, R. H., & Carnwell, R. (2001). The primary and secondary interface: The educational needs of nursing staff for the provision of seamless care. *Journal of Advanced Nursing, 34*(5), 629–638.

Wheaton, M. (1996). Cross-training: Meeting staffing needs in the ICU. *Nursing Management, 27*(11), 32B–33B.

Wilkinson, J. (1999). Implementing reflective practice. *Nursing Standard, 13*(21), 36–43.

Wood, I. (1998). The effects of continuing professional education on the clinical practice of nurses: A review of the literature. *International Journal of Nursing Studies, 35,* 125–131.

Woodley, A., & McIntosh, N. (1977). People who decide not to apply to the Open University. *Teaching at a Distance, 9* (July), 18–26.

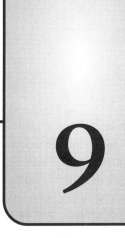

9

Scope of Nursing Leadership

Allison Patrick

Peggy White

9.1 Introduction

Nursing leadership is becoming increasingly scrutinized in a health care environment that is constantly changing and where there is an increased focus on balancing the costs and quality of health care. In nursing, leaders face the added challenge of recruiting and retaining the right mix of staff to produce quality outcomes. To accomplish this, the nursing profession requires leaders who can transform practice cultures so the "essence, uniqueness, and outcomes of professional practice can be realized" (Wesorick, 2002, p. 1).

As McCloskey and Molen noted in a 1987 review of nursing research, the topic of leadership in nursing does not have distinct boundaries and much of the published work is anecdotal and opinion based with some descriptive studies. Vance and

Larson (2002) reviewed 6,628 leadership citations in the health care and business literature and reported that only 4.4% were empirically data-based studies, while a significantly higher proportion of research-based citations were found in the business literature than in health care literature. The authors found that 3.3% of health care literature between 1970 and 1999 was original research and of this, only 51.6% involved nursing participants. Few studies examined the relationship between nursing leadership and patient outcomes. Most of the studies examining nursing leadership explored relationships between nurse leadership behaviors and nurse outcomes variables such as work environment, job satisfaction, productivity, intent to stay, and organizational commitment. Other studies collected data on nurse leaders' and staff nurses' perceptions of factors related to leadership success and effectiveness.

Nursing leadership is of central importance to the work environment of nurses. Havens and Aiken (1999) suggested that work environments that foster professional nursing practice in which nurses are encouraged to use their expertise and judgment are essential in increasing job satisfaction among clinical nurses. Nursing job satisfaction has been positively linked to quality patient outcomes (Gleason-Scott, Sochalski, & Aiken, 1999; McGillis Hall et al., 2001). A growing body of nursing research has identified that nurse leaders influence nurses' job satisfaction (Bratt, Broome, Kelber, & Lostocco, 2000; Irvine & Evans, 1995; McGillis Hall et al.; McNeese-Smith, 1995, 1997; Morrison, Jones, & Fuller, 1997), work empowerment (Klakovich, 1996; Laschinger, Wong, McMahon, & Kaufman, 1999), and work environments (Aiken et al., 2001; Clarke et al., 2001). Other studies suggest that nursing care affects patient outcomes (Scherb, 2002; Tourangeau, Giovannetti, Tu, & Wood, 2002), that nurses' work satisfaction relates to patient satisfaction (Weisman & Nathanson, 1985), and that nurses autonomy and participation in decision-making leads to improved patient outcomes (Aiken, Smith, & Lake, 1994; Anderson & McDaniel, 1999). However, few studies have explored the role of nursing leadership in shaping the environment to promote positive patient outcomes, although nursing leadership is critical in providing and managing the context, structure, human, and material resources that are necessary for effective patient care delivery systems (Fosbinder et al., 1999; Johnson, 1990; Perra, 2001). It is nursing leadership that creates the environment for professional practice (Dunham & Klafehn, 1990).

The criteria for selecting studies for this review included nursing leadership as an important variable in both patient and nursing related outcomes and the examination of nursing leadership as a distinct phenomenon. The keywords used in the search were *leadership*, *outcomes*, *managers*, and *administration*. These words were combined with the term *nurse* to limit the literature to sources relevant to nursing. A review of MEDLINE (1982-2003) and CINAHL (1982-2003) yielded a total of 171 relevant sources from which 97 theoretical and empirical studies were selected.

This chapter:

- Proposes a conceptual definition of *nursing leadership* based on the literature

- Presents the theoretical underpinnings of nursing leadership research

- Examines the way in which nursing leadership has been conceptualized, primarily relating to antecedent (external and internal environmental) factors that influence nursing leadership

- Critically examines the empirical evidence linking nursing leadership to specific interventions, focusing particularly on studies that relate nursing leadership to patient and nurse outcomes

- Discusses issues with the assessment of nursing leadership

- Reviews the approaches to measuring nursing leadership, giving consideration to the reliability, validity, and sensitivity of the nursing leadership instruments

- Recommends instruments to measure nursing leadership based on the research literature

- Identifies gaps in the literature and future research needs

9.2   Definition of the Concept of Leadership

"While the phenomenon of leadership has been extensively researched the concept of leadership remains elusive and definitions are difficult to obtain" (Holmes, 1991, p. 4). Vance and Larson (2002) found that the theoretical and operational definitions used in leadership studies were varied and frequently vague. Leadership has been described in various studies with a variety of conceptual models. As well, dimensions of leadership behaviors, leadership styles, and leadership practices are often used interchangeably by authors. Nursing leadership has been described as a set of learned behaviors comprising intrinsic traits and personalities inherent in the individual (Allen, 1998; Fagin, 1996). A number of studies examined leadership characteristics through the perceptions of leadership effectiveness (Dunham & Klafehn, 1990). Research has also indicated that nursing leadership is related to factors within an organization such as structure and culture (Stordeur, Vandenberghe, & D'hoore, 2000).

In the nursing literature, definitions of leadership have reflected either a focus on the leadership process or on the individual leader. Dunham & Klafehn (1990) defined leadership as an individual with decision-making capacity, shared values with nurses, a vision, and the ability to inspire others to work toward this vision. McCloskey and McCain (1987) and Huber et al. (2000) defined leadership as a process whereby the leader's role is to influence nurses to accomplish the goals of the organization. Dunham and Fisher (1990) defined nursing leaders as having excellent leadership attributes that included an administrative competence with adequate educational background, business skills, and clinical competence combined with a global understanding of leadership principles.

Fagin (1996) contended that nursing leaders are people who: (a) have demonstrated skill in managing, (b) influence others in the advancement of the profession, (c) possess interpersonal skills within and outside the discipline, (d) have impressive publications, and (e) maintain an imposing reputation. Cook (1999) defined a leader in nursing as a nurse directly involved in providing clinical care that continuously improves care and influences others.

The unique feature of the concept of nursing leadership is the complex relationship between leadership, nursing practice and patient care. Staff nurses identified that the most important characteristics of nursing leaders were experience, advanced knowledge, expertise, and clinical competence (Meighan, 1990). Dunham and Klafehn (1990) identified the need for nursing leaders to reflect on their leadership characteristics and be strategic with the application of their leadership style. McMillan and Conway (2002) contended that leadership resides in the ability to influence others and as such must be examined in terms of the person's capabilities, knowledge, and skills rather than specific behaviors of an individual.

9.3 Theoretical Underpinnings of Nursing Leadership

Many early theoretical models focused on individual characteristics or traits associated with effective leadership. Systematic research concerned with leadership theory first focused on the search for individual characteristics that universally differentiated leaders from nonleaders (House & Aditya, 1997). This attempt to identify universal traits associated with effective leadership led to the development of different theoretical perspectives related to traits. McClelland's Achievement Motivation Theory (McClelland, 1961), describes a high-achievement motivated individual as one who has the ability to set challenging goals, personally accepts responsibility for achieving goals, deliberately takes risks in pursuit of goals, and actively engages in performance evaluation through feedback. The theory implies that this behavior is innate in individuals and can be a predictor of effective leadership (House, 1991).

Taunton, Boyle, Woods, Hansen, and Bott (1997) included manager characteristics in a causal model of nurse retention and demonstrated that managers' consideration for staff, valuing their input, and supporting their personal development had a direct impact on retention. In a descriptive study, McNeese-Smith (1997) identified open communication, confidence, and a positive outlook as important nurse manager traits, which related positively to nurses' job satisfaction. The Charismatic Leadership Theory (House, 1977) described charismatic leadership traits as having extreme self-confidence, strong motivation to influence others, and a strong conviction in the moral correctness of their beliefs.

According to House and Aditya (1997), charismatic leaders are effective because they are associated with a sense of social responsibility and collective interests rather than with self-interest. Burns (1978) and Bass (1985) included charisma along with intellectual stimulation and individualized consideration as one of the major traits describing transformational leadership theory. While studies based on trait theories have identified a variety of traits contributing to effective leadership, the difficulties occur in the application of the theory to practice (House & Aditya). This may be due to the fact that leaders function in vastly different environments, and a variety of factors within these environments may influence a leader's effectiveness.

Following the trait theories, leaders were studied either by observing their behavior in laboratory settings or by asking individuals to describe the behavior of individuals in positions of authority and relating these descriptions to various criteria for leader effectiveness (House & Aditya, 1997). Fiedler's (1967) Contingency Theory of Leadership introduced situational variables as important influences on leadership characteristics and behaviors. Hersey and Blanchard (1988) developed a situational leadership theory that identified four leadership styles: telling, selling, participating, and delegating. The combinations of these behaviors produced either task or relationship behaviors. Task behaviors focus on providing direction about how to structure work whereas relationship behavior is characterized by two-way communication about work. The authors proposed that different situations required different styles. This leadership effectiveness model compared task versus relationship behavior of leaders, the environment in which leaders function, and the maturity of the group members. When nurses were given a list of 15 leadership traits in Meighan's (1990) descriptive study, the majority of traits they selected were traits of a relationship-oriented leader. Kouzes and Posner (1988) developed a theory of learned leader behaviors that explained how leaders achieved exceptional outcomes of follower motivation, loyalty, and performance. The Kouzes and Posner Leadership Model describes five competencies that correlate with leadership excellence including inspiring a shared vision, challenging the process, enabling others to act, modeling the way, and encouraging the heart. The popularity of this theoretical model is based on the principle that leadership is an observable and learned set of behaviors (Kouzes & Posner, 1988).

Leadership theories have primarily been concerned with the relationship between leaders and their immediate followers and have largely ignored the kind of organization and culture where leaders function, the relationships between leaders and superiors, external constituencies, peers, and the kind of product or service provided by the leaders' organization (House & Aditya, 1997). More recent research has attempted to study leadership within the context of organizational structure and culture. According to House and Aditya, leadership theories have focused excessively on superior–subordinate relationships to the exclusion of organizational and environmental variables that are crucial to effective leadership performance.

The ethnographic study conducted by Antrobus and Kitson (1999) used semi-structured interviews with 24 recognized nurse leaders to establish that effective nurse leaders operate as interpreters and translators—translating nursing issues between leadership domains and into a language of influence within an environmental context. According to Upenieks (2002), formal positional power along with informal power and access to resources within an organization contributed to leadership success. The results of Upenieks' (2003) qualitative study of recognized nurse leaders' perceptions of the value of their roles within organizations and the difference between roles and organizational settings suggested that organizations that focused on providing access to information, resources, support, and opportunity had the potential to enhance leadership. Upenieks (2003) suggested that nurse leaders could be more powerful and have more credibility if they learned how to think as professionals do in the business world.

Leatt and Porter (2003) believe that a strategic leadership style is critical for effective leadership. According to Leatt and Porter, important characteristics of a strategic leadership style include managing for tomorrow, not just today; involving people from all levels of the organization; building leaders throughout the organization; encouraging innovation and recognition of success; empowering and trusting others; and leading by example. Much of our understanding of leadership theory is not easily operationalized in the practical settings.

9.4 Factors that Influence Nursing Leadership

9.4.1 History

Nursing has a specific history and context that has influenced the development of nursing leaders. Nursing leadership has been strongly rooted in both religious and military backgrounds (Girvan, 1996a). Florence Nightingale was one of the first leaders in nursing and although she was widely acknowledged as having personal power, her ability to influence policy came from her close association with medicine (Girvan). Meighan (1990) contended that nursing's military roots supported leaders' use of control as a mechanism for achieving conformity in practice. The hierarchical structure of health care organizations has reinforced the need for this type of control resulting in the isolation of frontline nurses from decision-making related to patient care. Fosbinder et al. (1999) argued that the transition from command and control to new models of leadership has been a challenge. While nursing leadership has shifted from controlling nurses to empowering nurses to practice within the full scope of their profession, this has not been a simple process as it has occurred during times of tremendous change in health care organizations and ongoing concerns with the supply of and demand for nurses (Erickson, Hamilton, Jones, & Ditomassi, 2003).

Historically, nursing leaders were promoted from within organizations and while viewed as clinical experts, their management skills were often absent and, thus, their voices at the executive table were not often heard (Girvan, 1996a). Borman (1993) examined the positional and gender differences in hospital executives' role behaviors, values, and skills and reported that the socialization and mentoring experiences made available to nurses may have impacted on their exposure to and experience with the broad range of skills required at the executive level.

9.4.2 *Education*

Gelinas and Manthey (1997) identified that the learning needs and competencies required of nurse executives included having the ability to lead across cultural, functional, and departmental boundaries. Nursing leadership must facilitate change, be comfortable with constant change, have expertise in financial management, facilitate teamwork through team building, accept ambiguity, and manage personal growth (Gelinas & Manthey). Hartman and Crow (2002) conducted a survey of upper level managers to identify the strategic management skills and knowledge needs in health care organizations. Of the four major categories of learning needs identified, one related to the absence of skills required for strategic implementation, and another category identified the need for solid business and financial training.

The concept of future professional growth and mentoring of nurse leaders has been of considerable interest and concern. Stordeur et al. (2000) investigated the notion that when senior nursing leaders role-model transformational leadership behaviors in an organization, there is an increase in transformational leadership behaviors in lower level managers. The cascading effect of leadership behaviors was not supported in the study and suggested that there needed to be a purposeful and coordinated effort to provide leadership development and education to potential future nurse leaders. Dunham and Klafehn (1990) increased our awareness of the necessary balance between transformational and transaction leadership behaviors. The study identified the need for self-awareness and the need, as a nursing leader, to identify one's own learning needs, to improve upon one's leadership abilities, and to develop transformational leadership skills while reducing the dominance of transactional leadership behaviors. According to Fagin (1996), learning how to use one's leadership skills comes from testing various modes of behavior in small and large venues and finding what works, seeking to develop a new and wide repertoire of responses, and evolving a persona that has enough constancy to be recognizable as one's own individual leadership style while maintaining the flexibility to continue to develop.

Dunham-Taylor (1995) analyzed data collected from 1,990 nurse executive interviews exploring their perceptions of their strengths and weaknesses as leaders. The group that received the highest ranking identified themes of balance, always striving to improve, humility, and the description of leadership as a dynamic process. In comparison to the data collected from the other groups, the author suggested that there were stages of maturity that the nurse executives went through to develop competencies for transformational leadership behaviors. The results supported the idea that leadership competencies could be learned and suggested that preceptorship, mentoring, and education are key strategies for the development of future nursing leaders.

Weick, Prydun, and Walsh (2002) completed a study that identified desirable leadership traits as perceived by emerging and entrenched workforce members. The results suggested that the next generation of nursing leaders may have very different views on what constitutes effective leadership. As a workforce, Generation X has been well described in terms of career expectations, their emphasis on short-term employment, and their requirements for a positive work environment. Weick et al. suggested that leadership positions may not support the short-term career goals and lifestyle of the current generation of nurses. If this is true, there is an urgency for nurse researchers to identify effective leadership behaviors that can influence the learning environments that the emerging nursing workforce views as attractive places to work. If leadership positions are short-term goals then the development of leadership skills must begin earlier in undergraduate education programs. Mentoring must then become an important leadership behavior for nurse leaders in the 21st century.

9.4.3 Use of Self

In a study by Upenieks (2003), interviews were conducted with senior nursing executives who identified important "self" or personal traits for leadership effectiveness. The leaders in this study perceived that the ability to articulate the value of nursing to other organizational executive members and the ability to be a strong advocate for nursing was essential to leadership success. Upenieks established that a passion for nursing and the ability to articulate this passion to nurses and other administration team members were coupled with leadership effectiveness and support of nursing.

Other research has explored the characteristics of spirituality, emotional intelligence, and courage in relationship to leadership (Clancy, 2003; Goleman, 1995; Snow, 2001; Strack & Fottler, 2002; Wong & Law, 2002). Research has demonstrated a strong link between the success of an organization and the emotional intelligence of its leaders (Snow). Emotional intelligence (EI) is the capacity for recognizing our own feelings, others' feelings, and managing emotions in our relationships (Snow). Wong and Law reported that the EI of leaders affected worker satisfaction and extra role behaviors. This exploratory study was conducted using an EI measure developed by Wong and Law. The measure was tested on supervisor–subordinate dyads from a university setting and on 146 middle-level administrators in a government office. The authors contended that it was important for good leaders to have an understanding of their own emotions as well as the emotions of others. Leatt and Porter (2003) maintained that emotional competence directly impact on workplace characteristics and how people function in the workplace.

While there has been little research examining the influence of courage, Clancy (2003) argued that all leaders must have courage, as it is courage that allows leaders to hold true to their values and principles in decision-making. Cooper, Frank, Gouty, and Hansen (2003) surveyed the American Organization of Nurse Executives (AONE) about what they viewed as the ethical helps and challenges in their work environments. They rated their own personal moral values and standards as most helpful in dealing with ethical dilemmas (Cooper et al.). Clancy asserted that nurse executives faced ethical dilemmas around cost containment, safe staffing, and patient rights on a daily basis. Clancy also argued that courage may be an important link to ethical decision-making.

Strack and Fottler (2002) reviewed research examining the relationship between spirituality and leadership. Spirituality involves living according to one's beliefs, values, and practices. Consistency between beliefs and behaviors in leaders allows for effective relationships that are essential in today's environment. The research supported that effective leaders use spiritual wisdom, intelligence, and power to achieve organizational outcomes. Upenieks (2003) argued that there may be specific leader attributes that are more effective in creating environments that lead to positive outcomes for nurses.

9.4.4 *Organizational Structure and Power*

Structure and process variables within an organization are perceived by both staff nurses and nurse leaders to influence nursing leadership effectiveness. Stordeur et al. (2000) described the significant influences of organizational structure and culture on the leadership styles of nurse managers. The variation of leadership styles was explained primarily by the context of the organization. Upenieks' (2003) study of nurse leaders from both magnet and nonmagnet hospitals suggested that work environments that foster nurse satisfaction placed patients and nurses at the top of the hierarchical level. This study employed Kanter's Structural Theory of Organizational Behavior that depicted three sources of influence on the effectiveness of nursing leadership including: (a) the structure of power referring to access of information, support, and resources; (b) the structure of opportunity referring to increased role expectations, access to challenges, and advancement within the organization; and (c) the structure of proportion referring to the social arrangement of those in similar positions. Upenieks' study validated that access to power, opportunity, information, and resources created an empowered environment that produced a climate that fostered leadership success and enhanced levels of job satisfaction among nurses.

Upenieks' (2003) research provided excellent insight into the structures and behaviors of organizations and demonstrated how nursing leaders can use this knowledge to strategically increase their effectiveness. Upenieks suggested that nurse leaders could be more powerful and have more credibility among their peer executives if they learned how to think as professionals do in the business world. Wilson and Laschinger (1994) found that nurses' views about access to power and opportunity in their jobs depended on their perceptions of the nurse managers' influence within the organization.

Baumann et al. (2001) conducted a peer-reviewed research survey on nursing and work in addition to focus group interviews with managers, nurses, educators, government employees, and nursing association representatives. One of the purposes for this study was to identify effective solutions to improve the quality of the nursing work environment and ultimately patient outcomes. The authors concluded that nurses have limited power to influence change and limited participation in decision-making. Baumann et al. suggested that the reinstatement of formal nursing leadership positions with shared governance models and nursing practice committees would improve work environments.

A descriptive study by Manfredi (1996) concluded that the organization had a major influence on nursing leadership and described how the nurse manager operationalized leadership activities. Leadership activity has been influenced by the organization, and the priority for the organizational goals to be met has overshadowed the specific goals and interests of the nursing team. According to Manfredi, visions of nurse managers are a function of the organization and its existing circumstances.

9.4.5 *Organizational Redesign*

Nursing leadership has been greatly influenced by hospital restructuring in the 1990s. The role of nursing leadership in this restructured environment is dynamic, challenging, changing, and often uncertain (Davidson, 1996; Hartman & Crow, 2002). Gelinas and Manthey (1997) identified the impact of organizational redesign on nurse executive leadership, suggesting that nursing leaders have not only been changed by redesign but have been required to lead the redesign of clinical care, delivery systems, and integrated care. As health care organizations restructure, there is an increased emphasis on team-based interdisciplinary care. This necessitates the need for leaders who have the ability to work effectively across disciplines (Leatt & Porter, 2003).

The new leadership role requires new skill sets (Porter-O'Grady, 2003). Porter-O'Grady believes that there is a need for leaders who are able to help others see the need for change, challenge past practices, create a vision for the future, and construct new models of service delivery. In today's environment, nurse leaders require knowledge of nursing practice but also an understanding of regulatory issues as well as business skills, an understanding of risk and liability, strategic planning, and political acumen (Smith et al., 1994).

George, Farrell, and Brukwitzki (2002) argued that one of the key skills required by nurse leaders in restructured environments is the ability to cocreate a vision for the future. This requires leaders who are able to build trust within and among team members and across the organization (George et al.). The role of nursing leadership is to create an environment for professional nursing practice that supports positive client outcomes (Fosbinder et al., 1999; Upenicks, 2003). Leadership style, organizational context, and outcome performance need to be considered in any examination of leadership (Girvan, 1996b).

9.4.6 *Gender*

As nursing is a predominately female profession, gender may play a role in nursing leadership in health care organizations as the nurse executive is often the lone female on the executive team (Girvan, 1996b). Borman (1993) reported that there were gender differences in managerial values between male and female executives. Women do have a different approach to leading and affecting change. Borman and Biordi (1992) maintained that nurse administrators retain caring and connection as values. These are values that are at the core of nursing. They contend that these values are not part of the male value system. In Upenieks' (2003) review of the literature on the relationship between nursing leadership and gender, she reports that "significant levels of gender discord occur" (p. 142) in health care settings. Upenieks cited a study by Robinson and Walker in which 92% of respondents reported that gender plays a role in leadership and that it is easier for men to get promoted than for women. However, the majority of nursing leaders interviewed by Upenieks reported that they did not experience the effects of gender socialization and that their power was not less because they were female leaders.

In an ethnographic study, Rudan (2003) examined how men differ from women from the perspective of leader competence. He attended team meetings to observe leaders interacting with teams. His research supported that female leaders value relationships and connectedness, whereas men value individualism. He argued that the gender gap is narrowing; however, female leaders in health care must continue to communicate to others that they have the knowledge and skills required to lead.

It is clear that nursing leadership is affected by many complex and dynamic factors. However, Borman and Biordi (1992) argued that the health care environment is changing. In environments that are moving from bureaucratic structures to decentralized structures with an emphasis on quality patient care, nursing leaders with distinct knowledge of patient care and patient care issues become valuable members of the executive team (Borman & Biordi). Furthermore, nurse leaders practice from a caring value with a focus on relationship with people. This is paramount for leadership today and in the future.

9.5 Linking Nursing Leadership to Outcome Achievement

Much of the literature on nursing leadership is anecdotal with few qualitative studies and even fewer experimental studies (Cook, 1999; Girvan, 1996b). The studies that discuss the link between nursing leadership and patient outcomes are descriptive studies, as are the research studies examining the link between nursing leadership and nurse outcomes. Some of the current research examining this link includes correlational studies. Snow (2001) contended that nursing lags behind other industries in supporting research on the relationship between leadership and performance.

Researchers have begun to identify nursing leadership behaviors with a view of measuring these behaviors and linking them with nursing-sensitive patient outcomes. This has been an overwhelming challenge for nurse researchers due to the myriad of factors that influence patient care. In the current environment where there is an increased focus on the cost and quality of health care, nurses need to understand what is required of nursing leaders to promote positive patient outcomes. While there is increasing evidence linking nursing leadership with nurse outcomes, there is a dearth of research examining the role of nursing leadership and patient outcomes. Nevertheless, this type of research is essential as nursing leaders are ultimately accountable for the quality of patient care.

9.5.1 Nursing Leadership and Patient Outcome Achievement

George et al. (2002) described how the implementation of a shared leadership model led to increased staff leadership behaviors, autonomy, and improved patient outcomes. Shared leadership competencies include the ability to: (a) negotiate win-win solutions through team learning, (b) facilitate change and influence follower behaviors, (c) think and problem solve in a systems framework, (d) empower others to act responsibly through shared visioning, and (e) facilitate decision-making through a shared leadership paradigm. The intervention model used to demonstrate a direct link between the autonomous practice of nurses and the quality of patient outcomes was called the shared leadership concepts program (SLCP). The intervention was conducted on more than 700 nurses in one organized care delivery system. The program consisted of four 8-hour day modules delivered over a period of 2 months.

Three studies were completed between 1995 and 1999 to identify the outcomes of the SLCP intervention. The first study was a quasi-experimental pre-test–post-test design that examined the difference in self-perceptions of leadership behaviors among 30 expert nurses before and after the program (i.e., intervention). They reported that there was a significant difference in leadership behaviors following the program. The second descriptive pre-test–post-test study used

Kouzes and Posner's (1988) Leadership Practices Inventory to measure the use of leadership behaviors as perceived and observed by nurses preprogram and 6 months after the completion of the SLCP program. One hundred and forty nurses from more then five hospitals, off site clinics, and community programs in one organized care delivery system returned completed data. They reported statistically significant increases in both self-reported and observed leadership behaviors.

The third qualitative study utilized individual interviews with 24 randomly selected nurses during 1996 and 1997. The interviews were conducted at 3, 6, and 12 month intervals post completion of the SLCP program. Nurses reported increased personal self-growth as demonstrated by their acceptance of increased accountability for their practice. The nurses perceived that the leadership behaviors improved their ability to meet patient needs and promoted faster recovery, which improved the rapport and trust between nurse and patient and family and improved patient and family satisfaction with care. While nurses reported that increased workloads, high turnover, boring work, lack of responsibility, and insufficient management goal setting were barriers to utilizing their leadership skills, they also reported that they were more assertive in addressing these issues after participating in the SLCP program.

Houser (2003) used both qualitative and quantitative methodologies to study the contextual factors influencing the delivery of nursing care. The first component of the research consisted of a qualitative inquiry using focus group interviews with 36 nurses from an integrated delivery system. Transcripts of the focus groups were analyzed and interrater agreement of emerging themes was evaluated using Cohen's Kappa statistic for interrater agreement. The themes that emerged were leadership, staff expertise, staff stability, teamwork, financial resources, and workload. The nurses described elements of leadership style such as approachability, availability, role modeling, and inspirational behaviors. The most common desirable leadership behaviors were offering encouragement, excellent communication skills, ability to articulate clear expectations, and problem solving skills. There was also consensus regarding the need for a leader who is inspirational. Focus group participants identified a direct relationship between leadership effectiveness and low turnover of staff. Leadership was identified as a critical factor in the recruitment and retention of expert nurses (Houser).

Themes that emerged from the focus groups formed a factor model representing contextual effects on nursing-sensitive outcomes (Houser, 2003). This model was quantitatively tested in the second part of the study. The unit of analysis was the patient care unit. Forty-six patient care units in six nonteaching hospitals and three long-term care facilities were included in the sample population. Kouzes and Posner's (1988) Leadership Practices Inventory (LPI) was used to measure the leadership factors in the model. Nurse managers from each patient care unit and three randomly selected staff nurses reporting to each manager completed the LPI. Resulting scores indicated that strong leadership was related to higher levels of staff expertise and stability. Results also supported that there was an inverse relationship between strong levels of expertise and patient outcomes that included hospital-acquired pneumonia, hospital-acquired urinary tract infections, mortality, medication errors, and patient falls. The nurses in this study supported that strong leaders recruited and retained good nurses. Strong leaders contributed to positive patient outcomes by developing staff expertise and stability. As nursing staff become more competent and the number of competent and proficient nurses on a unit increases, the incidence of adverse events declines (Houser).

Anderson, Issel, and McDaniel (2003) examined the relationship between management practices and resident outcomes in 164 for-profit and nonprofit nursing homes in Texas. They surveyed directors of nursing (DONs) and registered nurses (RNs) about patterns of behavior in their organizations. Secondary data from the Medicaid Cost Reports and Texas Minimum Data Set were linked to primary data using a unique identifier. Anderson et al. hypothesized that open communication, participative decision-making, relationship-oriented leadership, and formalization in organizations would result in a lower prevalence of resident behavior problems as reflected by lower restraint use, decreased complications of immobility, and decreased fractures.

DONs and RNs completed a questionnaire about their perceptions of communication openness, participation in decision-making, and formalization (Anderson et al., 2003). RNs provided perceptions of relationship-oriented leadership. The resident outcomes examined were resident behavior, restraint use, complications of immobility, and fractures. The researchers found that larger facilities where there was an experienced DON with good communication skills resulted in lower use of resident restraints. Organizations where there was a DON with more experience, greater relationship-oriented leadership, and less formalization had a lower prevalence of complications of immobility. Organizations with a relationship-oriented leader had a lower prevalence of fractures.

The results suggested that certain characteristics of nursing leadership influenced resident outcomes (Anderson et al., 2003). The longer the director had been in the position, the lower the use of restraints within the organization. In addition, nursing leadership was related to lower prevalence of restraint use and complications of immobility. The authors suggested that the longer a person was in a position, the more knowledge and expertise they gained (Anderson et al.). This knowledge and expertise may impact on how nurse leaders communicate with staff and how this communication is received.

These studies support that there is a link between nursing leadership and patient outcomes; however, further research is required to extend our understanding of the link between nursing leadership and positive patient outcomes.

9.5.2 Nursing Leadership and Nurse Outcomes

Kramer and Schmalenberg (1988a, 1988b) found that one of the features that nurses cited as important to attract and retain nurses was having a chief nurse executive who had a strong position within the executive team. This feature along with nurse outcomes such as autonomy, control over practice, organization of clinical responsibilities at the unit-level, and a culture of valuing nursing knowledge has been supported by current research on the characteristics of magnet hospitals (Aiken et al., 2001).

McNeese-Smith (1995) discussed two studies that examined the perceptions of staff nurses regarding factors that they felt contributed to their job satisfaction, productivity, and commitment. This descriptive study was based on the results of earlier data collected by questionnaire that examined the impact of managers' leadership behavior on employee productivity, job satisfaction, and organizational commitment using the Kouzes and Posner's Leadership Model. The first study was conducted in two suburban, nonprofit, community hospitals, each with 250 beds. The second study was conducted in a large teaching hospital with 553 beds and many outpatient departments. In the first study, 41 managers and 610 employees who reported to the managers were invited to participate in a survey. The response rate was 77% (471). In the second study, 19 managers and 2,285 staff nurses were invited to participate in the study with a response rate of 77.5% (221). The results of the early data suggested that there were other factors besides leadership behaviors influencing the outcomes. Leadership behaviors accounted for only 9–15% of the variance for productivity, 11–27% of the variance for job satisfaction, and 16–29% for organizational commitment. In the second study, McNeese-Smith used semi-structured interviews of nurses in a large acute care teaching hospital to obtain responses related to the nurses' perceptions of factors influencing their job satisfaction, productivity, and commitment. Five nurses from each of six units for a total of 30 nurses were selected and interviewed individually. The most frequently discussed managerial behaviors that had a positive influence on the outcomes of job satisfaction, productivity, and commitment were recognition and thanks, meeting nurses' personal needs, mentoring, and the use of leadership skills such as sharing a vision, role modeling, empowering nurses, and open communication.

Medley and Larochelle (1995) conducted a descriptive study with staff nurses to examine if they were able to differentiate between transformational and transactional leadership and the relationship between leadership style and staff nurses' job satisfaction. They utilized the Multifactor Leadership Questionnaire to survey 278 randomly selected nurses from four acute care hospitals with bed capacities of 120–132. Results showed a significant positive relationship between head nurses exhibiting transformational leadership style and the job satisfaction of staff nurses. No significant relationship was demonstrated between transactional leadership style and job satisfaction.

Klakovich's (1996) work supported the findings of Kramer and Schmalenberg (1988a, 1988b). She found that registered nurses were more likely to be empowered if they perceived that there were higher levels of a constructive culture and if the leaders demonstrated a connective leadership style. The correlational study design explored combinations of relationships between variables using a registered nurse empowerment model to identify individual variables. Klakovich surveyed 113 RNs in an academic setting using the author-developed nurse empowerment model to determine the relative importance of each variable. Using stepwise regression; constructive culture, connective leadership, and defensive culture explained 45% of the variance in empowerment. Staff nurses were more likely to be empowered if they perceived high levels of constructive culture and low levels of defensive culture and if they were connective leaders.

Morrison and associates (1997) conducted a descriptive study in a regional medical center and invited 442 nursing department staff to participate. The response rate was 64% (275 staff). In this study, Bass' Multifactor Leadership Questionnaire was used to determine if transformational leadership influenced job satisfaction. The results of the study confirmed that leadership accounted for a significant amount of variance in job satisfaction, and transformational leadership behaviors were perceived by staff as empowering for them to work effectively. Transformational and transactional leadership styles were positively related to job satisfaction. Transformational leadership positively related to empowerment, and empowerment was positively correlated with job satisfaction. They also discovered that, regardless of the type of leadership style of nurse managers, nursing staff preferred that leaders take an active rather than passive leadership role. This study highlighted that leadership can be a significantly greater influence on job satisfaction than empowerment for specific nursing personnel.

Laschinger et al. (1999) conducted a descriptive study in a recently merged teaching hospital to test a model linking specific leader empowering behaviors to staff nurse perceptions of workplace empowerment. The authors surveyed a random sample of registered nurses. Staff nurses believed that their sense of workplace empowerment, job tension, and judgment of their ability to get their work done was related to their manager's use of empowering behaviors. Job stress was associated with absenteeism, errors in the workplace, poor quality care, lower productivity, and poor physical health.

Cook (1999) conducted a descriptive study involving semi-structured interviews with five nursing leaders who had been in director level positions for 5 to 15 years. One of the emerging themes was the unanimous agreement that effective leadership in nursing was a key factor for improving care. This research maintained that four factors impacted on and contributed to the dominant leadership style. These factors included experience, understanding, external environment, and internal environment.

In a cross-sectional survey study by Bratt et al. (2000), nursing leadership and job stress were the two most influential variables in the explanation of job satisfaction in pediatric intensive care unit nurses. The sample consisted of 1,973 staff nurses in pediatric critical care units in 65 institutions. Respondents stated that inadequate staffing coupled with high patient acuity compromised their ability to provide quality care.

Stordeur et al. (2000) completed a descriptive study using the Multifactoral Leadership Questionnaire to examine the impact of transformational leadership styles on nurses' satisfaction with their leader, extreme effort, and perceived unit effectiveness. The sample included 411 staff nurses, 41 head nurses, and 12 associate directors from eight hospitals. Only those hospitals whose respondents represented all hierarchical levels were included in the study. The results were significant and identified transformational leadership as a strong predictor of satisfaction with the leader, extra effort, and perceived unit effectiveness. Transformational leaders have a positive impact on nurses' perceptions by promoting autonomy and communicating a vision. This study supports the view that transformational leadership behaviors are associated with positive organizational outcomes.

Chiok Foong Loke (2001) examined the effect of leadership behaviors on employee outcomes using a descriptive study of nurses in one acute care hospital. The study explored the relationship between five leadership behaviors identified by Kouzes and Posner (1995) and the specific nurse outcome variables of job satisfaction, productivity, and commitment. Twenty nurse managers and 100 nurses were selected from a 1,600 bed acute care hospital in Singapore. Results showed that employee outcomes of productivity, job satisfaction, and organizational commitment were found to be statistically correlated with the manager's use of leadership behaviors. Regression analysis identified that leadership behaviors explained 9% of the variance for productivity, 29% of the variance for job satisfaction, and 22% of the variance for organizational commitment.

In a descriptive study by Upenieks (2003), 16 nurse leaders from four institutions were interviewed to determine nurse leaders' perceptions of the value of their role. Seven of the nurse leaders came from magnet hospitals with 300–400 beds and nine nurse leaders came from nonmagnet hospitals with 250–450 beds. Five factors contributing to leadership success emerged from the interviews including supportive organizational culture, organizational commitment to professional quality practice, leadership attributes of teamwork, business skills, and an ability to articulate the value of nursing. According to Upeniek, a positive magnet hospital culture does not naturally occur; it is created by a nurse leader who supports nursing excellence and professionalism. This study showed that the implementation of nursing practice models increased job satisfaction and, in addition, the successful implementation of nursing practice models was highly dependent on the manager's leadership skills in the change process.

Kramer and Schmalenberg (2003) described a study consisting of approximately 20 staff nurses from each of 14 magnet hospitals to: (a) ascertain staff nurses' concepts of autonomy, (b) empirically quantify autonomy, and (c) determine the relationship between degree of autonomy and staff nurses' rankings of quality of care on their units and their own job satisfaction. The results demonstrated a strong relationship between degree of autonomy and the nurses' rankings of job satisfaction and quality of care. Kramer and Schmalenberg suggested that autonomous nursing practice cannot exist without clinical competence and they identified nursing leadership as essential for the provision of opportunities for nurses to maintain clinical competence.

McGillis Hall et al. (2001) examined the impact of nursing staff mix models and organizational change strategies on patient, nurse, and system outcomes. This study was conducted in 19 teaching hospitals and included questionnaires, interviews, focus groups, and data collection from specific databases. Approximately 1,116 nurses were asked to provide their perceptions of the quality of nursing leadership in their organization. A subscale of Shortell et al.'s (1994) instrument was used to assess the degree to which unit nursing leadership sets and communicates clear goals and expectations and is responsive to changing needs and situations. Nursing leadership was found to have a statistically significant positive influence on nurses' job satisfaction and a statistically negative influence on nurses' perception of job pressure, job threat, and role tension.

Current multinational research provided further evidence that leadership along with sufficient resources and control over work environment was predictive of nurses' job satisfaction and retention and lead to better quality of care (Aiken et al., 2001; Clarke et al., 2001). This international collaborative utilized the Revised Nursing Work Index (NWI-R) to obtain measures about the practice environment of nursing and to explore other features of nurses' work (Aiken & Patrician, 2000; Sochalski, Estabrooks, & Humphrey, 1999). Embedded within this tool are questions about the presence of a chief nursing officer who is visible, accessible, and equal in power and authority to other top level executives (Aiken & Patrician; Lake, 2002).

In summary, the need for work environments that support nurses and promote positive patient outcomes has been articulated in the literature. In some studies, nursing leadership has been linked to several nurse outcomes including nursing job satisfaction, nurse empowerment, and a positive work environment. Nursing leadership has been widely discussed in terms of empowerment, job satisfaction, and work environments, and as a predictor of quality patient care. These research studies have confirmed the positive influence that effective leadership can have on nurses' performance and their subsequent impact on patient outcome achievement.

9.6   Issues in the Assessment of Nursing Leadership

The literature review identified several issues in the assessment of nursing leadership. These include the way in which models of leadership are conceptualized in nursing and the changing environment of nursing leaders.

9.6.1 Conceptual Models of Leadership

There are multiple constructs of the definition of nursing leadership that have made it difficult to measure the phenomenon. Some authors suggested that there were different outcomes of leadership and different aspects of leadership behavior that were more important than others. To date, assessment of nursing leadership has largely described the presence or absence of leadership characteristics, perceptions of the role of nursing leaders, and the impact of leadership on staff nurse job satisfaction, autonomy, and work environments.

According to Dunham and Klafehn (1990), transformational leadership has been characterized by the presence of charisma, individual consideration, and intellectual stimulation while transactional leadership has been characterized by contingent rewards and management by exception. The results of this study supported the view of Bass, Avolio, and Goodheim (1987), who stated that transformational leadership was not effective alone, but augmented the effects of transactional leadership.

McNeese-Smith (1995) examined the impact of managers' leadership behavior on employee productivity, job satisfaction, and organizational commitment. The study showed that the relationship between leadership behaviors and the outcomes of job satisfaction, productivity, and organizational commitment could not be separated. These results generated questions regarding the influence of factors other than leadership behaviors that influence outcomes.

Nursing leadership is a multifaceted construct and has been defined in relation to leadership behaviors, styles, and practices. Measurement based on one single model may not answer questions about the link between nursing leadership and patient outcomes.

9.6.2 *The Changing Environment for Nursing Leadership*

The dynamic nature of today's health care environment adds to the complexity of research on leadership. Health care has been identified as a complex business of relationships with providers, decision-makers, funders, and patients and their families (Mycek, 1998). In addition, technology and regulatory changes have involved ongoing adjustments in organizations (Hartman & Crow, 2002). In the current health care environment, there is a visible interdependence between administrative and clinical issues in health care as a result of economic pressures (Anderson & McDaniel, 2000). The effects of nursing leadership on patient outcomes have been shown to be indirect and multifactoral (Vance & Larson, 2002). Nursing leadership roles have changed and evolved with new titles and new reporting relationships (Gelinas & Manthey, 1997).

Weick, Prydun, and Walsh (2002) identified seven leadership characteristics that both entrenched and emerging nurses agreed were desirable in nursing leaders. Gleason-Scott et al. (1999) identified leadership traits in magnet hospitals that were very different from those found to be desirable in Weick et al.'s research. According to Weick et al., characteristics identified as desirable by the nursing staff in magnet hospital studies were found to be less important by current nursing staff. Although these results were from one study, the changing needs of the next generation of nurses highlights the imperative for researchers to establish positive significant links between leadership and outcomes.

Nursing leadership occurs in academic and practice settings. Nursing leadership is an important influence at all levels of the organization. The scope of nursing leadership roles are constantly expanding and evolving, which adds to the complexity of measuring nursing leadership and making comparisons across diverse settings.

9.7 Evidence Concerning Approaches to Measuring Leadership

There is a need to identify, quantify, develop, measure, and evaluate leadership competencies (Leatt & Porter, 2003). Huber et al. (2000) suggested that conducting "research and evaluating management interventions was problematic due to rapid changes; lack of staff with the capacity to design evaluation studies; and lack of reliable, valid, and practical measures of the salient independent and dependent variables for multiple and complex contextual variables" (p. 251). There is a need to examine the effect of important variables such as organizational structure, work environments, and the changing nursing workforce on the effectiveness of leadership performance. Conducting research on this indirect relationship in a changing, complex environment is challenging (Flood, 1994).

9.8 Nursing Measures of Leadership

The literature identified many instruments that have been used to measure leadership behaviors, but only those instruments that have been used with nurses are included in this review (see Table 9.1). While all leaders are required to influence people to achieve organizational goals, Leatt and Porter (2003) assert that health care environments are different due to the nature of client provider relationships, the complexity of patient care decisions, the impact of emerging technologies, patient safety, the issues associated with leading a professional workforce, the ongoing conflict between public–private funding, and the difficulty in measuring the success (outcomes) of care. Of the instruments used in research exploring nursing leadership, only a few were developed and tested for reliability and validity. Most of the research studies of nursing leadership have used interview techniques with author-developed questionnaires, self-report scales, and open-ended focus group discussions. The reliability and validity of these measurement tools have not been mentioned and they lack generalizabilty as they were developed to examine specific research questions. Many studies of nursing leadership have utilized a survey approach that elicits perceptions of leadership rather than leadership performance and effectiveness.

Table 9.1 Nursing Measures of Leadership

Instrument Author/Date of Publication	Target Population	Domains	Method of Administration	Reliability	Validity	Sensitivity to Nursing
LBDQ (Stogdill & Coons, 1957) (Stogdill, Goode & Day, 1962)	Group members in any organization.	40 item Likert-type scale with 12 subscales, describes the theory-based leaders behaviors along 2 dimensions: initiating structure and consideration.	Self-administered or administered to groups.	($\alpha = .83$ initiating structure, ($\alpha = .92$ consideration.	Construct: factor analysis supported 2 dimensions.	
LEAD self/other (Hersey & Blanchard, 1988a)	Leaders in any group.	Four types of theory-based leadership styles : telling, selling, participating & delegating along 2 dimensions – high/low task & high/low relationship; Consists of 12 situations and 4 optional actions.	Self-administered or administered to groups .	ITC – ranged from .11 to .52 (83% were above .25).	Criterion: each response met operationally defined criterion of < 80% with selection frequency. Face and content validity established.	Stability moderately strong over 2 administrations across 6-week interval.
Leadership Practices Inventory (LPI) (Kouzes & Posner, 1988)	Leaders in any group.	30 items, 10-point Likert scale with 5 categories: challenging the process, inspiring a shared vision, enabling others to act, modeling the way, & encouraging the heart. Assess actions and behaviors of leaders based on the theory.	Self-administered or observer assessment.	($\alpha = .73 - .79$ challenging the process; ($\alpha = .83 - .89$ inspiring a shared vision; ($\alpha - .70 - .86$ enabling others to act; ($\alpha = .72 - .81$ modeling the way; ($\alpha = .84 - .91$ encouraging the heart TRR = .93 challenging the	Construct: factor analysis supported 5 dimensions.	

ITC = item-total correlation (internal consistency)
α = Cronbach's alpha
TRR = test-retest reliability

Table 9.1 (continued)

Instrument Author/Date Publication	Target Population	Domains	Method of Administration	Reliability	Validity	Sensitivity to Nursing
				process; TRR = .94 inspiring a shared vision; TRR = .94 enabling others to act; TRR = .95 modeling the way; TRR = .93 encouraging the heart.		
Multifactoral Leadership Questionnaire (MLQ) (Bass & Avolio, 1990)	Leaders and managers in any group or organization.	Original instrument 80 item Likert-type 0-4, Updated version has 45 items and 12 subscales that measure leadership behaviors based on the theory: attributed charisma, idealized influence, inspirational leadership, intellectual stimulation, individual consideration, contingent reward, active management-by-exception, passive management-by-exception, laissez-faire leadership, extra effort, effectiveness and group satisfaction with the leader.	Self-administered or administered to groups.	α = .90 - .94	Construct: LISREL and partial least squares analysis – all reliabilities above .70.	

ITC = item-total correlation (internal consistency)
α = Cronbach's alpha
TRR = test-retest reliability

9.9 General Leadership Measures

9.9.1 *Leader Behavior Description Questionnaire (LBDQ)*

The Leader Behavior Description Questionnaire (LBDQ) was initially developed by Hemphill and Coons (1957) and was revised to reflect two dimensions of leadership behavior identified as consideration and initiation. Further revisions were made after the instrument was tested in empirical research in military organizations. New variables were identified based on the theory of role differentiation and group achievement (Stogdill, 1959). Stogdill, Goode, and Day (1962) revised the instrument a fourth time developing 12 subscales with component items representing a complex pattern of behaviors associated with the evolving leadership theory of role differentiation in social groups. The subscales were defined as representation, demand reconciliation, tolerance of uncertainty, persuasiveness, initiation of structure, tolerance of freedom, role assumption, consideration, production emphasis, predictive accuracy, integration, and superior orientation. The instrument can be self-administered or administered to groups. According to Stogdill (1963), reliability coefficients for the subscales were between .72 and .80 for initiating structure and .76 to .87 for consideration across nine separate nonnursing leader groups. For some subscales there was a greater range of reliability between leader groups. The lowest reliability coefficients appeared in corporation presidents in the representation, demand reconciliation, and role assumptions subscales—.54, .59, and .57 respectively. In a review of leadership instruments by McCloskey and Molen (1987), they reported that this instrument was the oldest and best-known measure of leadership; however, it has not been used in recent research studies of nursing leadership.

9.9.2 *Leader Effectiveness Adaptability Description (LEAD)*

The Leader Effectiveness Adaptability Description (LEAD) Instrument developed by Hersey and Blanchard (1988) employs 12 situations to assess leader behavior style, style range, and style adaptability (Hersey, Blanchard, & Johnson, 1996). This instrument is based on the situational leadership theory, which contends that no one leadership style is appropriate, but that effective leaders use leadership styles based on the abilities and willingness of employees. The four leadership styles reflect two dimensions including: (a) task behavior that involves one-way communication and (b) direction by the leader or relationship behavior that is characterized by two-way communication and encouragement and facilitation.

Hersey et al. (1996) asserted that all leaders have a primary style that is the behavior pattern that they use most frequently to influence others. In addition, some leaders have a secondary style that they use occasionally. There are two versions of the LEAD Instrument, the LEAD-Self and the LEAD-Other. The LEAD takes approximately 10 minutes to complete. Wolf (1996) reported that the internal consistency was reflected by 83% of the subscales items with a correlation of .25 or higher. The stability of the LEAD was moderately strong (Wolf).

Wolf (1996) utilized the LEAD-Self to evaluate a leadership training institute for nurse managers. Wolf found that participants in the 4-day program obtained short-term changes in primary leadership style and were more participative, follower-directed, and had improved two-way communication. However, the findings related to leadership adaptability were less clear. Participants who scored low on leadership adaptability on the pre-test experienced the greatest improvement following the training while participants who scored in the moderate range on admission demonstrated little improvement (Wolf).

9.9.3 *Multifactor Leadership Questionnaire (MLQ)*

The Multifactor Leadership Questionnaire (MLQ) was developed to assess leadership style and is based on the work of Bass (1985). The research found that successful leaders use a combination of transformational and transactional behaviors (Bass, Avolio, & Goodheim, 1987). The original instrument had 80 items. An updated version contains 45 items and 12 subscales (Huber et al., 2000). Leadership behaviors are measured using a 4-point Likert scale. The MLQ has an instrument for leader self-assessment as well as an instrument for completion by people who work with the leader. Five of the 12 leadership characteristics reflect transformational leadership qualities. These include attributed charisma, idealized influence, inspiration, intellectual stimulation, and individual consideration. Four characteristics are reflective of a transformational leadership style including contingent reward, active management by exception, passive management by exception, and laissez-faire (Cunningham & Kitson, 2000a). Morrison et al. (1997) cited a study where the MLQ had a high reliability with Cronbach alpha scores for the subscales of the instrument ranging from .67 to .93.

The MLQ has been widely used in research and recently it has been adapted and used for the assessment of nursing leadership in research studies (Cunningham & Kitson, 2000a, 2000b; Medley and Larochelle, 1995; Morrison et al., 1997). Medley and Larochelle (1995) utilized the MLQ to examine the relationship between transformational and transactional leadership style and staff nurses in an acute care setting. The MLQ was used by Morrison et al. (1997) to examine the relationship between nursing leadership style, empowerment, and job satisfaction in a regional medical center. Cunningham and Kitson (2000a, 2000b) reported on the use of the MLQ to evaluate a leadership development program aimed at improving clinical leadership capability for nurses. A pretest–post-test design was used and the MLQ was administered to leaders and persons reporting to that leader to detect changes in leadership capability. The authors reported that the MLQ was chosen because it offers a detailed breakdown of elements of transformational leadership (Cunningham & Kitson, 2000b). While they reported that problems were encountered with the length of the questionnaire and with the clarity of some of the questions, the tool was able to detect changes in the leadership behavior of nurses after the program (Cunningham & Kitson, 2000a). In this study the MLQ also showed that staff nurses reported a positive change in leadership styles.

9.9.4 Leadership Practices Inventory (LPI)

The Leadership Practices Inventory (LPI) was developed by Kouzes and Posner (1988) and is based on the theory that leadership is an observable and learnable set of practices. It was originally developed as an education tool for leadership development. More recently, it has been used to assess leadership practices in nursing research (Chiok Foong Loke, 2001; George, Burke, et al., 2002; Houser, 2003; McNeese-Smith, 1995; Tourangeau, Lemonde, Luba, Dakers, & Alksnis, 2003). The LPI has 30 items and measures leadership behaviors based on the leadership competencies of challenging the process, inspiring a shared vision, enabling others to act, modeling the way, and encouraging the heart. Six items measure each of the leadership practices using a 5-point Likert scale. This instrument takes approximately 10 minutes to complete. There are two versions of the LPI, a self-assessment and an observer assessment. Scores on the LPI have been relatively stable over time (Chiok Foong Loke; Tourangeau et al.). In addition, the scores have been found to be unrelated to demographic factors and organizational characteristics (Chiok Foong Loke). Kouzes and Posner (1995) reported Cronbach alpha scores on each of the subscales ranging from .71 to .85 for the LPI self-assessment and ranging from .82 to .93 for the LPI observer instrument.

The use of the LPI by Chiok Foong Loke (2001); George, Burke, et al. (2002); Houser (2003); and McNeese-Smith (1995, 1997) evaluated leadership behaviors that have been previously discussed in this chapter. Tourangeau et al. (2003) used the LPI to evaluate the effect of a 5-day residency program aimed at assisting aspiring and established nurse leaders to develop leadership knowledge, skills, and attitudes. Changes in leadership behaviors were more evident in observers' reports than self-reports. The authors maintained that it may take more time to see changes in our own behaviors.

9.9.5 Summary

Measurement of leadership represents a dilemma due to the lack of agreement about the meaning of the concept. Furthermore, the majority of instruments have been developed for use in fields other than nursing. The instruments presented in this review have established reliability and validity. In addition, the

MLQ, LPI, and LEAD instruments include both self and observer components. Hersey and colleagues (1996) contended that while self-perception is beneficial to leaders, in order to understand leadership style, information must be collected from the people who report to leaders so that leaders can understand how they influence people.

The leadership behaviors assessed in these instruments are behaviors that are required in nursing leaders. Wolf (1996) utilized the LEAD instrument and found that it may not be as effective in measuring the type of leaders that is required because of the focus on the two leader dimensions of task and relationships. The MLQ and the LPI may offer a more comprehensive approach to the measurement of the type of leadership behaviors and practices required of today's leaders.

It may be that the nursing profession does not require a unique tool to measure nursing leadership. The leadership behaviors and practices assessed in both the MLQ and LPI are behaviors that are required by nursing leaders to create work environments that promote nurse job satisfaction and empowerment. The evidence is beginning to demonstrate that these indicators produce positive patient outcomes. This is the goal of health care organizations.

9.10   Implications and Future Directions

Vance and Larson (2002) argued for the need for more research to inform the nursing profession on how leadership makes a difference in patient outcomes. There has been little research linking leadership styles and their effect on the quality of patient care and staff nurse effectiveness (Vance and Larson). Donabedian (1980) contended that structure is crucial in promoting the quality of care in organizations. Structure drives the process, which in health organizations is the delivery of care. Nursing leadership is a structural indicator that influences process variables within organizations and ultimately impacts on patient outcomes. Research on nursing leadership needs to capture leadership behaviors in relation to the process (nursing practice) and to patient outcomes. This review argues that it is difficult to operationalize leadership theories. For example, research has proven that educational interventions can increase the presence of leadership behaviors, but there is limited research to link these behaviors to improved patient outcomes. The LPI offers a more comprehensive approach to measuring leadership behaviors; however, further research is required to link these behaviors to positive outcomes that are sustainable over time.

Nursing leadership is responsible for establishing a strong nursing practice model, sustaining nurses as they learn to take accountability for their professional practice, building levels of trust, and improving communication among team members within organizations. Future research needs to establish clear links between effective nursing leadership and positive patient outcomes to ensure that the contribution of nursing to patient care is recognized.

9.11 References

Aiken, L. H., Clarke, S. P., Sloane, D. M., Sochalski, J. A., Busse, R., Clarke, H., et al. (2001). Nurses' report on hospital care in five countries. *Health Affairs, 20*(3), 43–53.

Aiken, L. H., & Patrician, P. A. (2000). Measuring organizational traits of hospitals: The revised nursing work index. *Nursing Research, 49*, 146–153.

Aiken, L. H., Smith, H. L., & Lake, E. T. (1994). Lower Medicare mortality among a set of hospitals known for good nursing care. *Medical Care, 32*, 771–787.

Allen, D. W. (1998). How nurses become leaders: Perceptions and beliefs about leadership development. *Journal of Nursing Administration, 28*(9), 15–20.

Anderson, R. A., Issel, L. M., & McDaniel, R. R. (2003). Nursing homes as complex adaptive systems: Relationship between management practice and resident outcomes. *Nursing Research, 52*, 12–21.

Anderson, R. A., & McDaniel, R. R. (1999). RN participation in organizational decision making and improvements in resident outcomes. *Health Care Management Review, 2*, 7–16.

Anderson, R. A., & McDaniel, R. R. (2000). Managing health care organizations: Where professionalism meets complexity science. *Health Care Management Review, 25*, 83–92.

Antrobus, S., & Kitson, A. (1999). Nursing leadership: Influencing and shaping health policy and nursing practice. *Journal of Advanced Nursing, 29*(3), 746–753.

Bass, B. M. (1985). *Multifactor Leadership Questionnaire.* Binghamton, NY: State University of New York.

Bass, B. M. & Avolio, B. J. (1990). *Transformational Leadership Development: Manual for the Multifactor Leadership Questionnaire.* Palo Alto, CA: Consulting Psychologists Press.

Bass, B. M., Avolio, B. J., & Goodheim, L. (1987). Biography and the assessment of transformational leadership at the world-class level. *Journal of Nursing Management, January,* 7–9.

Baumann, A., O'Brien-Pallas, L., Armstrong-Stassen, M., Blythe, J., Borbonnais, R., Cameron, S., et al. (2001). *Commitment and care: The benefits of a healthy workplace for nurses, their patients and the system.* A policy synthesis. Ottawa: Canadian Health Services Research Foundation and the Change Foundation.

Borman, J. S. (1993). Differences in hospital executives' leadership styles, managerial values, skills, and work–family conflict. *Nursing Administration Quarterly, 18,* 90–92.

Borman, J. S., & Biordi, D. (1992). Female nurse executives: Finally, at an advantage? *Journal of Nursing Administration, 22*(9), 37–41.

Bratt, M. M., Broome, M., Kelber, S., & Lostocco, L. (2000). Influence of stress and nursing leadership on job satisfaction of pediatric intensive care unit nurses. *American Journal of Critical Care, 9*, 307–317.

Burns, J. M. (1978). *Leadership.* New York: Harper & Row.

Chiok Foong Loke, J. (2001). Leadership behaviors: Effects on job satisfaction, productivity and organizational commitment. *Journal of Nursing Management, 9,* 191–204.

Clancy, T. R. (2003). Courage and today's nurse leader. *Nursing Administration Quarterly, 27*(2), 128–132.

Clarke, H. F., Laschinger, H. S., Giovannetti, P., Shamian, J., Thomson, D., & Tourangeau, A. (2001). Nursing shortages: Workplace environments are essential to the solution. *Hospital Quarterly, Summer,* 50–58.

Cook, M. J. (1999). Improving care requires leadership in nursing. *Nurse Education Today, 19,* 306–312.

Cooper, R. W., Frank, G. L., Gouty, C. A., & Hansen, M. M. (2003). Ethical helps and challenges faced by nurse leaders in the health care industry. *Journal of Nursing Administration, 33*(1), 17–23.

Cunningham, G., & Kitson, A. (2000a). An evaluation of the RCN clinical leadership development programme: Part 1. *Nursing Standard, 15*(12), 34–37.

Cunningham, G., & Kitson, A. (2000b). An evaluation of the RCN clinical leadership development programme: Part 2. *Nursing Standard, 15*(13), 34–40.

Davidson, D. R. (1996). The role of the nurse executive: In the corporation of health care. *Nursing Administration Quarterly, 20*(2), 49–53.

Donabedian, A. (1980). *Explorations in quality assessment and monitoring: Vol. 1. The definition of quality and approaches to its assessment.* Ann Arbor, MI: Health Administration Press.

Dunham, J., & Fisher, E. (1990). Nurse executive profile of excellent nursing leadership. *Nursing Administration Quarterly, 15,* 1–8.

Dunham, J., & Klafehn, K. A. (1990). Transformational leadership and the nurse executive. *Journal of Nursing Administration, 20*(4), 28–34.

Dunham-Taylor, J. (1995). Identifying the best in nurse executive leadership. Part 2: Interview results. *Journal of Nursing Administration, 25*(7/8), 24–31.

Erickson, J. I., Hamilton, G. A., Jones, D. E., & Ditomassi, M. (2003). The value of collaborative governance/staff empowerment. *Journal of Nursing Administration, 33*(2), 96–104.

Fagin, C. M. (1996). Executive leadership: Improving nursing practice, education and research. *Journal of Nursing Administration, 26*(3), 30–37.

Fiedler, F. E. (1967). *A Theory of Leadership Effectiveness.* New York: McGraw-Hill.

Flood, A. B. (1994). The impact of organizational and managerial factors on the quality of care in health care organizations. *Medical Care, 51,* 381–429.

Fosbinder, D., Parsons, R. J., Dwore, R. B., Murray, B., Gustafson, G., Daley, K., et al. (1999). Effectiveness of nurse executives: Measurement of role factors and attitudes. *Nursing Administration Quarterly, 23*(3), 52–62.

Gelinas, L. S., & Manthey, M. (1997). The impact of organizational redesign on nurse executive leadership. *Journal of Nursing Administration, 27*(10), 35–42.

George, V., Burke, L. J., Rodgers, B., Duthie, N., Hoffman, M. L., Koceja, V., et al. (2002). Developing staff nurse shared leadership behavior in professional nursing practice. *Nursing Administration Quarterly, 26*(3), 44–59.

George, V., Farrell, M., & Brukwitzki, G. (2002). Performance competencies of the chief nurse executive in an organized delivery system. *Nursing Administration Quarterly, 26*(3), 34–43.

Girvan, J. (1996a). Leadership and nursing: Part 1: History and politics. *Nursing Management, 3*(1), 10–12.

Girvan, J. (1996b). Leadership and nursing: Part 2: Styles of leadership. *Nursing Management, 3(2),* 20–21.

Gleason-Scott, J., Sochalski, J., Aiken, L. (1999). Review of magnet hospital research: Findings and implications for professional nursing practice. *Journal of Nursing Administration, 29*(1), 9–19.

Goleman, D. (1995). *Emotional Intelligence.* New York: Bantam Books.

Hartman, S. J., & Crow, S. M. (2002). Executive development in health care during times of turbulence. *Journal of Management in Medicine, 16,* 359–370.

Havens, D. S., & Aiken, L. H. (1999). Shaping systems to promote desired outcomes. The magnet hospital model. *Journal of Nursing Administration, 9*(2), 14–20.

Hemphill, J. K. & Coons, A. E. (1957). Development of the Leader Behavior Description Questionnaire. In R. M. Stogdill and A. E. Coons (Eds*). Leadership Behavior: Its Description and Measurement.* Columbus, OH: The Ohio State University.

Hersey, P., & Blanchard, K. (1988). *Leadership effectiveness and adaptability description.* San Diego, CA: Leadership Studies Inc.

Hersey, P., Blanchard, K. H., & Johnson, D. E. (1996). *Management of Organizational Behavior.* New Jersey: Prentice Hall.

Holmes, S. (1991). Clinical leadership: A role for the advanced practitioner. *Journal of Advances in Health and Nursing Care, 1*(3), 3–20.

House, R. J. (1977). A 1976 Theory of Charismatic Leadership. In J. G. Hunt and L. L. Larson (Eds). *Leadership: The Cutting Edge.* Carbondale, IL: Southern Illinois University Press.

House R. J. (1991). The distribution of power in organization: A MESO theory. *Leadership Quarterly 2*(1), 23–28.

House, R. J., & Aditya, R. N. (1997). The social scientific study of leadership: Quo vadis? *Journal of Management, 23*(3), 409–473.

Houser, J. (2003). A model for evaluating the context of nursing care delivery. *Journal of Nursing Administration, 33*(1), 39–47.

Huber, D. L., Maas, M., McCloskey, J., Scherb, C. A., Goode, C. J., & Watson, C. (2000). Evaluating nursing administration instruments. *Journal of Nursing Administration, 30*(5), 251–272.

Irvine, D. M., & Evans, M. G. (1995). Job satisfaction and turnover among nurses: Integrating research findings across studies. *Nursing Research, 44,* 246–253.

Johnson, L. J. (1990). Strategic management: A new dimension of the nurse executive's role. *Journal of Nursing Administration, 20*(9), 7–10.

Klakovich, M. D. (1996). Registered nurse empowerment. Model testing and implications for nurse administrators. *Journal of Nursing Administration, 26*(5), 29–35.

Kouzes, J. W., & Posner, B. Z. (1988). *The Leadership Challenge.* San Francisco, CA: Jossey-Bass.

Kouzes, J. W., & Posner, B. Z. (1995). *The Leadership Challenge: How to get Extraordinary Things Done in Organizations.* San Francisco, CA: Jossey-Bass.

Kramer, M., & Schmalenberg, C. (1988a). Magnet hospitals. Part 1: Institutions of excellence. *Journal of Nursing Administration, 18*(1), 13–24.

Kramer, M., & Schmalenberg, C. (1988b). Magnet hospitals. Part 2: Institutions of excellence. *Journal of Nursing Administration, 18*(2), 11–19.

Kramer, M., & Schmalenberg, C. (2003). Securing "good" nurse/physician relationships. *Nursing Management, 34*(7), 34–38.

Lake, E. T. (2002). Development of the practice environment scale of the nursing work index. *Research in Nursing and Health, 25,* 176–188.

Laschinger, H. K. S., Wong, C., McMahon, L., & Kaufman, C. (1999). Leader behavior impact on staff nurse empowerment, job tension, and work effectiveness. *Journal of Nursing Administration, 29*(5), 28–38.

Leatt, P., & Porter, J. (2003). Where are the healthcare leaders? The need for investment in leadership development. *Healthcare Papers, 4*(1), 14–31.

Manfredi, C. M. (1996). A descriptive study of nurse managers and leadership. *Western Journal of Nursing Research, 18,* 314–329.

McClelland, D. C. (1961). *The Achieving Society.* New York: Van Nostrand Reinhold.

McCloskey, J. C., & McCain, B. E. (1987). Satisfaction, commitment and professionalism of newly employed nurses. *Image, 19*(1), 20–24, 178.

McCloskey, J. C., & Molen, M. T. (1987). Leadership in nursing. In J. J. Fitzpatrick & R. L. Taunton (Eds.), *Annual Review of Nursing Research*, 5, 177–202.

McGillis Hall, L., Doran, D., Baker, G. R., Pink, G. H., Sidani, S., O'Brien-Pallas, L., et al. (2001). *A Study of the Impact of Nursing Staff Mix Models and Organizational Change Strategies on Patient, System and Nurse Outcomes.* Retrieved September 16, 2003, from www.nursing.utoronto.ca/lmcgillishall/research/completed-lead.html

McMillan, M., & Conway, J. (2002). Exploring nursing leadership. *Australian Journal of Advanced Nursing, 19*(4), 5–6.

McNeese-Smith, D. (1995). Job satisfaction, productivity, and organizational commitment, the result of leadership. *Journal of Nursing Administration, 25*(9), 17–26.

McNeese-Smith, D. K. (1997). The influence of manager behavior on nurses' job satisfaction, productivity and organizational commitment. *Journal of Nursing Administration, 27*(9), 47–55.

Medley, F. & Larochelle, D. R. (1995). Transformational leadership and job satisfaction. *Nursing Management, 26*(9), 64JJ–64NN.

Meighan, M. M. (1990). The most important characteristics of nursing leaders. *Nursing Administration Quarterly, 15,* 63–69.

Morrison, R. S., Jones, L., & Fuller, B. (1997). The relation between leadership style and empowerment on job satisfaction of nurses. *Journal of Nursing Administration, 27*(5), 27–34.

Mycek, S. (1998). Leadership for a healthy 21st century. *Health Care Forum Journal, July/August,* 26–30.

Perra, B. M. (2001). Leadership: The key to quality outcomes. *Journal of Nursing Care Quality, 15*(2), 68–73.

Porter-O'Grady, T. (2003). A different age for leadership, Part 2. *Journal of Nursing Administration, 33*(3), 173–178.

Rudan, V. T. (2003). The best of both worlds: A consideration of gender in team building. *Journal of Nursing Administration, 33*(3), 179–186.

Scherb, C. A. (2002). Outcomes research: Making a difference in practice. *Outcomes Management, 6*(1), 22–26.

Shortell, S. M., Zimmerman, J. E., Rousseau, D. M., Gillies, R. R., Wagner, D. P., Draper, E. A., et al. (1994). The performance of intensive care units: Does good management make a difference? *Medical Care, 32*(5), 508–525.

Smith, P. M., Parsons, R. J., Murray, B. P., Dwore, R. B., Vorderer, L. H., & Wallock Okerlund, V. (1994). The nurse executive, an emerging role. *Journal of Nursing Administration, 24*(11), 56–62.

Snow, J. L. (2001). Looking beyond nursing for clues to effective leadership. *Journal of Nursing Administration, 31*(9), 440–443.

Sochalski, J., Estabrooks, C. A., & Humphrey, C. K. (1999). Nurse staffing and patient outcome: Evolution of an international study. *Canadian Journal of Nursing Research, 31*(3), 69–88.

Stogdill, R. M. (1959). *Individual Behavior and Group Achievement.* New York: Oxford University Press.

Stogdill, R. M. (1963). *Manual for the Leader Behavior Description Questionnaire-Form XII: An experimental revision.* Columbus, OH: The Ohio State University.

Stogdill, R. M. & Coons. (1957). *Leader Behavior: Its Description and Measurement.* Bureau of Business Research, University of Ohio.

Stogdill, R. M., Goode, O. S., & Day, D. R. (1962). New leader behavior description subscale, *Journal of Psychology, 54,* 259–269.

Stordeur, S., Vandenberghe, C., & D'hoore, W. (2000). Leadership styles across hierarchical levels in nursing departments. *Nursing Research, 49,* 37–43.

Strack, G., & Fottler, M. D. (2002). Spirituality and effective leadership in health care: Is there a connection? *Frontiers of Health Services Management, 18*(4), 3–18.

Taunton, R. L., Boyle, D. K., Woods, C. Q., Hansen, H. E., & Bott, M. J. (1997). Manager leadership and retention of hospital staff nurses. *Western Journal of Nursing Research, 19*(2), 205–226.

Tourangeau, A. E., Giovannetti, P., Tu, J. V., & Wood, M. (2002). Nursing-related determinants of 30-day mortality for hospitalized patients. *Canadian Journal of Nursing Research, 33,* 71–88.

Tourangeau, A. E., Lemonde, M., Luba, M., Dakers, D., & Alksnis, C. (2003). Evaluation of a leadership development intervention. In press.

Upenieks, V. (2002). What constitutes successful nurse leadership? A qualitative approach using Kanter's theory of organizational behavior. *Journal of Nursing Administration, 32*(12), 622–632.

Upenieks, V. (2003). Nurse leaders' perceptions of what comprises successful leadership in today's acute care environment. *Nursing Administration Quarterly, 27,* 140–152.

Vance, C., & Larson, E. (2002). Leadership research in business and health care. *Journal of Nursing Scholarship, 32*(2), 165–171.

Weick, K. L., Prydun, M., & Walsh, T. (2002). What the emerging workforce wants in its leaders. *Journal of Nursing Scholarship, 34*(3), 283–288.

Weisman, C. S., & Nathanson, C. A. (1985). Professional satisfaction and client outcomes: A comparative analysis. *Medical Care, 23*(10), 1179–1192.

Wesorick, B. (2002). 21st century leadership challenge: Creating and sustaining healthy, healing work cultures and integrated service at the point of care. *Nursing Administration Quarterly, 26*(5), 18–32.

Wilson, B., & Laschinger, H. K. (1994). Staff nurse perception of job empowerment and organizational commitment. A test of Kanter's theory of structural power in organizations. *Journal of Nursing Administration, 24*(2), 39–47.

Wolf, M. S. (1996). Changes in leadership styles as a function of a four-day leadership training institute for nurse managers: A perspective on continuing program evaluation. *The Journal of Continuing Education in Nursing, 27*(6), 245–252.

Wong, C., & Law, K. S. (2002). The effects of leader and follower emotional intelligence on performance and attitude: An exploratory study. *The Leadership Quarterly, 13*, 243–274.

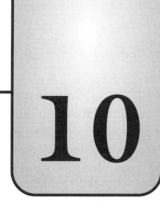

Overtime

Donna Thomson

10.1 Introduction

Overtime is a growing issue for both nurses and the organizations that employ them. Nurses have always been expected to work overtime during emergency situations but in recent times overtime has been used more frequently, often to cover known absences. The Canadian Labour and Business Centre (2002) reports that Canadian nurses work almost a quarter of a million hours of overtime every week. This is the equivalent of 7,000 full-time jobs per year (Canadian Nurses Advisory Committee [CNAC], 2002). This figure will increase significantly in the future unless strategies are implemented to address the predicted shortage of nurses.

Views on overtime vary depending on the particular discipline examining the issue. In general, nurses tend to view overtime negatively and the recommendations generated by the CNAC (2002) Report are aimed at reducing overtime hours for nurses. Increasing overtime is not unique to Canadian nurses. As early as 1979, Hollman reported that U.S. statistics indicated that one out of every four full-time American workers (27.4%) worked overtime. Hollman indicated that managers can not avoid the issue of overtime and must consider the impact of overtime on the quantity and quality of work and the effect on staff morale. He also suggested that improper assignment of overtime and excessive overtime can lead to grievances and poor management–employee relations.

In the United Kingdom, one in three nurses reported working the equivalent of one shift per month of unpaid overtime and one in six reported working more than two shifts per month (Wing, 1999). The American Nurses Association has been lobbying for legislation that prohibits the use of mandatory overtime (Whittaker, 2003). Whittaker indicates that several states have now enacted legislation that address overtime, although the approach may vary across states. For example, some American states limit the amount of overtime that nurses can work (e.g., New Jersey), some require that overtime be voluntary (e.g., Washington), and others simply require the development of policies and procedures regarding overtime utilization (e.g., Texas). In contrast to the perspective of nurses, economists and labor relations professionals sometimes view overtime positively as they view overtime in terms of maximizing productivity and reducing organizational costs.

This chapter:

- Provides an overview of the issues and challenges related to the measurement of overtime

- Reviews the factors that influence the use of overtime

- Discusses the impact of overtime on service cost and quality

- Examines the effect of overtime on the nurses who work overtime hours

The literature search included health care, economic, management, human resource, labor, and operations journals to find published literature on overtime from numerous perspectives. These searches produced 57 articles comprised of quantitative studies, several literature reviews, and meta-analysis. Many were opinion articles only. Sample sizes varied as some reported individual data and others used a group of workers as the study unit.

10.2   Definition of the Concept of Overtime

Overtime most often refers to hours worked in excess of 40 hours in an employee's regularly scheduled workweek. However, overtime can also be interpreted as hours above and beyond the planned workday. For example, a part-time nurse may be booked to work 8 hours but required to stay at work for an additional hour or two. While this nurse may not work more than 40 hours in a week, the unplanned extra work can still create havoc with her or his home life and add to the nurse's feelings of job strain due to loss of control.

10.3   Theoretical Underpinnings of Overtime

Economic models are often used to study overtime. Easton and Rossin (1997) argued that from an economic perspective overtime should be used when the prorated hourly per capita expense per employee exceeds the hourly premium for overtime. It is expected that the per capita cost will increase in the future and may contribute to the growing use of overtime. Easton and Rossin determined that the per capita cost was 26% at the time of their study as compared to 50% for premium pay and concluded that, for the moment, there must be other factors driving the use of overtime.

Hancock, Pollock, and Kim (1987) demonstrated that planned overtime in health care services could reduce labor costs and improve productivity. They suggested that overtime contributed to productivity by increasing the flexibility of scheduling models. Researchers have demonstrated using tour scheduling mathematical models that increased flexibility in the deployment of human resources can increase performance (Mabert & Showalter, 1990). The constraints imposed by full-time arrangements fall into three broad categories: shift constraints, day-off constraints, and tour constraints (Bechtold & Jacobs, 1990). Because overtime hours are not bound by these constraints, there is potential to increase performance through the use of planned overtime hours (Jacobs & Bechtold, 1993).

Economic theory examines overtime using supply, demand, and marginal cost theories. The Law of Demand states that as demand increases relative to supply the willingness to pay a higher price for a product or service will increase. In times of supply shortages such as the current state of the nursing profession, it is likely that employers will be more willing to pay for overtime than if the supply of nurses were not limited. Economists believe that most individuals will make rational maximizing decisions. That is, when there are alternate courses of action an individual will make the choice that provides them with the greatest utility. Marginal analysis looks at the additional cost of adding another unit. While the cost of adding another hour of care at overtime means that the marginal cost is increased, in comparison to the cost of adding more staff this may be acceptable.

While economic theory may have explained the rationale for the use of overtime, and mathematical models for staffing may have assisted in scheduling decisions, neither approach has incorporated the effect of overtime on employee fatigue, absenteeism, and accidents (Thomas, 1992). Overtime has been linked to lower productivity, high absenteeism, and fatigue (Akerstedt, Fredlund, Gillburg, & Jansson, 2002; Akerstedt, Knutsson et al., 2002), and high workers' compensation claims rates (Shamian et al., 2001). Overtime costs correlate highly with costs of sick time ($r = .928$, $p < .01$; O'Brien-Pallas, Thomson, Alksnis, & Bruce, 2001).

In order to fully understand the concept of overtime, it should be examined within a conceptual model. Many nurse researchers have used systems models that consider structure, process, and outcome in the context of external environments to explore the relationship between different constructs related to nurses and their work environment. Overtime can easily be examined within these models, but little formal research on overtime has been conducted to date. This approach would allow us to gain a greater understanding of the factors that determine overtime levels and the impact of overtime on multiple outcomes related to nurses, patients, and the health care system as a whole.

10.4   Factors that Influence the Use of Overtime

The Fair Labor Standards Act implemented in 1938 forms the legal foundation for overtime payments in the United States (King, 1997). This act was designed to ensure the fair distribution of work during a time when many were unemployed. Currently, the issue, at least within the nursing profession, is the limited number of nurses available to meet the demand for nursing services. As the supply of nurses decreases, the supply of overtime available for and demanded of nurses will increase.

10.4.1 Unpredictable Worker Demand–Supply

In the past, the use of overtime has generally been discouraged and viewed as a poor management practice. This has been largely due to the perception that overtime reduces productivity and increases costs. Overtime hours are generally paid at time and one-half or double time and tired workers are assumed to be less productive. In fact, there are many other factors that must be considered in relation to overtime utilization. Typically, overtime is considered a necessary buffer for short-term increases in demand or shortages in supply. The only way to avoid overtime completely is to always staff to a level that can meet the highest level of demand. Organizations can not afford to staff at these levels and even if the financial resources are available, human resources are currently scarce. Many organizations would have difficulty finding sufficient nurses to fill the number of full-time positions that would be required to meet these demands. In addition, this approach would be very inefficient and costly as staff would be underworked on many days. As a result, organizations use part-time workers to meet the known variations in supply such as predictable staff shortages (e.g., vacation, statutory holiday relief, and vacancies) and predictable demand variations (e.g., seasonal events and operating room schedules). Overtime is usually limited to unpredictable events related to supply (e.g., absenteeism) and unpredictable demand (e.g., sudden change in patient volume or acuity) when there is an imbalance for a short period of time. In some health care settings, such as the emergency department and labor and delivery suite, the demand will always be uneven and unpredictable. In these situations, overtime utilization is an accepted strategy as the demand for nursing services can not be delayed without sacrificing the quality of care. Unlike manufacturing organizations, service organizations cannot back-order demand requests.

10.4.2 Contractual Limitations

Although many union contracts provide explicit language on the payment and allocation of overtime, few address the maximum hours of overtime that can be required. Easton and Rossin (1997) suggested that this may be related to the desire of management to maintain staffing flexibility, and to some extent, employee's desire to have an opportunity to increase their income. Some contractual arrangements require a nurse to remain at work until relieved by another nurse. When an operating room case runs late, or the emergency department has a sudden influx of ill patients, staff are required to remain until it is considered safe to leave. Nurses have traditionally accepted this professional responsibility to work overtime despite their personal–family plans and individual wishes. However, in recent times the use of mandatory overtime has evolved to include situations where management has not been able to fill a known vacancy or to replace an absent nurse. Mandatory overtime has been a major factor in lengthy, high-profile nurses' strikes in Massachussetts, California, and New York (MassNurse, 2000).

10.4.3 Nurse Shortages

There are strong feelings that mandatory overtime should be used only as a last resort to provide patient care (Coughlin, 2001). When managers are not able to fill vacant positions or unpredictable absences with part-time staff, they should consider other alternatives such as the use of agency staff, part-time staff on other units, or posting of planned overtime. Staff who want to work voluntary overtime can select it, and this allows them to make appropriate arrangements to meet this demand. Full-time staff who are off duty should be offered the opportunity for voluntary overtime before those who are already at work are required to work mandatory overtime. In June 2000, the American Nurses Association House of Delegates overwhelmingly agreed that the use of overtime should be reserved for true emergencies and that refusal to work excessive overtime does not constitute patient abandonment (Worthington, 2001). One must consider that the use of planned overtime to reduce the need for human resources limits is affected by the amount of overtime each full-time worker is willing or able to work, and the fact that the organization's reserves to meet short-term demand fluctuations due to absenteeism and short-term unpredictable increases in demand will be depleted. However, managers are often reluctant to hire new employees until they are sure that the increased need will remain constant. They must weigh the cost of overtime against the costs associated with new hires and the potential for future overstaffing. Hiring new labor is not a perfect substitute for expanding the hours of existing workers as new workers are less productive due to lack of experience (Hollman, 1979). While overtime may raise the marginal cost of labor as many union contracts require payment at time and a half, firms may in fact benefit from greater short-term productivity as increases in demand can be met with less investment than the addition of extra workers.

10.4.4 Unpredictable Environment

A recent examination of Ontario hospital data for 1998/99 suggested that an estimated $171 million was spent on overtime hours for inpatient nurses, while close to $39 million was spent on inpatient nurses' sick time (O'Brien-Pallas et al., 2001). Overtime and absenteeism have diverted needed financial resources that could be reallocated to improve regular staffing and reduce the ratio of patients assigned to each nurse (O'Brien-Pallas et al.). This study was undertaken during a period when hospitals were downsizing staff. Gunderson (2001) stated that organizations will be reluctant to add full-time employees with high fixed costs when the market is unpredictable. He suggested that organizations will try to avoid hiring new employees due to the high cost associated with their hiring and potential layoffs. In addition, when there are cost constraints, organizations will attempt to amortize the fixed costs related to hiring new employees over a greater number of hours. Organizations may be willing to pay overtime premiums or pay high salaries for "commitment" even though others are unemployed or underemployed (Gunderson, p. 435). This is a plausible explanation for the high use of overtime during the restructuring period in Canada. The effect of this strategy on nurses was demonstrated in a quote from one of the surveys in the 1998 study of more than 8,000 Ontario nurses reported by Dunleavy, Shamian, and Thomson (2003), "People are working full-time and doing overtime and coming in on their days off and getting really sick" (p. 4).

10.4.5 Wage Levels

The demand for overtime by nurses is most likely related to wage levels. As the relative income of nurses decreases they may be more willing to work overtime. Idson and Robins (1991) suggested that economic incentives have a significant effect on workers' overtime decisions. A recent report on the income of nurses indicated that four nurses in one province earned more than $100,000 when the average wage was $52,000, and another 35 earned between $70,000 and $96,000 (CBC Saskatchewan, 2002). Carol Ringer of Regina Health District indicated that overtime allows nurses to achieve their financial goals (CBC Saskatchewan).

10.4.6 Inadequate Information

Unplanned overtime may occur when the information required to develop staffing patterns that meet demand is not readily available. Demand for nurses is generally a function of patient volume and acuity. The number of patients served by a nursing unit is general knowledge to all who work on the unit, but patient acuity is harder to define. Workload information can be extremely valuable in determining staffing needs as most workload measurement systems describe the volume of nursing resources required by measuring the patient needs for care, support, and case coordination. Unfortunately, few organizations produce workload information on a shift-by-shift, day-by-day basis in a format that can be used by nurse managers to adapt staffing schedules to meet known demand patterns. Management information systems providing relevant data to support decisions can provide nurse managers with a better understanding of the relationship between patient activity, staffing, and costs.

10.5 Linking Overtime Utilization to Outcome Achievement

10.5.1 Overtime Utilization and Nurse Outcomes

The amount of time people spend at work is an important measure of quality of life (Robinson & Bostrum, 1994). Sparks, Cooper, Fried, and Shirom (1997) found 21 studies with results that indicated significant positive mean correlations between overall health symptoms and hours of work. Duchon, Smith, Keran, and Koehler (1997) stated that overtime has been linked to three basic manifestations of fatigue: decrements in behavioral performance, physiological functioning, and subjective complaints. Worthington (2001) outlined three areas of concern related to overtime: prolonged exposure to hazards, fatigue, and stress. Fatigue can cause injuries. The odds of a high registered nurse (RN) lost-time claim rate increased by 70% for each quartile increase in the percentage of RNs reporting more than one hour of overtime per week (odds ratio [OR] = 1.70, $p < .01$) in a study involving more than 8,000 Ontario nurses (Shamian, O'Brien-Pallas, Thomson, Alksnis, & Kerr, Under Review). Hanecke, Tiedemann, Nachreiner, and Grzech-Suklo (1998) found exponentially increasing accident risk beyond the ninth hour and many nurses routinely work 12-hour shifts so overtime is well beyond this threshold.

In addition to accidents, work overload and long hours can lead to health problems such as smoking, high stress levels, and cardiovascular disease (Spurgeon, Harrington, & Cooper, 1997). In a Japanese study of men, weekly work hours were related to progressively increased odds ratios of acute myocardial infarction (Liu & Tanaka, 2002). In a previous study with similar findings this was attributed to the fact that the 24-hour high blood pressure of the overtime group was higher than for the control group (Hayashi, Koboyashi, Yamaoka, & Yano, 1996). Overtime is related to both sleep problems and fatigue (Akerstedt, Frelund, Gillberg, & Jansson, 2002). Overwork can also affect workers' stress levels. Workers who had higher levels of perceived constraints worked overtime or reported higher levels of job stress (Ettner & Grzywacz, 2001). These findings of physical and mental health relationships to overtime substantiate the significant correlations between health symptoms and the ability to refuse overtime reported by Schmitt, Colligan, and Fitzgerald (1980). However, Voss, Floderus, and Diderichsen (2001) found that overtime was linked to low levels of absence.

Babbar and Aspelin (1998) stated that overwork contributes not only to poorer worker health, but also disrupts family relationships. Overtime takes a toll not only on workers but on their families, their communities, and their clients. Longer hours of work make it difficult to balance the conflicting demands of home and work (Golden & Jorgensen, 2002). Sparks et al. (1997) found 12 qualitative studies that supported the link between long hours and both personal and family suffering. It is particularly worrisome when overtime is involuntary. Employees are the firm's most important resources and it is important that they not feel treated as prisoners at work (Babbar & Aspelin).

10.5.2 Overtime Utilization and Organizational Outcomes

Harrington (2001) suggested that evidence that longer work days translate into poorer performance and higher accident rates is lacking. In response to the European Community Directive related to the legal right to refuse more than 48 hours of work per week, the United Kingdom had also argued that there was no convincing evidence that hours of work should be limited on health and safety grounds. They suggested that most studies looked at health effects, primarily cardiac and mental health disorders, and there were few systematic investigations of performance effects or the effect of occupational exposure. Spurgeon and colleagues (1997) countered that the onset of fatigue is the most obvious direct result of working long hours. They cited a study from the manufacturing sector where the reduction in overtime showed no reduction in production and a fall in absenteeism, and in another study, there was a 3% rise in production. Numerous studies conducted during World War I showed a 6% increase in production from 10-minute rest periods. Spurgeon et al. indicated that these studies had been replicated many times and it was difficult to find evidence that long working hours are beneficial to either the employees or the efficiency of the organization.

Wruck (1990) argued that the current employment act reduced the scheduling flexibility that many organizations, like hospitals, needed to function efficiently. Similarly, Ruland and Ravn (2003) described how the use of an information system designed to provide decision support for nurse managers in financial management, resource allocation, and activity planning demonstrated a 41% reduction in overtime.

10.5.3 Overtime Utilization and Patient Outcomes

There are few documented studies specifically examining the effect of overtime utilization on patient outcomes. Most focus on the direct cost of overtime premium payments. During short periods of demand and supply imbalances, one might hypothesize that overtime would have a positive effect on patient outcomes. Nurses working overtime hours ensure that there are sufficient numbers of nurses to provide patient care and to avoid overwork for the nurses on that shift. In one study by Rosa (1995), in addition to increases in back injuries and a threefold increase in accident rates after 16 hours of work, there was also an increase in hospital outbreaks of bacterial infection associated with overtime. What we do not know is the level of overtime that will lead to errors that have a negative effect on patient outcomes or reduced productivity as nurses become overtired.

10.6   Issues in the Assessment of Overtime

10.6.1 Definitional Issues

Most overtime figures are derived from survey or payroll data that record the amount of overtime worked without providing a concise definition. In some employee surveys the total worked hours are requested and compared to a general standard. Overtime rates are most often calculated by comparing the amount of overtime to the expected number of worked hours per week. Due to the Fair Labor Standards Act, most U.S. articles define overtime as worked hours greater than 8 hours per day or more than 5 days per week (Easton & Rossin, 1997). From a cost perspective, overtime may be paid in other circumstances depending on union contracts. For example, a nurse may be paid overtime for consecutive weekends, less than defined turnover between shifts, and missed breaks. Health care organization need to address these aspects of overtime in order to avoid unproductive expenditures. From a nursing worklife perspective, this type of overtime contributes to nurse stress and dissatisfaction with working conditions even though the total hours may not be in excess of the usual standard for measuring overtime. In addition, secondary data does not capture unpaid overtime. Some organizations may report little paid overtime because nurses are working less than the amount of time defined for payment in their contract. However, 15 minutes per day of unpaid overtime each day can have a significant impact on the quality of worklife.

In all reports examined for this chapter the overtime data were viewed in aggregate form with no analysis of the distribution of overtime across individual respondents. When employers respond to surveys, they are likely using payroll data that would include only paid overtime whereas employees are more likely to include all overtime whether paid or not. As with all surveys, respondents may have hidden agendas that may bias the data in either direction. When nurse surveys are used to elicit the amount of overtime worked, the answers may be very different.

In a study by Shamian et al. (2001), RNs were asked to report separately how many hours per week, on average, that they worked paid and unpaid overtime. These two values were added together to create a "total overtime" variable. For those who reported no value for paid or unpaid overtime, zero hours were assumed. This item was converted to a hospital-level variable by calculating the percentage of RNs reporting more than 1 hour of total overtime per week at each hospital. The percentage of RNs reporting more than 1 hour of overtime per week was higher among hospitals with high claim rates. The regression showed that the probability of having a high RN lost-time claim rate increased by 70% for each quartile increase in the percentage of RNs reporting more than 1 hour of overtime per week. Similarly, the probability of having a high RN lost-time claim rate increased by 61% for each quartile increase in the percentage of RNs reporting more sick occasions than the national average. Consistent with Kristensen's (1999) model, the need to reduce demands that exceed the resources of the individual (e.g., workload, staffing, and overtime) and the need for a return to a basic degree of predictability (e.g., job security and freedom from injury and abuse in the workplace) take a high priority if lost-time claims of any type are to be reduced.

There is often no differentiation between voluntary and involuntary overtime. Some nurses may elect to work overtime in an effort to increase their income. This voluntary overtime may have very different effects than involuntary overtime where the nurse has no control over the decision. This differentiation cannot be captured in administrative databases and it is rarely asked in nurse surveys.

10.6.2 Measurement Issues

Routine collection of unpaid overtime would be excessively burdensome for health care organizations. These incidences are most often short and unrecorded. In addition, some organizations may have large amounts of paid overtime that are not captured. This occurs when employees elect to take time off in lieu of paid overtime. Often this information is recorded in a log book on the nursing unit, and when the staff take the time off it is simply recorded as regular worked hours.

Rones, Lig, and Gardner (1997) found that estimates of the length of the workweek from employer-based surveys count the number of jobs held by workers, so the averages are actually reported per job and not per worker. These databases typically lack demographic information that is critical to understanding workweek trends. Robinson and Bostrum (1994) found that a time diary approach to measuring time actually worked revealed fewer hours than estimated by the employee. Among workers claiming to work more than 55 hours per week, the gap was 10 hours; simply asking for estimates and taking them at face value would lead to serious overestimates.

10.7   Evidence Concerning Approaches to Overtime Utilization

Deleire, Bhattacharya, and Macurdy (2002) discussed the issues with comparing overtime across sectors and overtime within the same sector. They compared two large U.S. surveys that measured similar industries but used a different sampling methodology and set of exclusions. It was found that if a survey asked for the hours of overtime, the percentage of time that was overtime sometimes varied depending on the regular length of hours in a workday and the number of hours worked per week. The effect of overtime was also influenced by the distribution of overtime across employees within the organization. Only a few employees could account for a large proportion of overtime.

10.8   Nursing Measures of Overtime

Overtime is generally perceived by nurses as paid hours at a premium rate excluding shift differential, for example, working additional hours beyond the scheduled shift length on a given day or working on a scheduled day off. Nurses are often paid overtime rates for consecutive weekends or when time between shifts is less than mandated in their contractual agreement. These hours may not actually exceed the 40 hour per day or 5 day per week maximum, but may be reported as overtime due to the pay premium. Overtime utilization compared across hospitals may provide misleading results as some organizations have 8-hour shifts and others have 12-hour shifts. These factors can influence our perception of the effect of overtime on costs and staff behaviors.

10.9   Implications and Future Directions

Across Canada, nurses have reported that overtime expectations, whether mandatory or voluntary, are key worklife issues they face daily (Baumann et al., 2001).

Clearly, when overtime hours are used as a regular staffing strategy, particularly if the overtime is mandatory, nurses experience more job strain. As Baumann et al. summarized, research across occupations suggests that long periods of job strain affect personal relationships and increase sick time, conflict, job dissatisfaction, turnover, and inefficiency. The magnitude of the influence of overtime on high RN claim rates is important. Requesting staff to work overtime is a management decision but the findings of this and other studies suggests that the financial implications of these choices may be greater than previously identified (O'Brien-Pallas et al., 2001). Not only are employers facing the prospect of higher payrolls due to overtime premiums as well as pay for sick time and replacement staff but, as this study suggests, they may also be paying higher insurance premiums. Other negative consequences associated with high injury claim rates are the loss of productive hours of nursing care as well as the pain and suffering that nurses may experience.

Health care funders and professional organizations need to consider strategies to capture an accurate measurement of both voluntary and involuntary overtime on a regular basis. In 2001, the Ontario government added overtime reporting to the financial and statistical reporting requirement for public hospitals (Ontario Ministry of Health and Long-Term Care, 2002). This data is reported quarterly and will be available for researchers in the near future; however, this will be payroll data only, with the inconsistency noted above and a large amount of overtime unreported. Unpaid overtime may have a different effect than paid overtime on employees and organizations.

Few studies have examined overtime using theoretical models that incorporate all of the components of the work environment. Overtime must be examined in light of the internal and external factors using a theoretical framework to test hypotheses. A comprehensive cost–benefit analysis of overtime needs to be conducted. A study that includes the cost of absenteeism, orientation of additional staff, claims rates, and the relative productivity of overtime nurses and new nurses to full-time staff working regular hours needs to be conducted. It is important to determine whether there are differences in the effects of voluntary and involuntary overtime on the health and productivity of nurses. It is also important to determine what level of overtime shows a reduction in the cost of care and what level of overtime has an effect on the quality of care.

The definition of overtime might be more appropriately worded as, "Any hours that a nurse works beyond those which were originally scheduled whether paid or unpaid, voluntary or involuntary." While payroll systems accurately capture the total cost of overtime, these payroll systems need to create different pay codes to capture different types of overtime in order to truly understand their effect on the worklife of nurses and to develop strategies to reduce cost. Each type of overtime may require a different approach.

Future research on overtime should address the following issues:

- A more inclusive measure of overtime and differentiation between different types of overtime

- Measurement of overtime due to missed breaks

- A methodology to capture unpaid overtime and overtime paid in time off

- Contract overtime not related to excess hours

- The difference between voluntary and involuntary overtime on nurse outcomes

- A better understanding of the full cost of overtime and how it compares to the full cost of higher staffing levels

- The impact of overtime on patient outcomes

10.10   References

Akerstedt, T., Fredlund, P., Gillburg, M., & Jansson, B. (2002). Work load and work hours in relation to disturbed sleep and fatigue in a large representative sample. *Journal of Psychosomatic Research, 53,* 585–588.

Akerstedt, T., Knutsson, A., Westerholm, P., Theorell, T., Alfredsson, L., & Kecklund, G. (2002). Sleep disturbances, work stress and work hours—A cross-sectional study. *Journal of Psychosomatic Research, 53,* 741–748.

Babbar, S., & Aspelin, D. (1998). The overtime rebellion: Symptom of a bigger problem? *The Academy of Management Executive, 12*(1), 68–76.

Baker, A., Heiler, K., & Ferguson, S. (2003). The impact of roster changes on absenteeism and incidence frequency in an Australian coal mine. *Occupational and Environmental Medicine, 60,* 43–49.

Baumann, A., O'Brien-Pallas, L., Armstrong-Stassen, M., Blythe, J., Bourbonnais, R., Cameron, S., et al. (2001). *Commitment and care: The benefits of a healthy workplace for nurses, their patients and the system.* Ottawa: Canadian Health Services Research Foundation.

Bechtold, S., & Jacobs, L. (1990). Implicit modeling of flexible break assignments in optimal shift scheduling. *Management Science, 36,* 1339–1351.

Blaumol, W., Blinder, A., & Scarth, W. (1988). *Economics: Principles and policy* (2nd ed.). Toronto, Canada: Harcourt Brace Jovanovich.

Canadian Labour and Business Centre. (2002). *Full-time equivalents and financial costs associated with absenteeism, overtime, and involuntary part-time employment in the nursing profession.* Ottawa, Canada: Author.

Canadian Nurses Advisory Committee. (2002). *Our health, our future: Creating quality workplaces for Canadian nurses.* Ottawa, Canada: Author.

CBC Saskatchewan. (2002). *Nursing shortage leads to high overtime bills.* Retrieved May, 1, 2003 from CBC Saskatchewan Web Site: www.sask.cbc.ca

Coughlin, C. (2001). Professional responsibility versus mandatory overtime. *Journal of Nursing Administration, 31*(6), 290–292.

Deleire, T., Bhattacharya, J., & Macurdy, T. (2002). Comparing measures of overtime across BLS surveys. *Industrial Relations, 41,* 362–369.

Duchon, J., Smith, T., Keran, C., & Koehler, E. (1997). Psychophysiological manifestations of performance during work on extended shifts. *International Journal of Industrial Ergonomics, 20*, 39–49.

Dunleavy, J., Shamian, J., & Thomson, D. (2003). Handcuffed by cutbacks. *Canadian Nurse, 99*(3), 23–26.

Easton, F. F., & Rossin, D. F., (1997). Overtime schedules for full-time service workers. *Omega International Journal of Management Science, 25*, 285–299.

Ehrenberg, R. (1970). Absenteeism and overtime decision. American Economic Review, 60(3), 352–357.

Ehrenberg, R., & Schumann, P. (1984). Compensating for wage differentials for mandatory overtime. *Economic Inquiry, 22*, 460–477.

Employment Policy Foundation. (2000). *The true story behind overtime hours:* Issue Backgrounder, October, Washington DC: Author.

Ettner, S., & Grzywacz, J. (2001). Worker's perceptions of how jobs affect health: A social ecological perspective. *Journal of Occupational Health Psychology, 6*(2), 101–113.

Golden, L., & Jorgensen, H. (2002). *Time after Time: Mandatory overtime in the U.S. economy.* Briefing paper. Washington DC: Economic Policy Institute.

Gunderson, M. (2001). Economics of personnel and human resource management. *Human Resource Management Review, 11*, 431–452.

Hancock, W., Pollock, S., & Kim, M. (1987). A model to determine staffing levels, cost and productivity of hospital units. *Journal of Medical Systems, 11*, 319–330.

Hanecke, K., Tiedemann, S., Nachreiner, F., & Grzech-Suklo, H. (1998). Accident risk as a function of hours at work and time of day as determined from accident data and exposure models for the German working population. *Scandinavian Journal of Work and Environmental Health, 24*(3), 43–48.

Harrington, J. M. (2001). Health effects of shift work and extended hours of work. *Occupational and Environmental Medicine*, 58, 68–72.

Hayashi, T., Koboyashi, Y., Yamaoka, K., & Yano, E. (1996). Effect of overtime work on 24-hour ambulatory blood pressure. *Journal of Environmental Medicine, 10*, 1007–1011.

Hollman, R. (1979). Employee preferences for overtime. *Human Resource Management*, 24–31.

Idson, T., & Robins, P. (1991). Determinants of voluntary overtime decisions. *Economic Enquiry, 29*(1), 79–91.

Indran, S., Gopal, R., & Omar, A. (1995). Absenteeism in the workforce, Klang Valley, Malaysia: Preliminary report. *Asia Pacific Journal of Public Health, 8*(2), 109–113.

Jacobs, L., & Bechtold, S. (1993). Labour utilization effects of labour scheduling flexibility alternatives in a tour scheduling environment. *Decision Science, 24*, 148–166.

Jamal, M. (1986). Moonlighting: Personal, social, and organizational consequences. *Human Relations, 39*, 977–990.

Kawakami, N., Araki, S., Takatsuka, N., & Shimizu, H. (1999). Overtime, psychosocial working conditions, and the occurrence of noninsulin-dependent diabetes mellitus in Japanese men. *Journal of Epidemiology and Community Health, 53*, 359–363.

King, S. (1997). Oligopoly and overtime. *Labour Economics, 4,* 149–165.

Kristensen, T. (1999). Challenges for research and prevention in relation to work and cardiovascular diseases. *Scandinavian Journal of Work, Environment and Health, 25,* 550–557.

Liu, Y., & Tanaka, H. (2002). Overwork, insufficient sleep, and risk of non-fatal acute myocardial infarction in Japanese men. *Occupational and Environmental Medicine, 59,* 447–451.

Mabert, V., & Showalter, M. (1990). Measuring the impact of part-time workers in service organizations. *Journal of Operations Management, 9,* 209–229.

MassNurse. (2000). *MNA Labour Cabinet helps draft federal proposal bill would ban mandatory overtime for health care workers.* News article.

O'Brien-Pallas, L., Shamian, J., Thomson, D., Alksnis, C., Koehoorn, M., Kerr, M. et al. (Under Review). Work-related disability among nurses: Impact of job stress, hospital organizational factors, and individual characteristics.

O'Brien-Pallas, L., Thomson, D., Alksnis, C., & Bruce, S. (2001). The economic impact of nurse staffing decisions: Time to turn down another road? *Hospital Quarterly, 4,* 42–50.

Ontario Ministry of Health and Long-Term Care. (2002). *Ontario Hospital Reporting System Version 5.0.* Toronto, Canada: Author.

Pauly, M., Nicholson, S., Xu, J., Danzon, P., Murray, J., & Berger, M. (2002). A general model of the impact of absenteeism on employers and employees. *Health Economics, 11,* 221–231.

Proctor, S., White, R., Robins, T., Echeverria, D., & Rocskay, A. (1996). Effect of overtime on cognitive function in automotive workers. *Scandinavian Journal of Work Environment and Health, 22,* 124–132.

Robinson, J., & Bostrum, A. (1994). The overestimated workweek? What time diary measures suggest. *Monthly Labour Review, August,* 11–23.

Rones, P., Lig, R., Gardner, J. (1997). Trends in hours of work since the mid-1970s. *Monthly Labour Review, Apr.,* 3–12.

Rosa, R. (1995). Extended work shifts and excessive fatigue. *Journal of Sleep Research, 4*(2), 51–56.

Ruland, C. M., & Ravn, I. H. (2003). Usefulness and effects on costs and staff management of a nursing resource management information system. *Journal of Nursing Management, 11,* 208–215.

Schmitt, N., Colligan, M., & Fitzgerald, M. (1980). Unexplained physical symptoms in eight organizations: Individual and organizational analyses. *Journal of Occupational Psychology, 53,* 305–317.

Shamian, J., O'Brien-Pallas, L., Kerr, M., Koehoorn, M., Thomson, D., & Alknis, C. (2001). *Effects of job strain, hospital characteristics, and individual characteristics on work-related disability among nurses.* Toronto, Canada: Workman's Compensation and Insurance Board.

Shamian, J., O'Brien-Pallas L., Thomson D., Alksnis, C., & Kerr, M. S. (Under Review). Nurse absenteeism, stress and workplace injury: What are the contributing factors and what can–should be done about it? *Sociology and Social Policy.*

Smith, D. S., Rogers, S. H., Hood, E. R., & Phillips, D. M. (1998). Overtime reduction with the press of a button. An unexpected outcome of computerized documentation. *Nurse Case Management, 3*(6), 266–270.

Sparks, K., Cooper, G., Fried, Y., & Shirom, A. (1997). The effects of hours of work on health: A meta-analytic review. *Journal of Occupational and Organizational Psychology, 70,* 391–408.

Spurgeon, A., Harrington, J., & Cooper, C. (1997). Health and safety problems associated with long working hours: A review of the current position. *Occupational and Environmental Medicine, 54,* 367–375.

Thomas, R. (1992). Effects of scheduled overtime on labour productivity. *Journal of Construction Engineering and Management,* 118, 60–76.

Voss, M., Floderus, B., & Diderichsen, F. (2001). Physical, psychological and organizational factors relative to sickness absence: A study based on Sweden Post. *Occupational Environmental Medicine, 58,* 178–184.

Whittaker, S. (2003). From overtime to understaffing: The ANA works with states to secure nurse-friendly legislation. *American Journal of Nursing, 103*(2), 29.

Wing, M. (1999). Nursing makes you sick. *Nursing Times, 95*(7), 24–25.

Worthington, K. (2001). The health risks of mandatory overtime. *American Journal of Nursing, 101*(5), 96.

Wruck, E. (1990). Overhauling overtime standards. *Health Progress, Sept.,* 32–37.

Yaniv, G. (1995). Burnout, absenteeism, and the overtime decision. *Journal of Economic Psychology, 16,* 297–309.

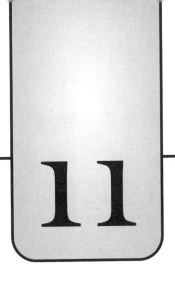

Absenteeism

Donna Thomson

11.1   Introduction

Little attention has been paid to the long-range effects of absenteeism on the effectiveness of the health care system. In the short run, absenteeism diverts essential financial resources away from the provision of patient care, thereby reducing our ability to meet the demand for nursing care. In the long run, an unhealthy work environment may drive some nurses to leave the nursing market to seek better employment opportunities and deter others from entering nursing as a profession. In the upcoming era of nurse shortages, these potential effects on recruitment and retention cannot be ignored. In addition, nurse absenteeism may have an effect on patient outcomes.

Absenteeism is one of the major contributors to rising health care costs. Johnson, Croghan, and Crawford (2003) conducted a review of sickness absence management in the context of the health care sector in the United Kingdom stating that employee absenteeism is an expensive and difficult problem for the National Health Service (NHS). They felt that the many and diverse causes of sickness absence need acknowledgement when devising strategies that can effectively provide solutions to the problems of sickness absence. Few countries maintain databases on absenteeism. In fact, without a public health system governments have no access to this information. In the years prior to cost containment efforts, both financial and human resources data were plentiful, and information on nurse absenteeism was kept within hospitals. More often than not, any absenteeism data has been based on employer or employee surveys. The impending shortage of nurses and the need to curtail health care expense has generated an interest in nursing absenteeism that has not been seen in the past. In some countries, nurses have the highest prevalence of illness and days lost among professionals and other working groups both within and outside the health care industry (Akyeampong, 1999b). The nature of this absenteeism varies from a single missed day to long-term disabilities. Nurses can experience both physical and stress-related illnesses. Some of the illnesses are work-induced and may trigger workers' compensation claims.

Despite the lack of quantitative absenteeism data, nurse researchers have focused on the cost and causes of absenteeism from an organizational and nurse perspective. In the United States there has been an interest in how governance and the organizational structure of nursing affect nurse absence behavior (Aiken, Clarke, & Sloane, 2002; Zelauskas & Howes, 1992). In Germany there have been studies on the effect of the nurses' perceptions of effort and reward (Bakker, Killmer, Siegrist, & Schaufeli, 2000). In the Scandanavian countries there has been a greater emphasis on the physical health related causes of absenteeism (Akerlind, Alexanderson, Hensing, Liejon, & Bjurulf, 1996; Boumans & Landeweerd, 1999, Ekberg & Wildhagan, 1996; Hemingway, Shipley, Stansfeld, & Marmot, 1997; Josephson, Lagerstrom, Hagberg, & Wigaeus Hjelm, 1997, Lagerstrom, Hansson, & Hagberg, 1998). In Canada, work environment and stress have been explored (Bruce, Sale, Shamian, O'Brien-Pallas, & Thomson, 2002; Laschinger, Shamian, & Thomson, 2001) along with the impact of restructuring (Burke & Greenglass, 2000) and cost (O'Brien Pallas, Thomson, Alksnis, & Bruce, 2001) as they relate to absenteeism. Downsizing and restructuring have been key drivers of absenteeism research in many countires. In Australia, the introduction of mandatory nurse–patient ratios has resulted in a decrease in absenteeism and turnover (Parish, 2002). In the Netherlands absenteeism was associated with the introduction of a 36-hour, 4-day workweek (Dzoljic, Zimmerman, Legemate, & Klazinga, 2003). In Germany a study of absenteeism focused on the difference between experienced nurses and trainees (Wenderlein, 2003) while another looked at the effect of low morale on absenteeism (Haw, Claus, Durbin-Lafferty, & Iversen, 2003).

This chapter will provide an overview of the issues and challenges related to the measurement of absenteeism, identification of the factors that contribute to absenteeism, and recommendations regarding future research.

The literature outlined in this chapter includes publications found in major databases, major publications in business management, human resources, psychology, sociology, and nursing. Review and meta-analytical articles were used to identify additional articles, and reference listings from retrieved publications were used to find additional articles. Overall, this literature search yielded 157 articles including 65 empirical studies that have been outlined. Both individual and group research studies were included as well as several theoretical papers. The articles were not restricted to nursing so that information could be learned from the findings in other fields.

11.2   Definition of the Concept of Absenteeism

Martocchio and Harrison (1993) defined absenteeism as the lack of a physical presence at a given setting and time when there is a social expectation to be there. *Days absent* and *occasions absent* are the most frequent measures of absenteeism (Hendrix & Spencer, 1989). Johns (1984) suggests that absenteeism is an observable behavior rather than a construct but that absenteeism may reflect constructs such as equity or withdrawal. There are two types of absenteeism noted in the literature: (a) innocent absenteeism and (b) culpable absenteeism. Innocent absenteeism refers to employees who are absent for reasons beyond their control, such as sickness and injury. Innocent absenteeism is not culpable, which means that the absence is blameless. In contrast, culpable absenteeism refers to employees who are absent without authorization for reasons that are within their control. For the large majority of employees, absenteeism is legitimate, innocent absenteeism, which occurs infrequently (Benefits Interface, Inc., 2000).

11.3   Theoretical Underpinnings of Absenteeism

The best discussion on the various theories used in absenteeism research was provided by Johns (1994). He describes eight distinct models for absence behaviors:

- The Withdrawal model describes absenteeism related to job satisfaction and organizational commitment.

- The Demographic model describes age, gender, and tenure associated with absenteeism.

- The Medical model describes how health behaviors such as smoking and alcoholism affect absence.

- The Stress model describes high work demands unrelated to job satisfaction.

- The Social and Cultural model describes how absence culture and norms influence individual absence rates.

- The Conflict model describes how absenteeism reflects unorganized conflict between management and employee.

- The Deviance model describes absenteeism as a product of negative traits at odds with the norm.

- The Economic model describes how individuals work only when the marginal rate of substitution of income for leisure is equal.

Few absenteeism researchers have conducted their research employing a conceptual framework, but many have defined the hypotheses about the relationships they expect to find. Several studies have tested components of the complex causal model presented by Brooke and Price (1989) that includes demographic and situational variables. Some researchers have studied absenteeism in the context of Karasek's (1979) job demands/decision latitude model (Blank & Diderichsen, 1995), Hackman and Oldham's (1975) job characteristics model (Landeweerd & Boumans, 1994), or a variation of Grey-Toft and Anderson's (1981) climate-stress model (Hemingway & Smith, 1999; Sui, 2002) to assess the effect of the workplace on absenteeism. Zboril-Bensen (2002) used Nicholson's degree of freedom model to assess individual decisions to be absent. Future research would benefit from a more formalized approach to the study of absenteeism. It must be considered in the context of the work environment and the external forces that can influence the behavior of the employee. For example, there have been anecdotal suggestions that some nurses are working in two locations and calling in sick at one location while working at the other in order to increase income.

11.4   Factors that Influence Absenteeism

From this review of the literature, the factors that contribute to absenteeism appear to be a combination of individual employee factors and characteristics of the workplace. Individual factors that have been cited include age, gender, experience, and nurses' health and stress. Organizational factors include job category, level of supervisor support, amount of overtime worked, the size and type of the organization, the type of nursing unit, the content of work, and organizational climate and controls.

11.4.1 Individual Factors

11.4.1.1 Demographic Information Including Age, Gender, and Experience

It has been postulated that the aging nurse workforce may be contributing to the current high rates of absenteeism; however, there is little information to support this hypothesis. Many of the studies on absenteeism, both in nursing and other sectors, controlled for age rather than using it as an independent variable. Few nursing studies were found that addressed the issue of age. A study of nurses in

Hong Kong suggested that age was a predictor of absenteeism in only one of the samples (Sui, 2002). In a study of hospital workers, Zavala, French, Zarkin, and Omachonu (2002) found that partial absenteeism (e.g., arriving late), but not total absenteeism, was a function of age and suggested that the longer the exposure to work, the more absenteeism events will occur.

There are a number of studies that link gender to absenteeism with females consistently having higher rates than men (Blank & Diderichsen, 1995; Philip, Taillard, Niedhammer, Guilleminault, & Bioulac, 2001). In one study of nurses in two hospitals, correlations were found between each absence-relevant event and the desire to be absent in all participants. However, ill health was the strongest correlate of absenteeism for both genders in the longitudinal phase of the study (Hackett, Bycio, & Guion, 1989). Nursing studies do not generally address the gender question as most nurses are female and the limited number of males precludes any comparisons based on gender.

In a study of four trusts in the United Kingdom, female staff that were predominately nurses were more likely than all of the other occupations to have experienced an absence (Ritchie, MacDonald, Gilmour, & Murray, 1999). Hackett's (1990) meta-analysis of individual studies in a variety of work settings found that age was inversely correlated with avoidable absences moderated by sex, with females having greater absences than males. Sharp and Watt's (1995) study of three occupational groups in the United Kingdom found that female absence occurrence rates compared to males were 1.2:1 and days absent were 1.5:1. Yet the differences in absence rates were removed by standardization of age and occupational status, with both men and women taking fewer but longer absences as age increased. In a study of postal workers in Sweden, Voss, Floderus, and Diderichsen (2001) found only a slightly higher incidence of illness in women relative to men. However, the population-based study in Sweden conducted by Akerlind, Alexanderson, Hensing, Liejon, and Bjurulf (1996) found that in all age categories women with children had more sickness (38%) than men with children (9%), and in a large study conducted in Malaysia, females had a higher severity of illness rates in all agencies (Indran, Gopal, & Omar, 1995). A more recent Swedish study by Akerstedt, Fredlund, Gillberg, and Jansson (2002) found that being a female of less than 50 years of age was a significant predictor of fatigue in a representative sample of the population. From these studies it would seem that being female does have an effect on absenteeism, but it is not clear whether older or younger females have more absences. To some extent it may depend on the measures of absenteeism in use, frequency or total days. Hackett (1990) summarized by stating that the impact of age and tenure are mixed; age has a moderate effect on avoidable absences, no effect on unavoidable absences, and sex was sometimes a moderator.

Hackett's (1990) meta-analysis found that a positive relationship between age or tenure and unavoidable absences was not supported and that age was more directly related to both absence types than tenure. Hakkanen, Viikari-Juntura, and Martikainen (2001) found that the effect of workload on sickness absence differed according to job experience, being highest for first-year workers and lowest among experienced (i.e., over 12 months) workers. It was suggested that the same effect might also be associated with job stress and older workers in their first year of employment. The Cohen (1991) meta-analysis of 41 studies demonstrated that career stage moderated the organizational commitment–outcomes relationship, and the relationship between commitment, performance, and absenteeism was stronger in the late-career stage. Gellatly's (1995) study in a chronic care hospital found organizational tenure positively related to continuance commitment, perceived absence norms, and total days absent.

11.4.1.2 Nurses' Physical and Mental Health

Ill health logically has an effect on the rates of absenteeism. Nurses may experience both physical and mental illness and injuries related to the work environment. Work in health care units is associated with considerable physical strain and many musculoskeletal complaints (Kant, de Jong, van Rijssen-Moll, & Borm, 1992). Work demands and expectations for efficiency have increased, effecting the levels of musculoskeletal pain and emotional exhaustion (Josephson, Lagerstrom, Hagberg, & Wigaeus Hjelm, 1997). Workers' compensation data indicate that musculoskeletal injuries are a major source of work-related disability among health care workers and that nurses have a higher risk of musculoskeletal sprain or strain claims compared to other occupational groups (Choi, Levitsky, Lloyd, & Stones, 1996; Workers' Compensation Board of British Columbia, 1998). In the past, musculoskeletal injury has primarily been associated with work-related physical factors. However, studies now implicate the role of job strain factors as predictors of musculoskeletal injury (Koehoorn, Kennedy, Demers, Hertzman, & Village, 1998; Lagerstrom, Hansson, & Hagberg, 1998).

In addition to physical illness caused by work, psychological effects have also been documented. Job strain has been shown to be predictive of absenteeism (Karasek & Theorell, 1990). Abu al Rub (2000) stated that nurses are under a great deal of distress related to a variety of work stressors and that work-related stress jeopardizes the mental and physical well-being of nurses, as well as the quality of care provided for clients. Fagin et al. (1996) found that 38% of mental health nurses were found to score at or above the criterion for emotional exhaustion. In a cross-sectional study of more than 500 staff, nurses reported high levels of psychological distress and the authors suggested that structural changes were required to increase job control and decrease demand (Araujo, Aquino, & Menezes, 1999). Stress has been associated with low satisfaction, poor quality of performance, increased absenteeism, and high turnover (Arsenault & Dolan, 1983). In a study of nurses in Sweden, stress was also associated with lower back pain (Ahlberg-Hulten, Theorell, & Sigala, 1995). Yet in a Quebec study, Bourbonnais, Comeau, Vezina, and Dion (1998) found that age, seniority, current position, and domestic load were not associated with high emotional exhaustion.

11.4.1.3 Job Dissatisfaction

Early absenteeism literature has examined absenteeism in terms of withdrawal behavior very similar in behavior to turnover (Chelius, 1981). Scott and Taylor (1985) found a strong relationship, although not causal in nature, between job satisfaction and absenteeism in a meta-analysis of 114 studies. The authors concluded that this was a withdrawal mechanism. This literature suggests that as nurses become more dissatisfied with their work environment their level of absenteeism will increase. Based on their research, Brooke and Price (1989) and Hackett (1989) each felt that job satisfaction was still the most important predictor of absenteeism. This relationship was confirmed in a more recent nursing study by Zboril-Bensen (2002), who found that higher rates of absenteeism were associated with the level of job satisfaction, longer shifts, working in acute care, and working full-time.

The role that nurse dissatisfaction plays in absenteeism has been explained by economists. Using economic theory, the utility associated with work reflects the individual's desire to work in terms of alternative options such as income and free time. As work becomes less desirable, actual worked hours may be used to bring absence into equality with the perceived utility (Chelius, 1981). Conversely, it has also been noted that when nurses are satisfied, this satisfaction does not mediate the relationship between situational and individual predictors and absenteeism (Goldberg & Waldman, 2000). In contrast to other researchers, Hackett and Guion (1985) found the correlation between absenteeism and job satisfaction was generally less than .40, and Matrunola (1996) did not find a relationship between job satisfaction and absenteeism.

11.4.1.4 Personality

Although Harrison and Martocchio (1998) identified personality as one of the five approaches to studying absenteeism, there were no studies related to nursing that investigated this cause. The dispositional approach assumes that staff are more likely to be absent if they have emotional instability, are anxious, have low achievement orientation, show aggression or impulsiveness, have social insensitivity, or demonstrate signs of alienation. Johns (1984) suggested that cross-situational absence would indicate a personality trait as a causal factor in absenteeism, but absenteeism studies do not explore absenteeism outside the work situation. Other researchers have considered absenteeism as a latent trait that can be linked to other types of negative behaviors such as lateness and poor performance. The grievance literature suggests that absenteeism increases post grievance and suggests that this is retribution for perceived inequities.

11.4.2 Organizational Factors

There have been numerous studies on organizational factors that affect absenteeism. The results suggest that organizational factors cannot be excluded when considering strategies to reduce absenteeism.

11.4.2.1 Job Strain

Short-term sick leaves have been associated with job strain in numerous studies (Bourbonnais, Comeau, Vezina, & Dion 1998; Bourbonnais & Mondor, 2001; Firth & Britton, 1989). Higher burnout levels were significantly associated with poorer self-rated and supervisor-rated job performance and more sick leave and reported absences for mental health reasons (Parker & Kulik, 1995). Felton (1998) stated that burnout is a health care professional's occupational disease that must be recognized early and treated.

There are many ways that managers can address burnout. Nurse stress has been associated with an imbalance between effort and reward. In a study of 204 German nurses, Bakker et al. (2000) found that nurses who experienced an effort–reward imbalance (ERI) reported higher levels on two of the three core dimensions of burnout (i.e., emotional exhaustion and depersonalization) than those who did not experience such an imbalance. Similar findings were found in a study of more than 8,000 nurses in Ontario (Shamian, Kerr, Laschinger, & Thomson, 2002). When focus groups were held with key health care stakeholders to explore the reasons for absenteeism, all groups agreed that psychosocial factors contributed to high absenteeism (Bruce, Sale, Shamian, O'Brien-Pallas & Thomson, 2002).

Ekberg and Wildhagen (1996) found that long-term sickness absence occurred when staff perceived higher physical and mental load in their jobs. They suggested that adequate levels of staffing that allow nurses to work safely and to relieve job stress related to the ability to provide quality care might reduce absenteeism. Workload was found to be the most important workplace satisfaction issue for Canadian nurses today (Thomson, 2002). Nurses who work in an environment that they perceive to be closer to their ideal experience have decreased levels of absenteeism and elevated nurse efficiency (Gregory, 1995).

11.4.2.2 Job Category

Several studies have found a strong inverse relationship between employment grade and the rate of absences due to back pain (Hemingway, Shipley, Stansfeld, & Marmot, 1997; Marmot, Feeney, Shipley, North, & Syme, 1995; Sharp & Watt, 1995). These studies specifically addressed the physical aspects of nursing work. However, nursing research has consistently shown a strong relationship between autonomy and job satisfaction, which often is associated with job grade and job satisfaction (Alexander, Weismann, & Chase, 1982; Blegen, 1993; Kramer & Hafner, 1989; McCloskey, 1990), and between job satisfaction and commitment (Acorn, Ratner, & Crawford, 1997). Higher level jobs tend to have more autonomy and control. Hendrix and Spencer (1989) found that absenteeism was associated with job involvement, commitment, burnout, and health. Farrell and Stamm (1988) also found work environment (i.e., task significance, variety, autonomy, identity, and feedback) and organization-wide correlates (i.e., pay, control policy, and shift) were better predictors of absenteeism than demographic (i.e., age, sex, tenure, and absence history) or psychological correlates (i.e., job satisfaction, commitment, job involvement, and stress). Zavala et al. (2002) found that employees with high decision latitude had lower absenteeism and days late, which confirmed the findings of the earlier studies.

Job category may also be examined from an economic perspective. Chelius (1981) suggested that as the pay rate increases, the price of free time increases, which may decrease absenteeism. However, this may be offset by the income effect, which posits that higher wage earners can afford more free time and therefore may want more. The income effect is only present when the wage per hour increases. When the compensation increase is in the form of fringe benefits there is no income effect as the compensation is not linked to hours worked. The author also stated that job satisfaction is a moderator of the wage income effect (Chelius). Those who are satisfied are less likely to be absent regardless of the wage rate.

11.4.2.3 Level of Supervisor Support

Michie and Williams (2003) found that the key work factors related to absenteeism were long hours of work, work overload, and pressure, but the effects of these factors on personal lives can be mediated by management style. Managers need to evaluate the rewards that are valued by nurses. Support by managers seems to be of great importance. Ahlberg-Hulten and colleagues (1995) found that in a study of Swedish nurses the lower the social support from supervisors, the greater the level of higher neck pain reported. Hoogendoorn et al. (2001), in a 3-year prospective study in the Netherlands, also concluded that low social support from either supervisors or coworkers appeared to be a risk factor for low-back pain. In a study of 49 neonatal nurses, perceptions of less supervisor support and less experience were associated with higher burnout subscale scores (Oehler, Davidson, Starr, & Lee, 1991). Firth and Britton (1989), in a study of nurses working in medical psychiatric units, found that perceived lack of support and emotional exhaustion predicted the frequency of absences. More recently, in a 3-month study of 5,563 Norwegian nurses' aides, the perceived lack of an encouraging and supportive culture in the work unit increased the likelihood (odds ratio [OR] = 1.73) that the employee would be absent (Eriksen, Bruusgaard, & Knardahl, 2003).

11.4.2.4 Work Hours

Both Shamian et al. (2002) and Burke and Greenglass (2000) found that full-time nurses had higher rates of self-reported absenteeism, and it was postulated that this may have been due to the greater number of hours worked in a poor work environment. The Shamian study involved more than 8,000 randomly selected nurses registered with the College of Nurses in Ontario in 1998; absences were self-reported in a mail-out survey. All respondents included demographic and work-related characteristics. Burke and Greenglass conducted their study around the same time, with more than 13,000 nurses selected from union membership lists.

11.4.2.5 Size and Type of Organization

Few studies were found on the effect of hospital size on absenteeism, but studies of absenteeism in nonnursing work environments found that there were significant linear relationships between hospital size and absenteeism (Markham, Dansereau, & Alutto, 1982; Philip et al., 2001). Markham et al. examined 66 high technology manufacturing firms in the United States over a 2-year period. The study by Philip et al. was also a longitudinal study over 2 years but was conducted in France with gas company employees. Shamian and colleagues (2002) found that teaching hospitals had higher rates of self-reported absenteeism. It is possible that this finding may be related to size rather than teaching status. This may have been related to the visibility of absenteeism and the relationships that are formed in smaller workplaces. Additional information on the relationship between hospital size and type became available in Ontario beginning in fiscal year 2002-2003 as Ontario hospitals became required to report sick hours (MOHLTC, 2002).

11.4.2.6 Nursing Unit Environment

The patients to whom nurses provide care may affect absence rates although little has been documented related to this concern. The Severe Acute Respiratory Syndrome (SARS) epidemic may have had a major effect on absence rates as nurses who cared for vulnerable patients made greater efforts to keep them free from possible infections. It is not known how large this effect may be, but it may be significant as nurses have been known to come to work even when sick. It is more important for nurses to stay away from work when they are sick than it is for other professions, and it may be more important for some nurses than for others. Those units who care for immuno-compromised patients such as those with HIV/AIDS must have stringent absenteeism policies that require that nurses stay home when ill.

Another aspect of the work environment that needs to be addressed is the area of workplace violence. Duncan et al. (2001) reported disturbing levels of violence primarily related to patient action in Alberta hospitals. This issue is more intense in mental health, emergency, and neurology units where patients do not know the consequences of their actions due to ill health. In a 3-year study of randomly selected workers in Finland, Kivimaki, Elovainio, and Vahtera (2000) found that sickness absence adjusted for age and sex was 51% greater in the victims of workplace bullying as compared to others. While patient abuse is not necessarily the same as workplace bullying, the findings suggest there may be an impact.

11.4.2.7 Content of Nursing Work

Nursing is very physical work requiring lifting, transferring, bending, and walking that may cause back injuries. One survey showed that nurses lost 750,000 working days per year as a result of back pain (Klauer-Triolo, 1989). The cost of ill health is not limited to those who are absent from work, but also those who present at work but cannot function with the same efficiency as those who are well. Harber and colleagues (1985) found that at least 15% of nurses reported that they had to stop work at least once during the day because of pain. Back pain is an expensive problem that is difficult to treat and quite prevalent in nursing. Studies have shown that workers with the greatest prevalence of back, shoulder, and knee injuries are employed in the health care industry. These injuries can be very costly (Cohen-Mansfield, Culpepper, & Carter, 1996); however, there are many strategies that have demonstrated positive results. Nurses who used mechanical lifting devices were less likely to have neck or back musculoskeletal disease and back injuries. Also, injuries were less likely when lifting teams were available (Trinkoff, Brady, & Nielson, 2003). Hospitals need to consider investment in back injury prevention programs for nurses (Blue, 1996; Venning, 1988; Yassi et al., 1995).

Hospitals need to address both the physical and emotional aspects of the workplace. A large Finnish study found that the adjusted sick absence rate was 1.2 times higher in women with low work-time control than in women with high work-time control (Ala-Mursula, Vahtera, Kivimaki, Kevin, & Pentti, 2002). High decision latitude was also found to be negatively and significantly related to both full and partial absenteeism in a U.S. study (Zavala et al., 2002). This study involved three annual and independent cross-sectional studies comprising 600 randomly selected employees at two sites including a hospital and an educational organization. Yet in a single hospital study, Dugan et al. (1996) found no significant relationships between stress and absenteeism, injuries, or turnover. More recently in a large Dutch study of many companies, Hoognedoorn and colleagues (2002) found that quantitative job demands, conflicting demands, decision authority, and skill discretion showed no relation to sickness absence due to low back pain.

11.4.2.8 Organizational Absence Climate and Policies

Morgan and Herman (1976) indicated that absenteeism is based on an expectancy model of behavior and organizations need to use motivators—both rewards and penalties. It has been suggested that organizational climate (i.e., tense or relaxed and supportive of new ideas or old modes) could be used as a research tool in attempts to reduce work-related absence (Piirainen, Rasanen, & Kivimaki, 2003) as organizational climate creates occupational stressors that result in positive behavioral outcomes (Hemingway & Smith, 1999). Bycio (1992) proposed that organizations should consider absenteeism in the selection process because employees with absentee patterns were rated as poor performers by supervisors using a variety of rating systems.

Markham and McKee (1995) examined group level effects on absence behavior and found that gender-controlled supervisory groups that had a perception of high external management standards and high internal personal standards had lower levels of absenteeism. Mathieu and Kohler (1990) found group level effect for the individual absence time-lost although not for the absence frequency, but the group had an absence policy for greater than 6 days absent. Martocchio and Judge (1994) found that illness explained the most absence variances, but several other factors varied across groups suggesting that the meaning of absence is not the same for all groups. Gellatly and Luchak (1998) found that hospitals' acceptable and expected absenteeism affects employees' normative perceptions but these were also influenced by their prior personal absence record, the absenteeism culture of their workplace, and the average level of absence. Perceived absence norms were found to influence future absence behavior 1 year later. Ostroff (1993) found a joint additive function of organizational climates and personal orientation.

Johns (1984) suggested that only 50% of absenteeism is controllable, and organizations need to consider the impact of interventions on cost versus the cost of the intervention. Robinson (2002) suggested that both absenteeism and presenteeism (being present) erode productivity and impact the bottom line. He reported that a survey found that the organizations with disability case management involving line supervisors in absence management and designating an internal absence manager had 74% lower rate of absence.

11.5   Linking Absenteeism to Outcome Achievement

Absenteeism can have an effect on nurses, patients and the organization. All would benefit from a greater understanding of absenteeism and strategies to reduce absenteeism in the future.

11.5.1 Absenteeism and Nurse Outcomes

It has been suggested that absenteeism occurs when turnover is low (Gray, Phillips, & Normand, 1996). This might be the effect of a tight marketplace. When there are other opportunities nurses leave, but when there are no available jobs, dissatisfied nurses call in sick. In 1993, Wise found that 306 out of 404 full-time nurses exhibited some type of withdrawal behavior. Termination accounted for 36%, systematic reduction in participation (SRP; i.e., working less than full-time) then termination accounted for 21%, and SRP without termination accounted for 19%. The relationship between absenteeism and both turnover and SRP was significant but opposite. In the study reported by Bruce et al. (2002), nurses reported moving to part-time as a way to cope with a stressful environment. A study of nurses in the United Kingdom by Firth and Britton (1989) demonstrated that lack of support and emotional exhaustion predicted the frequency of more than 4 days and more than 7 days respectively, but feelings of depersonalization predicted turnover. Similar to absenteeism, occupational stress (Dugan et al., 1996; Janssen, Jonge, & Bakker, 1999; Motowidlo, Packard, & Manning, 1986; Porter & Steers, 1973), workload (Jolma, 1990), leadership (Boyle, Bott, Hansen, Woods, & Taunton, 1999), social support (Cronin-Stubbs & Rooks, 1985), job satisfaction (Laschinger, Shamian, & Thomson, 2001; Lu, Lin, Wu, Hsieh, & Chang, 2002), and autonomy (Buchan, 1994; Porter & Steers, 1973) have been linked to turnover. Efforts to reduce absenteeism are likely to reduce turnover, another cost to the organization, as well. Rosse and Miller (1984) showed a relationship between absenteeism and lateness and turnover. They suggested that generally the relationship is not strong enough to suggest that they are surrogates for one another but that the three variables covariate, and all appear to share common routes in job-related affect (Rosse & Miller, p. 194).

11.5.2 Absenteeism and Patient Outcomes

Baumann et al. (2001) suggested that nurse absenteeism disrupts the continuity of patient care, but few studies have attempted to measure the extent of this effect. Taunton, Kleinbeck, Stafford, Woods, & Bott (1994) demonstrated that there was an increase in complication rates linked to increased absenteeism and hypothesized that this was related to loss of continuity of care and safety related to replacement of staff by nurses who are less skilled. Complications included nosocomial urinary tract and bloodstream infections. Dugan et al. (1996) found a strong relationship between nurse stress scale scores and the occurrence of patient incidents (i.e., patient falls and medication errors). The impact on patient outcomes depends on the overall rate of absenteeism and how the organization copes with the replacement of absent workers.

11.5.3 Absenteeism and Organizational Outcomes

Organizations incur additional costs when absenteeism rates are high. This may be in the form of lost productivity due to the absence of the worker or costs for replacement staff to maintain output levels. In addition, about 25% of respondents reported that they had experienced productivity losses before their absence, and 20% of respondents experienced productivity losses after absence. This suggests that there is an increase in estimated production losses of about 16% over previous estimates that did not consider productivity (Brouwer, van Exel, Koopmanchap, & Rutten, 2002). There may also be production losses when workers do not call in sick. Working instead of taking sick leave when ill was more prevalent in subjects with a high incidence of sickness (OR of 1.74 in women, OR of 1.60 in men; Voss et al., 2001). The highest level of presenteeism was found in the care, welfare, and education sectors and also in sectors that had to redo work after an absence (Aronsson, Gustafsson, & Dallner, 2000).

There are several components of overall expenses related to absenteeism. First, when staff are absent from work they are not productive; therefore, the expenses related to their compensation while away from work add to the cost of the product or service produced by the organization. Second, in hospitals where the demand for service cannot be controlled, direct care providers must be replaced. This adds an additional cost to that incurred due to the initial absence. Third, there is the cost related to staff time spent trying to replace the absent staff. When there is a shortage of relief staff, this can consume a considerable amount of productive time or may result in the use of highly paid agency staff or overtime rates for employees. Pauly et al. (2002) cautioned against assuming that the value in reducing absenteeism is the wage rate. The cost of absenteeism is larger when perfect substitutes are not available, especially when there is a team production or a penalty is associated with not meeting the output target.

Anecdotal evidence suggests that absenteeism programs are generally seen as punitive by nurses even if developed as a nondisciplinary process. However, as reflected in the comments obtained from hospital management, occupational health and safety personnel, and nurses in the focus groups, a punitive approach to absenteeism is likely to cause further deterioration in nurses' work environments (Shamian et al., 2001). This contrasts with Steers and Rhodes' (1978) model that suggests that employees consider the effects of strict absence policies, coworker relationships, work ethic, size of the work unit and the organization, opportunities for advancement, economic and market conditions, and pressures to attend before calling in sick. It must be recognized that absenteeism is only a symptom of a problem. Once the problem is addressed, the absenteeism will resolve itself.

11.6   Issues in the Measurement of Absenteeism

Measurements of absenteeism reported in this paper are primarily from one of two sources—administrative data and survey data. Harrison and Shaffer (1994) found that in seven studies, individuals reported roughly half the absenteeism of the perceived norm among peers regardless of attendance context, time interval, type of estimate, or administration condition. This suggests that survey data may not be very accurate and may result in underreporting personal absences and overreporting perceived norms.

Few studies are able to examine workload by time period, but in a hospital study Leonard, Dolan, and Arsenault (1990) found substantiated differences by month, season, and year, and this effect was more pronounced on frequency than on time lost with the peak frequencies occurring during the winter months. Johns (1984) cautioned to be wary of individual versus aggregate data. He also mentioned the need to consider absenteeism in light of job characteristics and external context as well in internal control measures in place.

Harrison and Hulin (1989) commented that measures of absence propensity are rarely normally distributed and often troublesome as the low base-rate of absenteeism, usually around 3%, is inadmissible in a linear regression. Also, product–moment correlations between aggregate absenteeism and some other variable are lowered by differences in the shapes of their respective distributions. They suggested using event history analysis to describe changes in state over time as previous absenteeism is a valuable predictor of future absenteeism. Other types of absences lower sick absenteeism (e.g., vacation) and all absences regardless of type have an effect. In Harrison and Hulin's study, those that paced their time away from work had less absenteeism. Employees who took a single day off were less likely to be off again soon. It was suggested that this was likely because of social norms and using hazard rate models for absence spells is useful for understanding the determinants of absenteeism.

11.7 Evidence Concerning Approaches to Measuring Absenteeism

Some of the factors that need to be considered when measuring absenteeism have been included in authors' comments on the limitations of their studies. When measuring absenteeism from administrative data only, the paid absences are included. In nursing, part-time staff who often make up a large portion of the workforce, are not paid for absences. Despite the fact that they are not paid, their absences generate work and costs related to finding replacements, disrupt the planned composition of the work team, and may affect the quality of patient care. The impact of predictable or unpredictable absences may be different. Predictable absences such as a long-term illness may include the number of occasions or number of days, reason for absence, paid or unpaid, replaced or not replaced, size of organization and work unit, demographics, employment status and experience of the employee, organizational absenteeism culture, linkage of absenteeism to performance appraisal, sick absences or all absences, and the effect of different sick plans and absenteeism monitoring programs.

11.8 Nursing Measures of Absenteeism

In nursing absenteeism studies, absences have been categorized as either short-term (i.e., less than 3 days) or medically certified (i.e., greater than 3 days; Bourbonnais, & Mondor, 2001; Eriksen et al., 2003). The definition of short-term absence does vary; for example, Hemingway and Smith (1999) used 2 days or less to define short-term, and Kivimaki et al. (2000) used 4 days as the break point between short- and long-term illness. Firth and Britton (1989) attempted to group absences in three categories: 1–3 days, 4–6 days, and 7 days or greater. The absence has been measured as a rate with the number of days or hours absent divided by the total number of days or hours paid. The denominator has also been designated as the number of days scheduled to work rather than total days paid, which includes scheduled days absent for vacation and statutory holidays.

11.9   Implications and Future Directions

Absenteeism is of great concern to the nursing community and the organizations that employ nurses. The cost of absenteeism is not just a dollar figure but the physical and emotional cost to nurses themselves who become ill due to the work environment. When absence rates increase, often the first reaction of management is to implement a monitoring system and set targets for absent occasions and/or days. What they often fail to realize is that absenteeism is often a symptom of organizational distress. If nurses are truly ill, no amount of monitoring will reduce absenteeism. If nurses are absent because the work environment is intolerable, then the organization must address the issues that are making nurses remain away from work. It is also important to understand the characteristics of nurses who are absent in order to understand the factors that affect their absenteeism and to develop strategies to address these issues. Absenteeism is most often studied at the aggregate level without looking at the characteristics of individual work environments. The research indicates that absenteeism can be influenced by work culture and the content of the work itself. There must be a concerted effort to clearly define how absenteeism is measured and studied as well as understanding the full costs associated with absenteeism. In addition, it must be recognized that the effect on patient outcomes may be associated with absenteeism when absentees are not replaced or when agency or part-time staff is used to replace sudden absences. It is likely that absenteeism cannot be cured with tighter disciplinary measures. These measures may reduce the rate of absenteeism in the short run, but if nurses are staying away from work due to poor working conditions then unhappy and perhaps unproductive nurses at the bedside will remain a problem. It is possible that stressed nurses may leave the organization instead of being absent.

Although the research conducted on nonnursing organizations may give us clues for understanding absenteeism in nursing, the very nature of the nurses and nursing work requires attention when considering nurse absenteeism. Nurses have always been predominantly women. Working shifts, the impact of home commitments, and the sleep effects of shift work are difficult for organizations to address. Nurses work in a team environment where the demand for work will not wait until the nurse returns. Absent nurses must be replaced yet it is difficult to find replacements that are perfect substitutes and, regardless of their competency, there are effects on the continuity of care and the care team that cannot be ignored. Because nurses work with vulnerable patients, nurses must stay away from work when they have illnesses that could be transmitted to their patients and in some instances the illness is transmitted from the patient to the nurse. Does this mean that nurse absenteeism targets should be different from those set in other work settings? Future research endeavors related to nursing absenteeism should address the following issues:

- What proportion of absenteeism is related to individual employee decisions related to nonwork condition versus work conditions and what proportion is due to ill health? How does the nurse–patient relationship affect illness?

- What are the different cost and quality effects between short-term and long-term absences? Do predictable absences have less effect that unpredictable absences?

- Do absent occasions and days of absenteeism really reflect culpable and inculpable absences or might the work environment be a precursor for both?

- Is there an effect of shift length and overall scheduling patterns on the frequency and cost of absenteeism?

- What are the relative differences between the cost of absenteeism and the cost of presenteeism?

- What is the full cost of absenteeism including effect of reduced productivity, turnover, time to replace absent nurses and the cost of absence monitoring?

- Are there differences in absence behavior across organizational and unit work settings and what is the distribution of absenteeism across employees? Are unique absence strategies required?

- Are there more appropriate approaches to analyzing absenteeism other than correlational and regression analysis?

- How do we capture unpaid absences and do unpaid absences also have a cost in terms of cost and quality for the organization?

11.10   References

Abu al Rub, R. (2000). Legal aspects of work related stress in nursing. Exploring the issues. *American Association of Occupational Health Nurses Journal, 48*(3), 131–135.

Acorn, S., Ratner, P., & Crawford, M. (1997). Decentralization as a determinant of job satisfaction and organizational commitment among Nurse Managers. *Nursing Research, 46,* 52–57.

Ahlberg-Hulten, G., Theorell, T. & Sigala, F. (1995). Social support, job strain and musculo-skeletal pain among female health care personnel. *Scandinavian Journal of Work Environmental Health, 21,* 435–439.

Aiken, L. H., Clarke, S. P., & Sloane, D. M. (2002). Hospital staffing, organization, and quality of care: Cross-national findings. *Nursing Outlook, 50*(5), 187–194.

Akerlind, I., Alexanderson, K., Hensing, G., Liejon, M., & Bjurulf, P. (1996). Sex differences in sickness absence in relation to parental status. *Scandinavian Journal of Social Medicine, 24,* 27–35.

Akerstedt, T., Fredlund, P., Gillberg, M., & Jansson, B. (2002). Work load and work hours in relation to disturbed sleep and fatigue in a large representative sample. *Journal of Psychosomatic Research, 53,* 585–588.

Akyeampong, E. B. (1999a). Missing from work in 1998: Industry differences. *Perspectives on Labour and Income, 11*(3), 30–36.

Akyeampong, E. B. (1999b). Work absence rates, 1987 to 1998. Catalogue #71-535-MPB99010, No 10. Ottawa, Ontario: Statistics Canada.

Ala-Mursula, L., Vahtera, J., Kivimaki, M., Kevin, M. V., & Pentti, J. (2002). Employee control over working times: Associations with subjective health and sickness absences. *Journal of Epidemiology and Community Health, 56,* 272–278.

Alexander, C. S., Weismann, C. S., & Chase, G.A. (1982). Determinants of staff nurses' perceptions of autonomy within different clinical settings. *Nursing Research, 31,* 48–52.

Allen, A. (1990). On-the-job injury: A costly problem. *Journal of Post Anesthetic Nursing, 5,* 367–368.

Araujo, T., Aquino, E., & Menezes, G. (1999). Psychosocial aspects of work and minor psychological disorders among nurses. *Abstract from the 4th International Conference on Occupational Health for Health Care Workers.* Montreal, Quebec: October TP–42.

Aronsson, G., Gustafsson, K., & Dallner, M. (2000). Sick but yet at work. An empirical study of sickness presenteeism. *Journal of Epidemiology and Community Health, 54,* 502–509.

Arsenault, A., & Dolan, S. (1983). The role of personality, occupation and organization in understanding the relationship between job stress, performance and absenteeism. *Journal of Occupational Psychology, 56,* 227–240.

Baker, A., Heiler, K., & Ferguson, S. (2003). The impact of roster changes on absenteeism and incidence frequency in an Australian coal mine. *Occupational and Environmental Medicine, 60,* 43–49.

Bakker, A., Killmer, C., Siegrist, J., & Schaufeli, W. (2000). Effort–reward imbalance and burnout among nurses. *Journal of Advanced Nursing, 31,* 884–891.

Barmby, T. A., Ercolani, M. G., & Treble, J. G. (2002). Sickness absence: An international comparison. *The Economic Journal, 112* (June), F315–F331.

Baumann, A., O'Brien-Pallas, L., Armstrong-Stassen, M., Blythe, J., Bourbonnais, R., Cameron, S., et al. (2001). *Investing in nurses' well-being: Ensuring patient care.* Ottawa, Canada: Canadian Health Services Research Foundation.

Benefits Interface, Inc. (2000, February). Introduction to attendance management. Retrieved August 18, 2003, from: http://www.benefits.org/interface/cost/absent.htm

Blank, N., & Diderichsen, F. (1995). Short-term and long-term sick-leave in Sweden: Relationships with social circumstances, working conditions and gender. *Scandinavian Journal of Social Medicine, 23*(4), 265–272.

Blegen, M. (1993). Nurses' job satisfaction: A meta-analysis of related variables. *Nursing Research, 42,* 36–41.

Blue, C. L. (1996). Preventing back injury among nurses. *Orthopaedic Nursing, 15,* 9–20.

Boedeker, W. (2001). Associations between workload and diseases rarely occurring in sickness absence data. *Journal of Environmental and Occupational Medicine, 43,* 1081–1088.

Boumans, N., & Landeweerd, J.A. (1999) Nurses' well-being in a primary nursing care setting in the Netherlands. *Scandinavian Journal of Caring Science, 13,* 116–122.

Bourbonnais, R., Comeau, M., Vezina, M., & Dion, G. (1998). Job strain, psychological distress, & burnout in nurses. *American Journal of Industrial Medicine, 34,* 20–28.

Bourbonnais, R., & Mondor, M. (2001). Job strain and sickness absence among nurses in the province of Quebec. *American Journal of Industrial Medicine, 39,* 194–202.

Boyle, D. K., Bott, M. J., Hansen, H. E., Woods, C. Q., Taunton, R. L. (1999). Managers' leadership and critical care nurses' intent to stay. *American Journal of Critical Care, 8*(6), 361–371.

Brooke, P., & Price, J. (1989). The determinants of employee absenteeism: An empirical test of a causal model. *Journal of Occupational Psychology, 62,* 1–19.

Brouwer, W. B. F., van Exel, N. J. A., Koopmanchap, M. A., & Rutten, F. F. H. (2002). Productivity costs before and after absence from work: As important as common? *Health Policy, 61*(2), 173–187.

Bruce, S., Sale, J., Shamian, J., O'Brien-Pallas, L., & Thomson, D. (2002). Musculoskeletal injuries, stress and absenteeism. *Canadian Journal of Nursing, 98*(9), 12–17.

Buchan, J. (1994). Lessons from America? US magnet hospitals and their implications for UK. *Journal of Advanced Nursing, 19,* 373–384.

Burke, R. J., & Greenglass, E. R. (2000). Effects of hospital restructuring on full-time and part-time nursing staff in Ontario. *International Journal of Nursing Studies, 37*(2), 163–171.

Burton, R. (1992). Tackling absenteeism. *Nursing Standard, 7*(3), 37–40.

Bycio, P. (1992). Job performance and absenteeism: A review and meta-analysis. *Human Relations, 45*(2), 193–220.

Canadian Labour and Business Centre. (2002). *Full-time equivalents and financial costs associated with absenteeism, overtime, and involuntary part-time employment in the nursing profession.*

Cascio, W. (1982). Costing the effects of smoking in the workplace. Chapter 4 in *Costing human resources: The financial impact of behavior in organizations.* Boston, MA: Kent Publishing Co.

Cascio, W. (1982). The hidden costs of absenteeism. Chapter 3 in *Costing human resources: The financial impact of behavior in organizations*. Boston, MA: Kent Publishing Co.

Chelius, J. (1981). Understanding absenteeism: The potential contribution of economic theory. *Journal of Business Research, 9*, 409–418.

Choi, B., Levitsky, M., Lloyd, R., & Stones, I. (1996). Patterns and risk factors for sprains and strains in Ontario, Canada 1990: An analysis of the workplace health and safety agency database. *Journal of Occupational and Environmental Medicine, 38*(4), 379–389.

Cohen, A. (1991). Career stage as a moderator of the relationships between organizational commitment and its outcomes: A meta-analysis. *Journal of Occupational Psychology, 64*, 253–268.

Cohen, A. (2000). The relationship between commitment forms and work outcomes: A comparison of three models. *Human Relations, 53*(3), 387–417.

Cohen-Mansfield, J., Culpepper, W. J. 2nd, Carter, P. (1996). Nursing staff back injuries: Prevalence and cost in long term care facilities. *American Association of Occupational Health Nurses Journal, 44*, 9–17.

Coleman, S., & Hansen, S. (1994). Reducing work-related back injuries. *Nursing Management, 25*(11), 58–61.

Collins, J. W., & Owen, B. D. (1996). NIOSH research initiatives to prevent back injuries to nursing assistants, aides, and orderlies in nursing homes. *American Journal of Industrial Medicine, 29*, 424.

Coutts, J. (2001). Healthy workplaces mean more satisfied nurses. *Hospital Quarterly, Summer*, 57–58.

Cronin-Stubbs, D., & Rooks, C. A. (1985). The stress, social support, and burnout of critical care nurses: The results of research. *Heart and Lung, 14*(1), 31–39.

Dugan, J., Lauer, E., Bouquot, Z., Dutro, B., Smith, M., & Widmeyer. (1996). Stressful nurses: The effect on patient outcomes. *Journal of Nursing Care Quality, 10*(3), 46–58.

Duncan, S. M., Hyndman, K., Estabrooks, C. A., Hesketh, K., Humphrey, C. K., Wong, J. S., et al. (2001). Nurses' experience of violence in Alberta and British Columbia hospitals. *Canadian Journal of Nursing Research, 32*(4), 57–78.

Dzoljic, M., Zimmerman, M., Legemate, D., Klazinga, N. S. (2003). Reduced nurse working time and surgical productivity and economics *Anesthesia & Analgesia, 97*(4), 1127–1132.

Ehrenberg, R. (1970). Absenteeism and overtime decision. *The American Economic Review, 60*(3), 352–357.

Ekberg, K., & Wildhagen, I. (1996). Long-term sickness absence due to musculoskeletal disorders: The necessary intervention of work conditions. *Scandinavian Journal of Rehabilitation Medicine, 28*(1), 39–47.

Eriksen, W., Bruusgaard, D., & Knardahl, S. (2003). Work factors as predictors of sickness absence: A three month prospective study of nurses' aides. *Occupational and Environmental Medicine, 60*, 271–280.

Fagin, L., Carson, J., Leary, J., De Villiers, N., Bartlett, H., O'Malley, P., et al. (1996). Stress, coping and burnout in mental health nurses: Findings from three research studies. *International Journal of Social Psychiatry, 42*(2), 102.

Farrell, D., & Stamm, C. (1988). Meta-analysis of the covariates of employee absence. *Human Relations, 41*, 211–227.

Felton, J. S. (1998). Burnout as a clinical entity: Its importance in health care workers. *Occupational Medicine, 48*(4), 237–250.

Firth, H., & Britton, P. (1989). Burnout, absence and turnover amongst British nursing staff. *Journal of Occupational Psychology, 62*, 55–59.

Gauci Borda, R., Norman, I. J. (1997). Factors influencing turnover and absence of nurses: A research review. *International Journal of Nursing Studies, 34*(6), 385–394.

Gellatly, I. (1995). Individual and group determinants of employee absenteeism: A test of a causal model. *Journal of Organizational Behavior, 16*, 469–485.

Gellatly, I., & Luchak, A. (1998). Personal and organizational determinants of absence norms. *Human Relations 51*(8), 1085–1102.

Goldberg, C., & Waldman, D. (2000). Modeling employee absenteeism: Testing alternative measures and mediated effects based on job satisfaction. *Journal of Organizational Behavior, 21*, 665–676.

Gray, A., Phillips, V. L., & Normand, C. (1996). The costs of nursing turnover: Evidence from the British National Health Service. *Health Policy, 38*, 117–138.

Gregory, G. D. (1995). Using a nursing performance information system. *Nursing Management, 26*(7), 74–77.

Grey-Toft, P. & Anderson, J. G. (1981). Stress among hospital nursing staff: Its causes and effects. *Social Science Medicine, 15A*, 639–647.

Hackett, R. (1989). Work attitudes and employee absenteeism: A synthesis of the literature. *Journal of Occupational Psychology, 62*, 235–248.

Hackett, R. (1990). Age, tenure and employee absenteeism. *Human Relations, 43*(7), 601–619.

Hackett, R., & Bycio, P. (1996). An evaluation of employee absenteeism as a coping mechanism among hospital nurses. *Journal of Occupational and Organizational Psychology, 69*, 327–338.

Hackett, R., Bycio, P., & Guion, R. M. (1989). Absenteeism among hospital nurses: An idiographic-longitudinal analysis. *Academy of Management Journal, 32*, 424–453.

Hackett, R., & Guion, R. (1985). A re-evaluation of the absenteeism–job satisfaction relationship. *Organizational Behavior and Human Relation Processes, 35*, 340–381.

Hackman, J. R., & Oldham, G. R. (1975). Development of the job diagnostic survey. *Journal of Applied Psychology, 60*(2), 159–170.

Hakkanen, M., Viikari-Juntura, E., & Martikainen, R. (2001). Job experience, workload, and risk of musculoskeletal disorders. *Occupational and Environmental Medicine, 58*(2), 129–135.

Harber, P., Billet, E., Gutowski, M., SooHoo, K., Lew, M., & Roman, A. (1985). Occupational low-back pain in hospital nurses. *Journal of Occupational Medicine, 27*, 518–524.

Harrison, D., & Hulin, C. (1989). Investigations of absenteeism: Using event history models to study the absence-taking process. *Journal of Applied Psychology, 74*(2), 300–316.

Harrison, D., & Martocchio, J. (1998). Time for absenteeism: A 20-year review of origins, and outcomes. *Journal of Management, 24*(3), 305–350.

Harrison, D., & Shaffer, M. (1994). Comparative examinations of self-reports and perceived absenteeism norms: Wading through Lake Wobegon. *Journal of Applied Psychology, 79*(2), 240–251.

Haw, M. A., Claus, E. G., Durbin-Lafferty, E., & Iversen, S. M. (2003). Improving work morale of nurses despite insurance cost cutting. Program planning *Pflege, 16*(3), 161–167.

Hemingway, H., Shipley, M. J., Stansfeld, S., & Marmot, M. (1997). Sickness absence from back pain, psychosocial work characteristics and employment grade among office workers. *Scandinavian Journal of Work and Environmental Health, 233*(2), 121–129.

Hemingway, M., & Smith, C. (1999). Organizational climate and occupational stressors as predictors of withdrawal behaviors and injuries in nurses. *Journal of Occupational and Organizational Psychology, 72*, 285–299.

Hendrix, W., & Spencer, B. (1989). Developmental and test of a multivariate model of absenteeism. *Psychological Reports, 64*, 923–938.

Hensing, G., Alexanderson, K., Allebeck, P., & Bjurulf. (1998). How to measure sickness absence? Literature review and suggestion of five basic measures. *Scandinavian Journal of Social Medicine, 26*(2), 133–144.

Hinshaw, A. S. Smeltzer, C. H., & Atwood, J. R. (1987). Innovative retention strategies for nurse staffing. *Journal of Nursing Administration, 17*(6), 6–17.

Hoogendoorn, W. E., Bongers, P. M., de Vet, H. C., Houtman, I. L., Ariens, G. A., van Mechelen, W., et al. (2001). Psychosocial work characteristics and psychological strain in relation to low-back pain. *Scandinavian Journal of Work Environmental Health, 27*(4), 258–267.

Hoognedoorn, W. E., Bongers, P. M., de Vet, H. C., Ariens, G. A., van Mechelen, W., & Bouter, L. M. (2002). High physical work load and low job satisfaction increase the risk of sickness absence due to low back pain: Results of a prospective cohort study. *Occupational and Environmental Medicine, 59*(5), 323–328.

Indran, S., Gopal, R. & Omar, A. (1995). Absenteeism in the workforce, Klang Valley, Malaysia—preliminary report. *Asia Pacific Journal of Public Health, 8*(2), 109–113.

Jamal, M. (1990). Relationship of job stress and type A behavior to employee's job satisfaction, organizational commitment, psychosomatic health problems and turnover motivation. *Human Relations, 43*(8), 727–738.

Jamal, M., & Crawford, R L. (1981). Consequences of extended work hours: A comparison of moonlighters, over-timers, and modal employees. *Human Resource Management, 20*(3), 18–23.

Janssen, P. P., Jonge, J. D., & Bakker, A. B. (1999). Specific determinants of intrinsic work motivation, burnout and turnover intentions: A study among nurses. *Journal of Advanced Nursing, 29*(6), 1360–1369.

Johns, G. (1984). Unresolved issues in the study and management of absence from work. In P.S. Goodman & S. Atkin (eds). *Absenteeism: New approaches to understanding, measuring and managing employee absence*, pp. 360–390. San Fransisco: Jossey–Bass.

Johns, G. (1994). How often were you absent? A review of the use of self-reported absence data. *Journal of Applied Psychology, 79*(4), 574–591.

Johns, G. (1997). Contemporary research on absence from work: Correlates, causes and consequences. *International Review of Industrial and Organizational Psychology, 12*, 115–173.

Johnson, C. J., Croghan, E., & Crawford, J. (2003). The problem and management of sickness absence in the NHS: Considerations for nurse managers. *Journal of Nursing Management,.11*(5), 336–342.

Jolma, D. J. (1990). Relationship between nursing workload and turnover. *Nursing Economics, 8*(2), 110–114.

Josephson, M., Lagerstrom, M., Hagberg, M., & Wigaeus Hjelm, E. (1997). Musculoskeletal symptoms and job strain among nursing personnel: A study over a three year period. *Occupational and Environmental Medicine, 54*, 681–685.

Kant, I. J., de Jong, L. C., van Rijssen-Moll, M., & Borm, P. J. (1992). A survey of static and dynamic work postures of operating room staff. *International Archives of Occupational and Environmental Health, 63*(6), 423–428.

Karasek, R. A. (1979). Job demands, job decision latitude and mental health: Implications for job redesign. *Administrative Science Quarterly, 24*, 284–307.

Karasek, R., & Theorell, T. (1990). *Healthy work: Stress, productivity, and the reconstruction of working life*. New York: Basic Books.

Kim, J. S., & Campagna, A. F. (1982). Effects of flextime on employee attendance and performance: A field experiment. *Academy of Management Journal, 24*, 729–741.

Kivimaki, M., Elovainio, M., & Vahtera, J. (2000). Workplace bullying and sickness absence in hospital staff. *Occupational and Environmental Medicine, 58*, 656–660.

Klauer-Triolo, P. (1989). Occupational health hazards of hospital staff nurses. Part II: Physical, chemical, and biological stressors. *American Association of Occupational Health Nurses Journal, 37*(7), 274–279.

Klauer-Triolo, P., Allgeier, P. A., & Schwartz, C. E. (1995). Layoff survivor sickness: Minimizing the sequelae of organizational transformation. *Journal of Nursing Administration, 25*(3), 56–63.

Koehoorn, M., Kennedy, S., Demers, P., Hertzman, C., & Village, J. (1998). *Risk factors for musculoskeletal disorders among health care workers*. Report to the Worker's Compensation Board of British Columbia: Richmond, British Columbia.

Kovach, K. A. (1979). Is it time to amend the overtime provisions of the Fair Labor Act? *Human Resource Management, 18*(3), 23.

Kramer, M., & Hafner, L. (1989). Shared values: Impact on staff nurse job satisfaction and perceived productivity. *Nursing Research, 38*(3), 172–176.

Lagerstrom, M., Hansson, T., & Hagberg, M. (1998). Work-related low back problems in nursing. *Scandinavian Journal of Work, Environment and Health, 24*(6), 449–464.

Landeweerd, J., & Boumans, N. (1994). The effect of work dimensions and need for autonomy on nurses' work satisfaction and health. *Journal of Occupational and Organizational Psychology, 67*, 207–217.

Laschinger, H. K., Shamian, J., & Thomson, D. (2001). Impact of nursing work environment characteristics on staff nurse organizational trust, burnout, nurse-assessed quality of care and work satisfaction. *Nursing Economics, 19*(5), 209–219.

Leonard, C., Dolan, S., & Arsenault, A. (1990). Longitudinal examination of the stability and variability of two common measures of absence. *Journal of Occupational Psychology, 63*, 309–316.

Libet, J., Frueh, C., Pellegrin, K., Gold, P., Santos, A., & Arana, G. (2001). Absenteeism and productivity among mental health employees. *Administration and Policy in Mental Health, 29*(1), 41–50.

Lu, K. Y., Lin, P. L., Wu, C. M., Hsieh, Y. L., & Chang, Y. Y. (2002). The relationships among turnover intentions, professional commitment, and job satisfaction of hospital nurses. *Journal of Professional Nursing, 18*(4), 214–219.

Markham, S., & McKee, G. (1995). Group absence behavior and standards: A multilevel analysis. *Academy of Management Journal, 38*(4), 1174–1190.

Markham, S. E., Dansereau, F. Jr., & Alutto, J. A. (1982). Group size and absenteeism: A longitudinal analysis. *Academy of Management Journal, 25*, 921–927.

Marmot, M., Feeney, A., Shipley, M., North, F., & Syme, S. L. (1995). Sickness absence as a measure of health status and functioning: from the UK Whitehall II study. *Journal of Epidemiology and Community Health, 49*, 124–130.

Martocchio, J. (1994). The effects of absence culture on individual absence. *Human Relations, 47*(3), 243–261.

Martocchio, J., & Harrison, D. (1993). To be there or not to be there? Questions, theories, and methods in absenteeism research. *Research in Personnel and Human Resources Management, 11*, 259–328.

Martocchio, J., & Judge, T. (1994). A policy-capturing approach to individuals' decisions to be absent. *Organizational Behaviors and Human Decision Processes, 57*, 358–386.

Mathieu, J., & Kohler, S. (1990). A cross-level examination of group absence influences on individual behavior. *Journal of Applied Psychology 75*(2), 217–220.

Matrunola, P. (1996). Is there a relationship between job satisfaction and absenteeism? *Journal of Advanced Nursing, 23*(4), 827–834.

McCloskey, J. (1990). Two requirements for job contentment: Autonomy and social integration. IMAGE: *Journal of Nursing Scholarship 22*(3), 140–142.

McLaughlin, A. M., & Erdman, J. (1992). Rehabilitation staff stress as it relates to patient acuity and diagnosis. *Brain Injuries, 6*(1), 59–64.

Michie, S., & Williams, S. (2003). Reducing work related psychological ill health and sickness absence: A systematic literature review. *Occupational and Environmental Medicine, 60*, 3–9.

Mitchell, P. H., Armstrong, S., Forshee Simpson, T., & Lentz, M. (1989). ANA American Association of Critical-Care Nurses Demonstration Project: Profile of excellence in critical care nursing. *Heart & Lung, 18*(3), 219–237.

MOHLTC. (2002). *Ontario Hospital Reporting System User Guide*. Toronto: Author.

Morgan, L. & Herman, J. (1976). Perceived consequences of absenteeism. *Journal of Applied Psychology, 61*(6), 738–742.

Motowidlo, S. J.., Packard, J. S., & Manning, M. R. (1986). Occupational Stress: Its causes and consequences for job performance. *Journal of Applied Psychology 71*, 618–629.

O'Brien-Pallas, L., Thomson, D., Alksnis, C., & Bruce, S. (2001). The economic impact of nurse staffing decisions: Time to turn down another road? *Hospital Quarterly, 4*(3), 42–50.

Oehler, J. M., Davidson, M. G., Starr, L. E., & Lee, D. A. (1991). Burnout, job stress, anxiety, and perceived social support in neonatal nurses. *Heart and Lung, 20*, 500–505.

Ostroff, C. (1993). The effects of climate and personal influences on individual behavior and attitudes in organizations. *Organizational Behavior and Human Decision Processes, 56*, 56–90.

Parish, C. (2002). Stem the tide. *Nursing Standard, 17*(8), 12–13.

Parker, P. A., & Kulik, J. A. (1995). Burnout, self, and supervisor-rated job performance, and absenteeism among nurses. *Journal of Behavioral Medicine, 18*, 581–599.

Pauly, M., Nicholson, S., Xu, J., Danzon, P., Murray, J., & Berger, M. (2002). A general model of the impact of absenteeism on employers and employees. *Health Economics, 11*, 221–231.

Philip, P., Taillard, J., Niedhammer, I., Guilleminault, C. & Bioulac, B. (2001). Is there a link between subjective daytime somnolence and sickness absenteeism? A study in a working population. *Journal of Sleep Research, 10*, 111–115.

Piirainen, H., Rasanen, K., & Kivimaki, M. (2003). Organizational climate, perceived work-related symptoms and sickness absences: A population-based survey. *Journal of Occupational and Environmental Medicine, 45*(2), 175–184.

Porter, L. W., & Steers, R. M. (1973). Organization, work and personal factors in employee turnover and absenteeism. *Psychological Bulletin, 80*, 151–176.

Proper, K. I., Staal, B. J., Hilebrandt, V. H., van der Beek, A. J., & van Mechelen, W. (2002). Effectiveness of physical activity programs at worksites with respect to work-related outcomes. *Scandinavian Journal of Work and Environmental Health, 28*(2), 75–84.

Rasanen, K., Notkola, V., & Husman, K. (1997). Perceived work conditions and work-related symptoms among employed Finns. *Social Science Medicine, 45*(7), 1099–1110.

Rentsch, J., & Steel, R. (1998). Testing durability of job characteristics as predictors of absenteeism over a six-year period. *Personnel Psychology, 51*(1), 165–189.

Ritchie, K. A., MacDonald, E. B., Gilmour, W. H., & Murray, K. J. (1999). Analysis of sickness absence among employees of four NHS trusts. *Occupational and Environmental Medicine, 56*(10), 702–708.

Robinson, E. (2002). An integrated approach to managing absence supports greater organizational productivity. *Employee Benefits Journal, 27*(2), 7–11.

Rosse, J., & Miller, H. (1984). Relationship between absenteeism and other behaviors. In P. S. Goodman & R. S. Atkin (eds.), *Absenteeism: New approaches to understanding, measuring and managing employee absence*, pp. 194–228. San Fransisco: Jossey–Bass.

Scott, D., & Markham, S. (1982). Absenteeism control methods: A survey of practices and results. *Personnel Administrator,* June, 73–84.

Scott, K., & Taylor, G. (1985). An examination of conflicting findings on the relationship between job satisfaction and absenteeism: A meta-analysis. *Academy of Management Journal, 28*(3), 599–612.

Shamian, J., Kerr, M., Laschinger, H., & Thomson, D. (2002). Work environment and work environment health indicators for Registered Nurses. *Canadian Journal of Nursing Research, 33*(4), 35–50.

Shamian, J., O'Brien-Pallas, L., Thomson, D., Alksnis, C., & Kerr, M. S. (submitted). Nurse absenteeism, stress and workplace injury: What are the contributing factors and what can/should be done about it? *Sociology and Social Policy.*

Shamian, J., O'Brien-Pallas, L., Kerr, M., Loehoorn, M., Thomson, D., & Alksnis, C. (2001). *Effects of job strain, hospital organizational factors and individual characteristics on work-related disability among nurses.* Toronto, ON: Workplace Safety and Insurance Board (WSIB).

Shannon, H., Mayr, J., & Haines, T. (1997). Overview of the relationship between organizational and workplace factors and injury rates. *Safety Science, 26,* 201–217.

Sharp, C., & Watt, S. (1995). A study of absence rates in male and female employees working in occupations of equal status. *Occupational Medicine, 45*(3), 131–136.

Siegrist, J. (1996). Adverse health effects of high-effort/low rewards conditions. *Journal of Occupational Health Psychology, 1*(1), 27–41.

Spector, P. (1986). Perceived control by employees: A meta-analysis of studies concerning autonomy and participation at work. *Human Relations, 39*(11), 1005–1016.

Spence Laschinger, H. K., Shamian, J., & Thomson, D. (2001). Impact of nursing work environment characteristics on staff nurse organizational trust, burnout, nurse-assessed quality of care, and work satisfaction. *Nursing Economics, 19*(5), 209–220.

Steers, R., & Rhodes, S. (1978). Major influences on employee attendance: A process model. *Journal of Applied Psychology, 63*(4), 391–407.

Sui, O. (2002). Predictors of job satisfaction and absenteeism in two samples of Hong Kong nurses. *Journal of Advanced Nursing, 40*(2), 218–229.

Taunton, R.L., Kleinbeck, S. V. M., Stafford, R., Woods, C. Q. & Bott, M. J. (1994). Patient outcomes: Are they linked to registered nurse absenteeism, separation or work load? *Journal of Nursing Administration, 24*(45), 48–55.

Tholdy Doncevic, S., Romelsjo, A., & Theorell, T. (1998). Comparison of stress, job satisfaction, perception of control and health among district nurses in Stockholm and prewar Zagreb. *Scandinavian Journal of Social Medicine, 26*(2), 106–114.

Thomson, D. (2002). *Nurse job satisfaction: Factors relating to nurse satisfaction in the workplace.* Report commissioned by Health Canada.

Timmins, F., & Kaliszer, M. (2002) Absenteeism among nursing students: Facts or fiction? *Journal of Nursing Management, 10,* 251–264.

Trinkoff, A. M., Brady, B., & Nielson, K. (2003). Workplace prevention and musculoskeletal injuries in nurses. *Journal of Nursing Administration, 33*(3), 153–158.

Vahtera, J., Kivimaki, M., & Pentti, J. (2001). The role of extended weekends in sickness absenteeism. *Occupational and Environmental Medicine, 58*(12), 818–822.

Venning, P. J. (1988). Back injury prevention among nursing personnel: The role of education. *American Association of Occupational Health Nurses Journal, 36,* 327–333.

Voss, M., Floderus, B., & Diderichsen, F. (2001). Physical, psychosocial, and organizational factors relative to sickness absence: A study based on Sweden Post. *Occupational and Environmental Medicine, 58*(3), 178–184.

Wenderlein, F. U. (2003). Work satisfaction and absenteeism of nursing staff: Comparative study of 1021 nurse trainees and nurses. *Gesundheitswesen, 65*(11), 620–628.

Williams, G., & Slater, K. (2000). Absenteeism and the impact of the 38-hour week, rostered day off option. *Australian Health Review, 23*(4), 89–95.

Wise, L. C. (1993). The erosion of nursing resources: Employee withdrawal behaviors. *Research in Nursing and Health, 16*(1), 67–75.

Workers' Compensation Board of British Columbia (1998). *Health care industry: Focus report on occupational injury and disease.* Vancouver, British Columbia: Workers' Compensation Board of British Columbia.

Wright, M. E. (1997). Long-term sickness in an NHS teaching hospital. *Occupational Medicine, 47*(7), 401–406.

Xie, J., & Johns, G. (2000). Interactive effects of absence culture salience and group cohesiveness: A multi-level and cross-level analysis of work absenteeism in the Chinese context. *Journal of Occupational and Organizational Psychology 73,* 31–52.

Yaniv, G. (1995). Burnout, absenteeism, and the overtime decision. *Journal of Economic Psychology 16,* 297–309.

Yassi, A., Khokhar, R., Tate, R., Cooper, J., Snow, C., & Vallentyne, S. (1995). The epidemiology of back injuries in nurses at a large Canadian tertiary care hospital: Implications for prevention. *Occupational Medicine, 45,* 215–220.

Zavala, S. K., French, M. T., Zarkin, G. A., & Omachonu, V. K. (2002). Decision latitude and workload demand: Implications for full and partial absenteeism. *Journal of Public Health Policy, 23*(3), 344–361.

Zboril-Bensen, L. (2002). Why nurses are calling in sick: The impact of health-care restructuring. *Canadian Journal of Nursing Research, 33*(4), 89–107.

Zelauskas, B. & Howes, D. G. (1992). The effects of implementing a professional practice model. *Journal of Nursing Administration, 22*(7/8), 18–23.

Zerwekh, J. (1992). The practice of empowerment and coercion by expert public health nurses. *Image: Journal of Nursing Scholarship, 24*(2), 101–105.

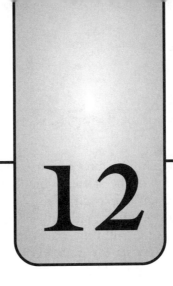

Conclusions

Linda McGillis Hall

12.1 Overview

This report outlines findings from a critical review and analysis of the literature on variables in work environments that can be considered indicators of the quality of nurses' worklife in health care settings. The indicators include: nurse staffing; educational background of nursing staff; experience of nursing staff; team functioning; organizational climate and culture; span of control of unit manager; workload/productivity; level of autonomy and decision-making experienced by nurses; professional development opportunities; scope of the nursing leadership role; use of overtime hours and agency staff; absenteeism hours; and number of grievances. A summary of the key findings for each of the worklife concepts follows.

12.1.1 Nurse Staffing

Nurse staffing and the care provided by nursing personnel are central to the provision of quality patient care in the health care system. Substantial theoretical evidence suggests that nurse staffing is an important parameter to capture in the study of outcomes research. Measures of nurse staffing include those that focus on numerical assessments of the staffing complement as well as measures that capture the mix of the staff employed in the organization (e.g., proportion of RNs, nursing hours per patient day, ratio of RNs to patients, and staff mix), how these staff are employed (e.g., full-time, part-time, and casual) and demographic characteristics of the nursing staff (e.g., level of experience and education).

This review of the literature of nurse staffing concludes with the following implications and suggestions for future work. First, measures of nurse staffing should capture the proportion of RNs; the staffing mix; the proportion of full-time, part-time, and casual staff; and the level of education and experience of the nursing staff. This can enable the health care leader or researcher to capture the full impact of nurse staffing on patient clinical and system quality outcomes. Second, research that predicts estimates of the staffing changes necessary to achieve more positive patient outcomes should be pursued. For the nursing health services manager it is essential to have a more actionable mechanism to assess nurse staffing complements in the work setting. Third, further refinement of the unit of measurement for nurse staffing is needed. Unit-level measures of nurse staffing that are accurately adjusted for patient complexity should be employed in future research in this area. Finally, recent research has begun to examine the impact of nurse staffing in relation to the intended effects of nursing care. Further work is needed to determine the potentially positive contributions that nurses make to patient outcomes such as functional status, self-care ability, and self-management of pain symptoms.

12.1.2 Team Functioning

The quality of health care depends on how well members of the team communicate, coordinate care, and negotiate their interdependencies in practice to achieve a cohesive treatment plan for patients. Teamwork has been assessed with multidimensional measures that target multiple concepts such as communication, coordination, and decision-making, as well as measures that target one component of teamwork, such as questionnaires that assess only coordination or communication.

This review of approaches to the assessment of teamwork in health care concludes with the following implications and suggestions for future work. First, to better understand teamwork in health care, finding methods to assess it and effectively intervene to improve it are going to be increasingly important because of the complexity of patient care today. Therefore, the investigation of interprofessional teamwork is needed through studies that evaluate interprofessional interventions that promote effective teamwork. Second, measures such as the Organizational Assessment Inventory/Team Interaction Questionnaire (Shortell et al., 1994), which have demonstrated good reliability and validity in a number of studies, warrant further evaluation in settings outside of hospitals for which they were developed. Finally, several team assessment instruments, such as the Relational Coordination Instrument (Gittell, 2000) have been adapted for use in health care from other industry settings. These instruments show promise, but have only had limited testing in the health care context, primarily in the acute care setting. Further testing of instruments that have demonstrated good reliability and validity in other settings or have had only limited testing in health care is needed.

12.1.3 Organizational Culture and Climate

Organizational climate and culture are not strongly differentiated, and represent different but overlapping interpretations of the same phenomena. Organizational climate and culture are influenced by individual, organizational, and external factors. Much of the research on climate and culture focuses on nursing outcomes, especially job and work satisfaction. Several instruments for measuring organizational climate and culture are available. The instruments capture various domains on climate and culture and demonstrate acceptable reliability; however, there is limited evidence to support validity. Sensitivity to Nursing varies across these instruments.

This review of approaches to the assessment of organizational culture and climate in health care has identified two suggestions for future work. First, there are limitations in the ability to compare climate and culture across settings, and the impact on outcomes caused by variation in measures and analytical approaches may be of concern. Further work is required to improve the validity and nursing sensitivity of some of the instruments described in this book related to the measurement of organizational culture. Second, the overlapping interpretations of the climate, culture, and practice environment constructs found in this review are cause for concern. It is evident that a content analysis of the instruments examined in this review (e.g., Organizational Culture Inventory, Nursing Unit Culture Assessment Tool–2, and the culture component of the Nursing Assessment Survey) is needed, as well as a comparison of these with elements explored in the practice environment measures (e.g., Revised Nursing Work Index).

12.1.4 Span of Control of Unit Managers

Unit managers have been found to have an impact on staff outcomes. Factors in the work environment that influence the span of control of unit managers need to be examined and taken into consideration. Some of these factors include similarity and complexity of the workers' functions, unit unpredictability, and number of staff providing support for the unit. The challenge lies in developing a tool to measure span of control of the unit manager based on all of these factors including the numerical measure.

The review of the literature of span of control has identified three areas for future work. First, there is a need to develop guidelines regarding the number of staff a nurse manager may effectively support to consistently provide positive leadership on a daily basis. Second, a tool to measure span of control is required. The challenge is for researchers to develop a tool that includes the various factors influencing span of control. Finally, studies that examine the relationships between span of control and patient outcomes will advance our understanding of the important role of unit-based nurse managers in the health care system.

12.1.5 Workload and Productivity

Nursing workload and productivity are important concepts relative to patient outcomes, quality of care, nurse outcomes, and health system costs. This literature review identifies that although workload management systems have been in use for a number of years in the acute care sector, the conceptual adequacy of these measures and their psychometric properties have been relatively unexplored until the last two decades. A paucity of research exists in measuring nursing workload and productivity in nonacute care sectors including community, long-term, and chronic care.

The review of the literature of nursing workload and productivity has highlighted three key areas of future study. First, workload systems should involve multiple measures that capture the complexity of patient conditions, the decisions that providers make, environmental complexity, as well as the factors that influence processes and patient, nurse, and system outcomes. Second, further research to enable the development of quality-adjusted measures of productivity that are sensitive to the multiple factors that influence inputs, throughputs, and outputs of the system are needed. Finally, in the community sector, standardized collection of data elements related to the number, type, and length of visits, as well as characteristics of and outcomes for clients, providers, and agencies are needed.

12.1.6 Autonomy and Decision-Making

Autonomy is extensively addressed in the literature as a key indicator of quality work environments; yet the definition, measurement, and interpretation of research findings have complicated the effective integration and promotion of this key indicator into nursing work environments. The opportunity exists to build upon the detailed descriptive work that exists in this area.

The review of the literature of autonomous nursing practice concludes with the following implications and suggestions for future work. First, measures of autonomy need to be of relevance within the various domains in nursing (e.g., practice, leadership, and education) and across various roles. Autonomous practice needs to be explored within the context of the nurses' work environments. Professional nurse autonomy should be reflected in professional nursing behaviors and actions and tools developed to measure such. Second, based on the instruments reviewed, the NWI-R (Aiken, Havens, & Sloane, 2000) along with the ranking of the autonomous clinical behavior scale recently tested by Kramer and Schmalenberg (2003) should be used and tested in future research studies. Finally, understanding and measuring professional nurse autonomy from an organizational perspective in relation to patient outcomes should be a priority on the research agenda. There is an urgent need to measure and define the characteristics of organizations and units that demonstrate autonomous nursing practice and the impact of autonomous nursing practice on patient outcomes.

12.1.7 Professional Development Opportunities

"Professional development" is a term that covers a wide variety of educational activities ranging from formal professional requirements to informal, individual actions. Continuing professional development is a complex multifaceted concept whose definition and measurement should incorporate stakeholder perspectives (e.g., employer, regulatory body, and individual) in relation to specific learning contexts. Attributes of the professional identified in the literature include knowledge, critical thinking ability, communication skills, leadership ability, participation and use of research in practice, involvement in professional nursing organizations, and reflection skills.

The review of the literature of professional development opportunities for nurses concludes with suggestions. Future research that draws on the perspectives of all three stakeholders set in specific contexts, considering structured and unstructured professional development, and examining the impact of professional development on practice and nurse-sensitive patient outcomes is needed.

12.1.8 Scope of Nursing Leadership

Much of the literature on nursing leadership is descriptive with few qualitative studies and even less experimental studies. The literature review identified several issues in the assessment of nursing leadership including the way in which models of leadership are conceptualized in nursing and the changing environment of nursing leaders. There has been little research linking leadership styles and their effect on the quality of patient care and staff nurse effectiveness.

The review of the literature of nursing leadership concludes with the following suggestion. Future research on nursing leadership needs to capture leadership behaviors in relation to the process of nursing practice and to patient outcomes. The Leadership Practices Inventory offers a comprehensive approach to measuring leadership behaviors; however, further research is required to link these behaviors to positive outcomes that are sustainable over time. As well, clear links between effective nursing leadership and positive patient outcomes is needed to ensure that the contribution of nursing to patient care is recognized.

12.1.9 Overtime

Overtime is a growing issue for both nurses and the organizations that employ them. There are few documented studies specifically examining the effect of overtime utilization on patient, nurse, or organizational outcomes. The review of the literature of overtime concludes with the following two suggestions for future work. First, health care funders and professional organizations need to consider strategies to capture an accurate measurement of both voluntary and involuntary overtime on a regular basis. Second, few studies have examined overtime using theoretical models that incorporate all of the components of the work environment. Overtime must be examined in light of the internal and external factors using a theoretical framework to test hypotheses.

12.1.10 Absenteeism

Absenteeism is one of the major contributors to rising health care costs. Research indicates that absenteeism can be influenced by work culture and the content of the work itself. There must be a concerted effort to clearly define how absenteeism is measured and studied as well as understanding the full costs associated with absenteeism. In addition, it must be recognized that the effect on patient outcomes may be associated with absenteeism when absences are not replaced or when agency or part-time staff is used to replace sudden absences. Although the research conducted on nonnursing organizations may give us clues for understanding absenteeism in nursing, the very nature of the nurses and nursing work requires attention when considering nurse absenteeism. Future research endeavors related to nursing absenteeism should address issues specific to nursing work and the context in which it occurs.

12.2   Conclusion

This comprehensive review of the literature has provided evidence that the following indicators of nurse staffing and quality nursing work environments should be explored in future work:

- Nurse staffing
  - The proportion of RNs
  - The staffing mix
  - The proportion of full-time, part-time, and casual staff
  - The level of education and experience of the nursing staff

- Quality nursing work environment
  - Teamwork (communication and coordination)
  - Organizational culture and climate
  - Span of control of nurse manager
  - Nursing workload and productivity
  - Autonomy and decision-making
  - Professional development
  - Overtime utilization
  - Absenteeism

As well, earlier work in this area has identified the need to assess nurses' job satisfaction as a key variable of the quality of nurses' work environments (McGillis Hall, 2003).

The findings of this comprehensive literature review are consistent with those identified in the most recent report released from the Institute of Medicine (IOM)—*Keeping Patients Safe: Transforming the Work Environment of Nurses* (Page, 2003). This report from the IOM Committee on the Work Environment for Nurses and Patient Safety sought to identify factors in the nursing work environment that can impact patient safety as well as ways of improving working conditions to increase patient safety (Page). Recommendations related to four components of health care organizations were advanced: (a) leadership and management, (b) workforce, (c) work processes, and (d) organizational culture.

One of the key issues identified in the 1996 Institute of Medicine report on nurse staffing was the importance of considering nurses' worklife in future research efforts (Wunderlich, Sloan, & Davis, 1996). It is of interest to note that the majority of work to date has focused on determining the relationship between nurse staffing and patient outcomes, while little attention has been paid to issues in the nursing work environment. Future work should focus on aspects of the nurses' worklife and the nursing work environment that can influence patient and organizational outcomes.

12.3   References

Aiken, L. H., Havens, D. S., & Sloane, D. M. (2000). The Magnet Nursing Services Recognition Program: A comparison of two groups of magnet hospitals. *American Journal of Nursing, 100,* 26–36.

Gittell, J. H. (2000). Organizing work to support relational co-ordination. *International Journal of Human Resource Management, 11*(2), 517–539.

Kramer, M., & Schmalenberg, C. E. (2003). Magnet hospital staff nurses describe clinical autonomy. *Nursing Outlook, 51,* 13–19.

McGillis Hall, L. (2003). Nursing outcome: Nurses' job satisfaction. In D. Doran (Ed). *Nursing-sensitive outcomes: State of the science,* pp. 283–318. Mississauga, ON: Jones and Bartlett Publishers.

Page, A. (2003). *Keeping patients safe: Transforming the work environment of nurses.* Washington DC: National Academy Press.

Shortell, S. M., Zimmerman, J. E., Rousseau, D. M., Gillies, R. R., Wagner, D. P., Draper, E. A., et al. (1994). The performance of intensive care units: Does good management make a difference. *Medical Care, 32*(5), 508–525.

Wunderlich, G. S., Sloan, F. S., & Davis, C. K. (1996). *Nursing staff in hospitals and nursing homes: Is it adequate?* Washington DC: National Academy Press.

Index